Fundamentals of High-Resolution Lung CT

Common Findings, Common Patterns,
Common Diseases, and Differential Diagnosis

SECOND EDITION

T0337492

Fundamentals of High-Resolution Lung CT

Common Findings, Common Patterns, Common Diseases, and Differential Diagnosis

SECOND EDITION

Brett M. Elicker, M.D.
Professor of Clinical Radiology and Biomedical Imaging
Chief, Cardiac and Pulmonary Imaging
University of California—San Francisco
San Francisco, California

W. Richard Webb, M.D.
Professor Emeritus of Radiology and Biomedical Imaging
Emeritus Member, Haile T. Debas Academy of Medical Educators
University of California—San Francisco
San Francisco, California

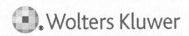

. Wolters Kluwer

Philadelphia • Baltimore • New York • London
Buenos Aires • Hong Kong • Sydney • Tokyo

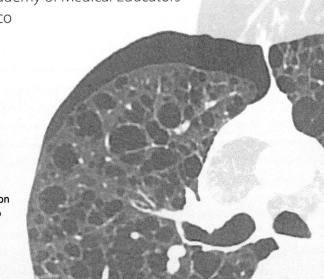

Acquisitions Editor: Sharon Zinner
Editorial Coordinator: Lindsay Ries
Manufacturing Coordinator: Beth Welsh
Marketing Manager: Julie Sikora
Production Project Manager: Marian Bellus
Designer: Teresa Mallon
Production Service: TNQ Technologies

2nd Edition
Copyright © 2019

Library of Congress Cataloging-in-Publication Data

Names: Elicker, Brett M., author. | Webb, W. Richard (Wayne Richard), 1945-author.
Title: Fundamentals of high-resolution lung CT : common findings, common patterns, common diseases, and
    differential diagnosis / Brett M. Elicker, W. Richard Webb.
Description: Second edition. | Philadelphia: Wolters Kluwer, 2018. | Includes bibliographical references and index.
Identifiers: LCCN 2018035606 | ISBN 9781496389923 (paperback)
Subjects: | MESH: Lung—diagnostic imaging | Tomography, X-Ray Computed | Radiography | Diagnosis, Differential |
    Lung Diseases—diagnostic imaging
Classification: LCC RC756 | NLM WF 600 | DDC 616.2/4075—dc23 LC record available at https://lccn.loc.gov/2018035606

Dedication

To my sons, Jack and Cole, from your dad
To my grandson Teddy, a new addition for the new edition

PREFACE

The accurate interpretation of high-resolution CT (HRCT) in patients with diffuse lung disease is fundamentally based on (1) the recognition of specific HRCT findings; (2) an understanding of what they mean and their relationship to differential diagnosis; (3) a basic knowledge of the lung diseases that most commonly result in diffuse lung disease; and (4) the typical constellation of findings associated with each of these diseases.

Although interpreting HRCT can seem to be a complicated task, an understanding of these four basic principles often leads to the recognition of a typical or classic "pattern" of lung disease and the correct diagnosis or a list of diagnostic possibilities. On the other hand, it is important to understand that some HRCT patterns are necessarily nonspecific and should lead to further evaluation and correlation with clinical findings or lung biopsy.

This second edition is fully updated to provide the most up-to-date information on new knowledge, new diseases, and new guidelines for diagnosis. In addition, many images have been updated, and two new features are included.

First, a two-page summary of each chapter is included at the beginning of the book. These summaries distill the fundamental concepts and typical findings of common diseases from each chapter into an outline form. Additionally, six images are included in each chapter summary that demonstrate classic imaging appearances. These chapter summaries are intended to provide a quick reference of the key points and typical imaging appearances.

Second, within each of the chapters, typical examples of common diseases are specifically designated as "Classic Images". These also provides a quick visual reference for those wishing to review typical imaging appearances of various HRCT patterns and diseases.

In some sense, this book is "HRCT Lite." It is intended to provide a simple and easily understandable approach to diagnosis and differential diagnosis. However, it is also important to emphasize that we do not consider this book to be an oversimplification of the HRCT principles and diagnosis of diffuse lung disease. The chapters and illustrations in this book are based on, and demonstrate, the fundamental observations, rules, shortcuts, thought patterns, and differential diagnoses we use in everyday clinical practice and have built up over a period of years of HRCT-pathologic correlation. It also is intended to review our basic and practical understanding of the lung diseases commonly assessed using HRCT.

It is our intention that this book provides the fundamental insights and facts necessary to interpret HRCT in most clinical settings, in an easily understood and digestible format. Although it is not comprehensive, it is our hope that it provides a practical and useful understanding of HRCT and its use in the diagnosis of diffuse lung disease.

Brett M. Elicker
W. Richard Webb
San Francisco, California

CONTENTS

Chapter 1 Summary: HRCT Indications, Technique, Radiation Dose, and Normal Anatomy

1) Indications for HRCT
   a) Detection of disease
      i) High sensitivity for most diseases
      ii) Often able to detect disease at an early stage
      iii) Normal HRCT excludes most diffuse diseases
   b) Characterization
      i) Interstitial, airways, or alveolar disease
      ii) Predicts inflammatory versus fibrotic disease
   c) Differential diagnosis
      i) HRCT is key in multidisciplinary diagnosis
      ii) HRCT + clinical can be highly specific
      iii) When HRCT + clinical does not suggest a single disease, pathology is required
   d) Follow-up over time
      i) Particularly helpful when pulmonary function tests are inaccurate
      ii) Evaluating new symptoms and distinguishing worsening disease or a superimposed process
2) Techniques and protocols
   a) Key components of HRCT
      i) Thin slices (≤1.25 mm sections)
      ii) Reconstructed with sharp algorithm
      iii) Scanning at full inspiration
   b) Axial versus volumetric scanning
      i) Advantages of axial scanning
         (1) Sampling of lung anatomy usually adequate for diagnosis
         (2) Slightly sharper images
         (3) Relatively low radiation dose
      ii) Advantages of volumetric scanning
         (1) Faster
         (2) Evaluation of the entire lung
   c) Prone imaging
      i) Normal patients may have dependent opacity in the posterior subpleural lung
      ii) Interstitial disease often begins in the subpleural lung
      iii) Posterior, subpleural opacity that persists on the prone images likely represents real interstitial lung disease
   d) Expiratory imaging
      i) Used to detect air trapping
      ii) Sensitive for diagnosis of airways disease
      iii) Static or dynamic techniques may be used
      iv) Often acquired at three levels: aortic arch, tracheal carina, and above diaphragm
3) Radiation
   a) Yearly exposure is 2.5 milliSieverts (mSv)
   b) Axial HRCT: spaced (q 10 mm) 100 mA slices ~0.7 mSv
   c) Volumetric HRCT
      i) ~4 to 7 mSv using 300 mA
      ii) ~1 to 2 mSv using 100 mA

4) Normal anatomy (see figure below)
   a) Large bronchi and arteries
      i) Bronchoarterial ratio (BAR)
         (1) Ratio of diameter of bronchial lumen to the size of adjacent artery
         (2) BAR > 1 is often abnormal; however, it may be seen as a normal finding in certain patients (e.g., elderly)
   b) Peribronchovascular (axial) interstitium
      i) Accompanies the arteries, bronchi, and lymphatics as they radiate from hila
      ii) Lymphatic diseases (e.g., sarcoidosis) commonly are peribronchovascular
   c) Pulmonary lobule (secondary pulmonary lobule)
      i) Smallest unit of the lung delineated by connective tissue septa
      ii) Polygonal in shape, measuring 1 to 2.5 cm
         (1) Interlobular septa
            (a) Marginate the periphery of the lobule
            (b) Contain veins and lymphatics
            (c) Only a few seen in normal patients
         (2) Centrilobular structures
            (a) The lobular artery and bronchiole
            (b) Artery visible as a dot or as Y-shaped
            (c) Site of airway and vascular diseases
         (3) Subpleural interstium
            (a) Contiguous with the interlobular septa
            (b) Pleural or fissural thickening
         (4) Intralobular interstitium: the connective tissue within the pulmonary lobule

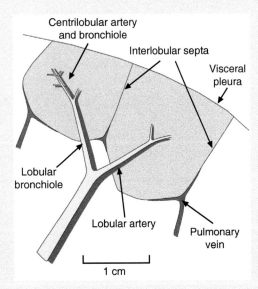

Centrilobular artery and bronchiole

Interlobular septa

Visceral pleura

Lobular bronchiole

Lobular artery

Pulmonary vein

1 cm

1) Interlobular septal thickening (**Fig. A**)
   a) Key features
      i) Linear opacities outline pulmonary lobules
      ii) Linear opacities 1 to 2.5 cm in length
      iii) Centrilobular artery (dot) within lobules
   b) Ignore unless it is the predominant feature
   c) Differential diagnosis (when predominant)
      i) Smooth morphology (**Fig. A**)
         (1) Pulmonary edema (may be associated with cardiomegaly, effusions, etc.)
         (2) Lymphangitic spread of neoplasm (usually a history of cancer is present)
      ii) Nodular morphology (**Fig. B**)
         (1) Lymphangitic spread of neoplasm (usually a history of cancer is present)
         (2) Sarcoidosis (young patient, no or mild symptoms)
      iii) Irregular morphology: usually indicates lung fibrosis (see below)
2) Honeycombing (HC) (**Fig. C**)
   a) A specific sign of fibrosis
   b) Key features (must be present to make a confident diagnosis of honeycombing)
      i) Air-density lucencies (black holes)
      ii) Relatively thick wall
      iii) Involves immediate subpleural lung
      iv) One or more layers
      v) Other sign of fibrosis usually present
      vi) Usually indicates UIP
   c) Findings associated with a UIP pattern
      (1) Honeycombing (HC)
      (2) Reticulation
      (3) Subpleural/basilar distribution
      (4) Absence of features atypical for UIP
   d) Differential diagnosis of a UIP pattern
      (1) Idiopathic pulmonary fibrosis
      (2) Connective tissue disease
      (3) Drugs
      (4) Asbestosis
   e) Other causes of honeycom bing when not associated with a UIP pattern
      i) Fibrotic NSIP (HC minimal if present)
      ii) Hypersensitivity pneumonitis (variable distribution; may have mosaic perfusion/air trapping or centrilobular nodules)
      iii) Sarcoidosis (upper lobe predominant)
      iv) Post-ARDS fibrosis (anterior distribution)

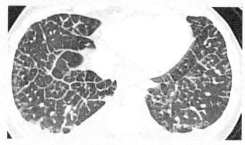

FIGURE A. Interlobular septal thickening: pulmonary edema, smooth, 1 to 2.5 cm long, reticular opacities outline pulmonary lobules

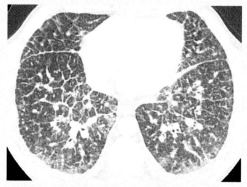

FIGURE B. Interlobular septal thickening: lymphangitic spread of neoplasm, both nodular and smooth septal thickening, history of lung cancer

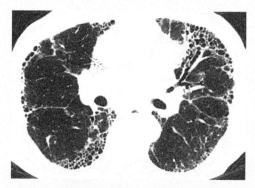

FIGURE C. Honeycombing from UIP: subpleural distribution, both single and multiple layers, associated reticulation, and traction bronchiectasis

3) Intralobular interstitial thickening (IIT) (**Figs. D–F**)
   a) Features
      i) Reticular opacities within pulmonary lobules
      ii) Smaller than interlobular septa
      iii) Varying morphology (thick, thin, fine coarse)
   b) Significance depends on associated features
      i) If associated with HC, see 2, above
      ii) If associated with traction bronchiectasis but no HC (**Fig. D**)
         (1) Fibrosis very likely present
         (2) Differential diagnosis
            (a) Sarcoidosis (upper lobe predominant)
            (b) Hypersensitivity pneumonitis (variable distribution; some have mosaic perfusion/air trapping or centrilobular nodules)
            (c) NSIP (basilar and subpleural distribution, subpleural sparing very suggestive)
            (d) UIP (HC not always present)
         (3) Biopsy usually required for diagnosis in the absence of known connective tissue disease
      iii) If associated with ground glass opacity (**Figs. E, F**)
         (1) Often represents inflammatory or infiltrative disease
         (2) Differential diagnosis
            (a) Acute symptoms (**Fig. E**)
               (i) Pulmonary edema
               (ii) Infection
               (iii) Diffuse alveolar damage
               (iv) Hemorrhage
            (b) Chronic symptoms (**Fig. F**)
               (i) Hypersensitivity pneumonitis
               (ii) NSIP
               (iii) UIP (rare to have significant GGO)
      iv) If seen as an isolated abnormality (e.g., without honeycombing, traction bronchiectasis or GGO)
         (1) Nonspecific finding
         (2) Broad differential diagnosis
         (3) Biopsy usually required for diagnosis
4) Nonspecific reticulation
   a) Reticular opacities that do not represent interlobular septal thickening, honeycombing, or intralobular interstitial thickening
   b) Often referred to as reticulation, irregular reticulation, or reticular pattern
   c) Nonspecific finding
   d) Approach the same as with intralobular interstitial thickening

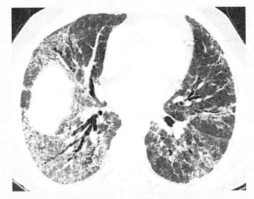

FIGURE D. Intralobular interstitial thickening (IIT) with traction bronchiectasis: myositis, IIT representing fibrosis

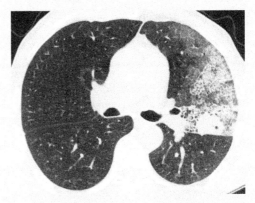

FIGURE E. Intralobular interstitial thickening (IIT): ground glass opacity and IIT from hemorrhage around a cavitary malignancy

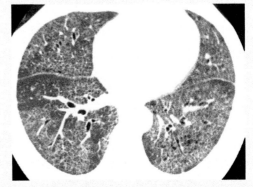

FIGURE F. Intralobular interstitial thickening: connective tissue disease, associated with ground glass opacity and cysts, representing cellular NSIP

Chapter 3 Summary: Nodular Lung Disease

1) Features of pulmonary nodules and their distribution determines the differential diagnosis
2) Most useful approach is to determine the distribution of the nodules in relation to normal lung structures
3) Three distributions of nodules are described
4) Perilymphatic distribution of nodules (**Figs. A, B**)
   a) Key features
      i) Lung structures involved include
         (1) Peribronchovascular interstitium (key feature)
         (2) Subpleural intersititium (key feature)
         (3) Interlobular septa (usually not the predominant feature except with lymphangitic spread of neoplasm and occasionally sarcoidosis)
         (4) Centrilobular region (usually not the predominant feature)
      ii) Appear patchy or nonuniform
   b) Differential diagnosis
      i) Sarcoidosis (most common, young patient with no or mild symptoms)
      ii) Lymphangitic spread of neoplasm (common, older patient with history of malignancy)
      iii) Pneumoconiosis (uncommon, exposure history important)
      iv) Lymphoid interstitial pneumonia (rare, history of immunosuppression or connective tissue disease)
      v) Amyloidosis (rare, may have history of myeloma)
5) Random distribution of nodules (**Fig. C**)
   a) Key features
      i) Diffuse, uniform lung involvement
      ii) NOT clustered around any specific lung structures
      iii) Subpleural nodules are present
   b) Differential diagnosis
      i) Tuberculosis (common, signs and symptoms of infection present except sometimes in elderly)
      ii) Fungal infection (common, signs and symptoms of infection present, travel to endemic region)
      iii) Malignancy (common, history of malignancy usually present)
      iv) Sarcoidosis (rare to give a random distribution, consider in young patients with no or mild symptoms)

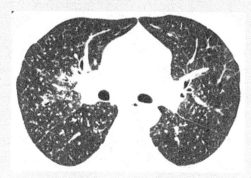

FIGURE A. Perilymphatic nodules: sarcoidosis, clustered peribronchovascular and subpleural nodules

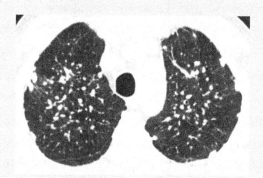

FIGURE B. Perilymphatic nodules: silicosis in a bricklayer, subpleural and peribronchovascular nodules

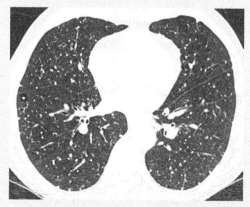

FIGURE C. Random nodules: histoplasmosis, diffuse distribution, not clustered, subpleural nodules present

6) Centrilobular distribution of nodules (**Figs. D–F**)
   a) Key features
      i) Subpleural nodules are NOT present
      ii) Center of nodules at least 5 mm from the subpleural lung
      iii) Even distance between nodules
      iv) Large nodules will eventually touch the pleura
   b) Causes: airways and vascular diseases
   c) Broad differential diagnosis that may be narrowed by the presence of other features:
      i) Attenuation (ground glass or soft tissue)
      ii) Distribution (symmetric or asymmetric)
      iii) Tree-in-bud opacities (branching, tubular opacities with nodules)
   d) Differential diagnosis
      i) Ground glass attenuation (**Fig. E**)
         (1) Hypersensitivity pneumonitis (common, bird or mold exposure in 50% of patients)
         (2) Respiratory bronchiolitis (common, cigarette smoking history)
         (3) Infection (common, usually viral, signs and symptoms of infection present)
         (4) Follicular bronchiolitis (rare, history of immunosuppression or connective tissue disease)
         (5) Pneumoconiosis such as siderosis (rare)
         (6) Vascular causes such as edema, hemorrhage, pulmonary hypertension, metastatic calcification (common or rare depending on etiology, symmetric distribution, pleural effusions or other CT features present)
      ii) Soft tissue attenuation
         (1) Infection (common, acute symptoms)
         (2) Aspiration (common, acute symptoms)
         (3) Invasive mucinous adenocarcinoma (uncommon, chronic symptoms)
         (4) Langherhans cell histiocytosis (rare, cigarette smoking, cysts and cavitary nodules also present)
      iii) Tree-in-bud opacities (**Fig. F**)
         (1) Infection (common)
         (2) Aspiration (common)
         (3) Invasive mucinous adenocarcinoma (rare, chronic symptoms)
         (4) Follicular bronchiolitis (rare, history of immunosuppression or connective tissue disease)
         (5) Asthma and allergic bronchopulmonary aspergillosis (rare, central bronchiectasis, high-density mucous)
         (6) Panbronchiolitis (rare, chronic symptoms, often seen in Asian patients)

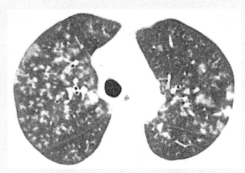

FIGURE D. Centrilobular nodules: viral infection, ground glass and soft tissue attenuation, tree-in-bud, larger nodules touch pleura

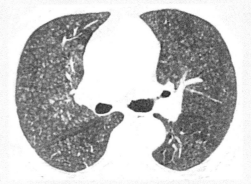

FIGURE E. Centrilobular nodules: hypersensitivity pneumonitis, ground glass attenuation, diffuse distribution

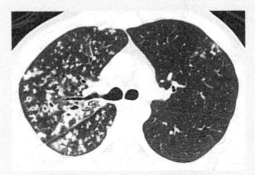

FIGURE F. Tree-in-bud opacities: tuberculosis, branching tubular opacities, soft tissue attenuation centrilobular nodules, asymmetric distribution

Chapter 4 Summary: Increased Lung Attenuation: Ground Glass Opacity and Consolidation

1) Ground glass opacity (GGO) (**Figs. A–C**)
   a) Key features
      i) Homogeneous regions of increased opacity
      ii) Vessels still visible in abnormal lung
   b) Reflects abnormalities below resolution of HRCT
   c) May be due to alveolar filling, interstitial abnormalities, or both
   d) Acute versus chronic symptoms most important clinical information
   e) Differential diagnosis
      i) Acute symptoms
         (1) Infection (most commonly viral) (**Fig. A**) or aspiration
         (2) Acute lung injury (diffuse alveolar damage)
         (3) Pulmonary edema (associated smooth interlobular septal thickening, cardiomegaly, or pleural effusions)
         (4) Hemorrhage (hemoptysis)
         (5) Rare causes: acute hypersensitivity pneumonitis (exposure history) and acute eosinophilic pneumonia (smokers)
      ii) Chronic symptoms
         (1) Hypersensitivity pneumonitis (exposure history, may be associated with air trapping or centrilobular nodules)
         (2) Nonspecific interstitial pneumonia (peripheral/basilar distribution, subpleural sparing)
         (3) Desquamative interstitial pneumonia (cystic lucencies, peripheral/basilar distribution) (**Fig. B**) and respiratory bronchiolitis (centrilobular nodules) in smokers
         (4) Follicular bronchiolitis (connective tissue disease or immunosuppression, centrilobular nodules)
         (5) Invasive mucinous adenocarcinoma (consolidation more common)
         (6) Organizing pneumonia or chronic eosinophilic pneumonia (consolidation more common)
         (7) Sarcoidosis (perilymphatic nodules usually seen)
         (8) Lipoid pneumonia (presence of fat)
         (9) Alveolar proteinosis (rare)
   f) Crazy paving (**Fig. C**)
      i) Combination of GGO and interlobular septal thickening
      ii) Acute setting: differential, the same as GGO
      iii) Chronic setting: differential, the same as GGO except that alveolar proteinosis is more likely

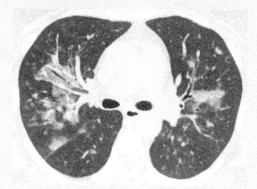

FIGURE A. Ground glass opacity from viral infection: acute symptoms, symmetric bilateral distribution

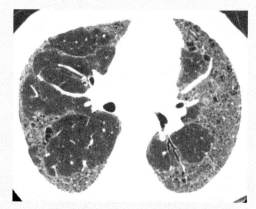

FIGURE B. Ground glass opacity from desquamative interstitial pneumonia: peripheral distribution, associated cysts

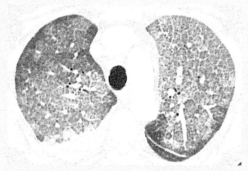

FIGURE C. Crazy paving from pulmonary edema: acute symptoms.

2) Consolidation (**Figs. D–F**)
  a) Key features
    i) Homogeneous regions of increased opacity
    ii) Vessels obscured in abnormal lung
    iii) Associated with air bronchograms
  b) May be due to alveolar filling, confluent interstitial abnormalities, or both
  c) Acute versus chronic symptoms most important clinical information
  d) Differential diagnosis
    i) Acute symptoms (same as GGO)
      (1) Infection (**Fig. D**) or aspiration
      (2) Acute lung injury (diffuse alveolar damage)
      (3) Pulmonary edema (associated smooth interlobular septal thickening, cardiomegaly, or pleural effusions)
      (4) Hemorrhage (hemoptysis)
    ii) Chronic symptoms
      (1) Organizing pneumonia (OP) and chronic eosinophilic pneumonia (CEP) (most common)
      (2) Invasive mucinous adenocarcinoma (**Fig. E**)
      (3) Sarcoidosis (peribronchovascular distribution, nodules also present)
      (4) Lymphoma
      (5) Lipoid pneumonia (fat attenuation)
  e) Additional helpful features that may be present
    i) Atoll or revered halo sign (**Fig. F**)
      (1) Ring of consolidation surrounding central area of GGO or normal lung
      (2) Most commonly due to OP or disease associated with OP on pathology (e.g., CEP)
      (3) Other (non-OP) causes of this sign
        (a) Infarcts (peripheral, wedge-shaped, only one or a few atolls)
        (b) Infection (invasive fungal infection in neutropenia, paracoccidioidomycosis in South America)
        (c) Sarcoidosis (perilymphatic nodules usually seen)
        (d) Granulomatosis with polyangiitis (other systemic manifestations)
    ii) Galaxy sign
      (1) Consolidaton due to confluent granulomas with adjacent nodules
      (2) Most commonly due to sarcoidosis
      (3) Other causes include pneumoconiosis, granulomatous infections
    iii) Low-attenuation consolidation
      (1) Fat attenuation (<–30 HU) in consolidation
      (2) Suggestive of lipoid pneumonia

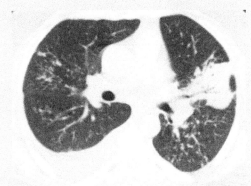

FIGURE D. Consolidation from fungal pneumonia: air bronchograms, associated clustered small nodules

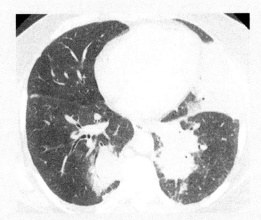

FIGURE E. Consolidation from invasive mucinous adenocarcinoma: chronic symptoms

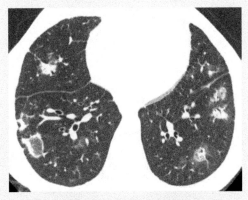

FIGURE F. Atoll or reversed halo sign from organizing pneumonia: chronic consolidation and ground glass opacity

Chapter 5 Summary: Decreased Lung Attenuation: Emphysema, Mosaic Perfusion, and Cystic Lung Disease

1) Emphysema
   a) Represents lung destruction
   b) Three types depending on mechanism of injury
   c) Centrilobular emphysema
      i) Common, associated with smoking
      ii) Most severe around centrilobular bronchiole
      iii) Features
         (1) Focal air-attenuation lucencies
         (2) No visible walls in most
         (3) Typically upper lobe and central predominant
         (4) Dots may be seen at the center of lucencies (centrilobular artery)
   d) Panlobular emphysema (Fig. A)
      i) Rare; associated with alpha-1 antitrypsin deficiency, smoking, or oral Ritalin injection
      ii) Involves the entire pulmonary lobule
      iii) Features
         (1) Generalized lung lucency
         (2) Small vessels in abnormal regions
         (3) Diffuse or lower lobe predominant
   e) Paraseptal emphysema (Fig. B)
      i) May be idiopathic or associated with smoking
      ii) Features
         (1) Focal, air-attenuation cysts
         (2) Thin wall
         (3) Subpleural location, in a single layer
2) Mosaic perfusion (Fig. C)
   a) Geographic areas of varying lung attenuation (lucent lung is abnormal)
   b) Reflects decreased blood flow to specific areas
   c) Reduced blood flow results in lucent lung
   d) Causes: airways disease (reflex vasoconstriction from hypoxia) or vascular disease
   e) Features of mosaic perfusion (to distinguish it from ground glass opacity)
      i) Geographic, sharp borders between opaque and lucent lung
      ii) Smaller vessels in lucent lung
      iii) Air trapping in lucent lung on expiratory imaging
      iv) Stability over time (ground glass opacity usually changes)
   f) Differential diagnosis (only used when mosaic perfusion is the predominant finding)
      i) Constrictive bronchiolitis (aka bronchiolitis obliterans)
      ii) Asthma
      iii) Hypersensitivity pneumonitis
      iv) Vascular diseases (primarily chronic thromboembolic disease)

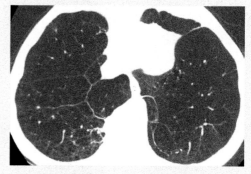

FIGURE A. Panlobular emphysema: alpha-1 antitrypsin deficiency, diffuse lung lucency with attenuated vascularity

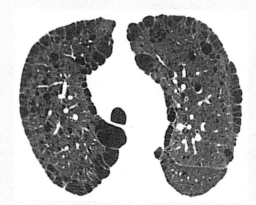

FIGURE B. Paraseptal emphysema: single layer in subpleural lung, thin walls, associated with centrilobular emphysema

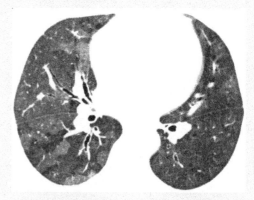

FIGURE C. Mosaic perfusion: constrictive bronchiolitis, geographic regions of lucent lung with sharp borders

3) The headcheese sign (**Fig. D**)
   a) Reflects mixed obstruction (airways disease) and infiltration (usually interstitial disease)
   b) Features (must have all of these in significant amounts)
      i) Mosaic perfusion (lucent lung)
      ii) Ground glass opacity (opaque lung)
      iii) Normal lung (intermediate attenuation)
   c) Differential diagnosis
      i) Hypersensitivity pneumonitis (accounts for the large majority of cases)
      ii) Respiratory bronchiolitis and/or desquamative interstitial pneumonia (smoking history)
      iii) Viral infection (acute symptoms)
      iv) Follicular bronchiolitis and/or lymphoid interstitial pneumonia (connective tissue disease or immunosuppression)
      v) Sarcoidosis (nodules usually present)
      vi) Two separate processes (e.g., asthma and edema)
4) Cystic lung disease (**Figs. E, F**)
   a) Rare, cysts can resemble other air-attenuation findings (e.g., honeycombing, traction bronchiectasis, emphysema)
   b) Features
      i) Round, air-attenuation lesion
      ii) >1 cm in diameter (by definition)
      iii) Thin wall
   c) A few cysts are a normal finding
   d) Differential diagnosis
      i) Lymphangioleiomyomatosis (extensive cysts, women of childbearing age or tuberous sclerosis, round shape, involve entire lung, usually no nodules)
      ii) Langerhans cell histiocytosis (extensive cysts, smokers, irregular shape, spare lung bases, nodules also present)
      iii) Lymphoid interstitial pneumonia (history of immunosuppression or connective tissue disease)
      iv) Pneumatoceles from prior infection (e.g., pneumocystis)
      v) Treated cystic metastases
      vi) Birt–Hogg–Dubé (lower lobe, adjacent to vessels, skin lesions, and other manifestations)
      vii) Neurofibromatosis
      viii) Papillomatosis
      ix) Amyloidosis and light-chain deposition disease (myeloma)

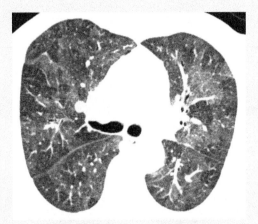

FIGURE D. Headcheese sign: hypersensitivity pneumonitis, ground glass opacity, and mosaic perfusion, both in significant amounts

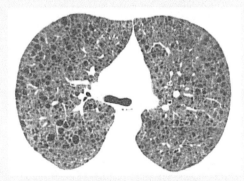

FIGURE E. Lymphangioleiomyomatosis: young woman, diffuse round cysts without nodules

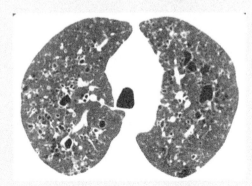

FIGURE F. Langerhans cell histiocytosis: smoking history, irregular cysts and nodules

1) Large airways diseases
   a) Key findings
      i) Airways dilatation (bronchoarterial ratio >1 to 1.5 is borderline, >1.5 is usually abnormal)
      ii) Irregular or saccular morphology
      iii) Wall thickening and mucous impaction
   b) Three types of inflammatory bronchiectasis
      i) Cylindrical: mild, regular, and smooth walls
      ii) Varicose: more severe and longstanding, irregular areas of dilation intermixed with narrowing
      iii) Cystic: severe, saccular dilation, air/fluid levels
   c) Differential diagnosis of mild to moderate bronchiectasis is very broad, a few common causes include
      i) Acute infection
      ii) Chronic infection (e.g., atypical mycobacterial infection: right middle lobe and lingular predominant, atelectasis often present) **(Fig. A)**
      iii) Chronic bronchitis
      iv) Asthma
      v) Aspiration
      vi) Any of the causes of severe bronchiectasis may be detected at an earlier stage
   d) Differential diagnosis of severe (cystic) bronchiectasis
      i) Mid-upper lobe distribution
         (1) Cystic fibrosis (bilateral and symmetric)
         (2) Tuberculosis (usually asymmetric)
         (3) ABPA (asthma and cystic fibrosis patients, central/parahilar location, high-attenuation mucous >100 HU) **(Fig. B)**
      ii) Lower lobe distribution
         (1) Constrictive bronchiolitis (only when longstanding and severe, severe childhood viral infection most common cause)
         (2) Immunodeficiency (agammaglobulinemia, hypogammaglobulinemia, and common variable immunodeficiency)
         (3) Primary ciliary dyskinesia (sinus disease and infertility, 50% have situs inversus)
         (4) Williams–Campbell or tracheobronchomegaly (abnormalities of airway cartilage, usually lack significant airways thickening or impaction) **(Fig. C)**

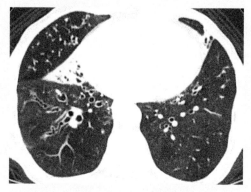

FIGURE A. Atypical mycobacterial infection: varicose bronchiectasis, right middle lobe and lingular collapase

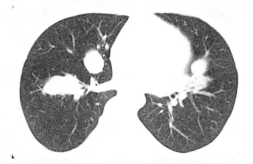

FIGURE B. Allergic bronchopulmonary aspergillosis: central/parahilar cystic bronchiectasis

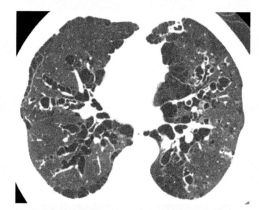

FIGURE C. Tracheobronchomegaly: cystic bronchiectasis with only minimal airways thickening or impaction

2) Small airways disease
  a) Key findings
     i) Bronchiolectasis
     ii) Tree-in-bud opacities
     iii) Centrilobular nodules
     iv) Mosaic perfusion and air trapping
  b) Bronchiolitis with centrilobular nodules of ground glass opacity (**Fig. D**)
     i) Inflammation ≫ fibrosis
     ii) Differential diagnosis
        (1) Hypersensitivity pneumonitis (exposure in 50%, primarily birds and molds)
        (2) Respiratory bronchiolitis (smoking)
        (3) Follicular bronchiolitis (connective tissue disease or immunosuppression)
        (4) Pneumoconioses (e.g., siderosis)
        (5) Atypical infections (viral most common)
  c) Bronchiolitis with centrilobular nodules of soft tissue attenuation (**Fig. E**)
     i) Bronchiolar impaction with consolidation of peribronchiolar alveoli
     ii) Usually patchy and heterogeneous
     iii) Differential diagnosis
        (1) Infection (acute symptoms)
        (2) Aspiration (acute or chronic symptoms)
        (3) Invasive mucinous adenocarcinoma (chronic symptoms)
  d) Bronchiolitis with tree-in-bud opacities
     i) Tubular branching opacities with nodules
     ii) Differential diagnosis
        (1) Acute infection
        (2) Chronic infection (e.g., atypical mycobacterial infection, cystic fibrosis, primary ciliary dyskinesia, immunodeficiency)
        (3) Aspiration
        (4) Rare causes (panbronchiolitis, sarcoidosis)
  e) Bronchiolitis with mosaic perfusion and/or air trapping (**Fig. F**)
     i) Bronchiolar narrowing or occlusion with reflex vasoconstriction
     ii) If other findings are present (e.g., tree-in-bud opacities), mosaic perfusion is nonspecific
     iii) Differential diagnosis (when seen in isolation)
        (1) Constrictive bronchiolitis (pattern of injury with various causes: postviral, connective tissue disease, drugs, toxic inhalation, graft versus host disease, chronic rejection in lung transplant)
        (2) Asthma
        (3) Hypersensitivity pneumonitis

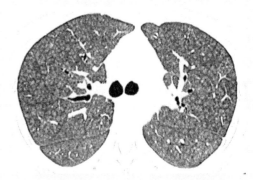

FIGURE D. Bronchiolitis with centrilobular nodules of ground glass opacity from hypersensitivity pneumonitis: diffuse distribution.

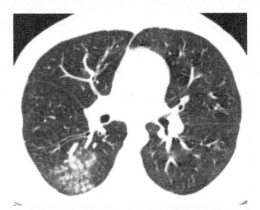

FIGURE E. Bronchiolitis with centrilobular nodules of soft tissue attenuation from infection, asymmetric, heterogeneous

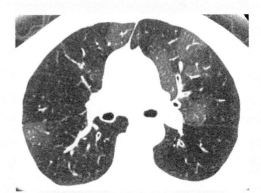

FIGURE F. Bronchiolitis with mosaic perfusion from constrictive bronchiolitis: sharp borders, smaller vessels in lucent lung

Pulmonary Vascular Diseases and Pulmonary Hemorrhage

1) Pulmonary hypertension (PH)
   a) Nice (France) classification (five groups)
      i) Group 1: pulmonary arterial hypertension (PAH; PH due to pulmonary artery disease)
      ii) Group 1´: pulmonary venoocclusive disease and/or pulmonary capillary hemangiomatosis
      iii) Group 2: PH due to left-sided heart disease
      iv) Group 3: PH due to lung diseases or hypoxia
      v) Group 4: chronic thromboembolic PH
      vi) Group 5: PH with unclear and/or multifactorial mechanisms
   b) HRCT findings of PH
      i) Enlarged main pulmonary artery (>3.3 cm or larger than aorta)
      ii) Increased size of right ventricle/atrium and superior/inferior vena cava
      iii) Mosaic perfusion (lucent lung usually peripheral and nonlobular)
      iv) Centrilobular nodules (reflect edema, hemorrhage, or cholesterol granulomas)
   c) Key diseases that cause PH
      i) Parenchymal lung disease
         (1) Causes: emphysema and fibrotic lung diseases > airways and cystic lung diseases
         (2) Lung disease correlates with severity of PH, although connective tissue disease and sarcoidosis may have superimposed vascular disease
         (3) PA size is less accurate as a sign of PH in this setting
      ii) Chronic thromboembolic PH (CT-PH) (**Fig. A**)
         (1) Contrast-enhanced CT is insensitive
         (2) HRCT: mosaic perfusion
            (a) Peripheral distribution, nonlobular
            (b) More severe in CT-PH than other causes of PH
      iii) Idiopathic PAH (**Fig. B**)
         (1) Diagnosis of exclusion
         (2) Young women
         (3) Enlarged PA seen in >90%
         (4) Centrilobular nodules often present
      iv) Pulmonary venoocclusive disease (PVOD) (**Fig. C**)
         (1) Obliterated pulmonary venules
         (2) May worsen on vasodilators
         (3) Smooth interlobular septal thickening in the absence of left-sided heart disease
      v) Pulmonary capillary hemangiomatosis
         (1) Overlapping features with PVOD
         (2) Centrilobular nodules typical
      vi) Many other causes of PH exist that are not usually evaluated with HRCT

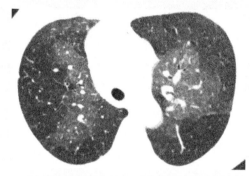

FIGURE A. Chronic thromboembolic PH: mosaic perfusion, large peripheral areas of lucent lung with smaller vessels

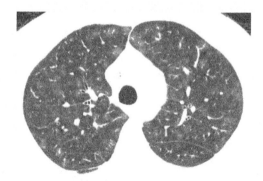

FIGURE B. Idiopathic pulmonary arterial hypertension: centrilobular nodules reflect edema, hemorrhage, or cholesterol granulomas

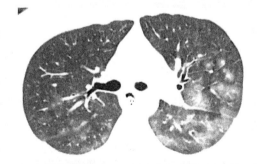

FIGURE C. Pulmonary venoocclusive disease and capillary hemangiomatosis overlap: interlobular septal thickening, centrilobular nodules, ground glass opacity from acute pulmonary edema on vasodilators

2) Vasculitis
  a) Classified by size of vessel involved
    i) Large vessels: giant cell arteritis, Takayasu arteritis, Behçet's disease
    ii) Medium vessels: polyarteritis nodosa and Kawasaki disease (rare to affect pulmonary arteries or lungs)
    iii) Small vessels: granulomatosis with poly-angiitis, eosinphilic granulomatosis with polyangiitis, and microscopic polyangiitis
  b) Key diseases
    i) Giant cell and Takayasu arteritis
      (1) Typical ages: giant cell arteritis (>40 years), Takayasu arteritis (<40 years)
      (2) Wall thickening, stenosis, and aneurysms of large thoracic arteries (systemic arteries > pulmonary arteries)
      (3) Mosaic perfusion due to pulmonary arterial stenoses and reduced blood flow
    ii) Behçet's disease
      (1) Clinical features: oral/genital ulcers, uveitis, skin lesions
      (2) Pulmonary arterial aneurysms and thrombus with hemorrhage
      (3) Systemic venous thrombosis
    iii) Granulomatosis with polyangiitis (Wegener's granulomatosis) **(Fig. D)**
      (1) Most common vasculitis to affect lungs
      (2) C-ANCA in >90%
      (3) HRCT
        (a) Nodules/masses: variable size but can be large, often cavitary (representative of infarcts and inflammation)
        (b) Ground glass opacity: focal or diffuse (representative of pulmonary hemorrhage)
        (c) Consolidation: patchy, bilateral (representative of organizing pneumonia)
    iv) Esoinophilic granulomatosis with polyangiitis **(Fig. E)**
      (1) Asthma, hypereosinophilia, and necrotizing vasculitis
      (2) HRCT
        (a) Lobular ground glass opacity and consolidation (most typical)
        (b) Other findings: nodules/masses, airway thickening, and impaction
    v) Microscopic polyangiitis **(Fig. F)**
      (1) Middle-aged men
      (2) Pulmonary hemorrhage most common manifestation

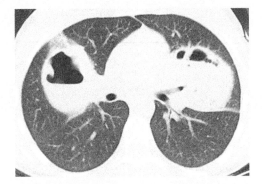

FIGURE D. Granulomatosis with polyangiitis: large cavitary masses

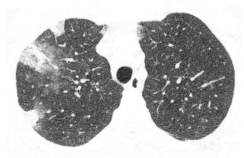

FIGURE E. Esoinophilic granulomatosis with polyangiitis: peripheral and lobular ground glass opacity and consolidation

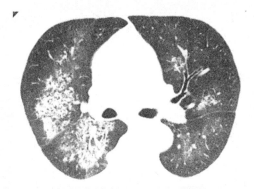

FIGURE F. Microscopic polyangiitis: alveolar hemorrhage, bilateral consolidation, and ground glass opacity

Chapter 8 Summary: Pulmonary Edema, Acute Lung Injury, Diffuse Alveolar Damage, and the Acute Respiratory Distress Syndrome

1) Hydrostatic pulmonary edema
   a) Mechanisms
      i) Increased hydrostatic pressure in the pulmonary veins (pulmonary venous hypertension most commonly from left-sided heart failure or valvular disease)
      ii) Reduced oncotic pressure (rare, e.g., low albumin)
   b) Interstitial edema: HRCT findings (**Fig. A**)
      i) Smooth interlobular septal thickening (ILS), this is particularly suggestive of edema
      ii) Subpleural edema (fluid adjacent to fissures)
      iii) Peribronchovascular interstitial thickening
      iv) Distribution typically bilateral and symmetric but asymmetry is not uncommon
      v) Differential diagnosis
         (1) Lymphangitic spread of neoplasm (when ILS is the predominant feature)
         (2) Inflammatory airways disease (when peribronchovascular thickening is the predominant feature)
   c) Alveolar edema: HRCT findings (**Fig. B**)
      i) Ground glass opacity (GGO) and consolidation
      ii) Crazy paving (GGO + ILS)
      iii) Centrilobular nodules
      iv) Distribution is usually symmetric; however, asymmetric causes of edema include (**Fig. C**):
         (1) Patient positioning
         (2) Asymmetric emphysema/bullous disease
         (3) Mitral regurgitation (right upper lobe edema)
         (4) Pulmonary embolism (edema spares areas with reduced perfusion)
         (5) Neurogenic edema (often upper lung predominant)
      v) Often coexists with interstitial edema
      vi) Differential diagnosis: infection, acute lung injury, and hemorrhage
2) Increased permeability edema without diffuse alveolar damage (DAD)
   a) Mechanism: injury to capillary endothelial injury
   b) Rare as an isolated abnormality; most cases of permeability edema are associated with DAD
   c) Causes: drugs, transfusion, toxic shock syndrome, air embolism, Hantavirus
   d) HRCT: same as hydrostatic pulmonary edema

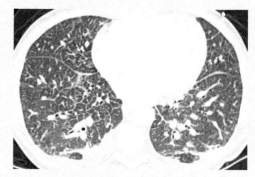

FIGURE A. **Pulmonary edema:** interstitial, interlobular septal, and peribronchovascular interstitial thickening.

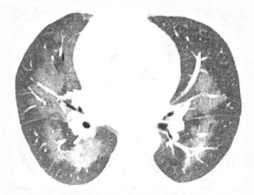

FIGURE B. **Pulmonary edema:** alveolar, symmetric ground glass opacity, parahilar distribution

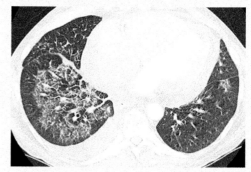

FIGURE C. **Pulmonary edema, asymmetric:** predominantly right-sided ground glass opacity, interlobular septal thickening, and pleural effusion.

3) Increased permeability edema with DAD
   a) Definitions of terms
      i) *DAD*: a histologic diagnosis with alveolar and capillary injury, permeability edema, hemorrhage, necrosis, and sometimes fibrosis
      ii) *Acute lung injury*: a clinical syndrome associated with DAD
      iii) *Acute respiratory distress syndrome (ARDS)*: a clinical syndrome with specific criteria
         (1) Acute onset
         (2) Bilateral opacities on chest radiographs
         (3) Exclusion of cardiac failure of fluid overload as a cause
         (4) Reduced ratio of partial pressure of oxygen in arterial blood to fraction of inspired oxygen (Pao_2/Fio_2)
            (a) *Mild ARDS*: Pao_2/Fio_2 $\leq$300 mm Hg but >200 mm Hg
            (b) *Moderate ARDS*: Pao_2/Fio_2 $\leq$200 mm Hg but >100 mm Hg
            (c) *Severe ARDS*: Pao_2/Fio_2 $\leq$100 mm Hg
   b) Common causes
      i) Systemic processes
         (1) Sepsis and/or shock
         (2) Disseminated intravascular coagulation
         (3) Drugs
         (4) Pancreatitis
         (5) Burns
      ii) Direct insult to the lungs
         (1) Pneumonia or aspiration
         (2) Trauma
         (3) Toxic inhalations
         (4) Exacerbation of diffuse lung disease
   c) HRCT findings (**Figs. A–C**)
      i) Bilateral, symmetric ground glass opacity and consolidation
      ii) Gradient of opacity from anterior (normal) to posterior (confluent consolidation) is common (**Fig. D**)
      iii) Patchy, nondependent consolidation suggests a superimposed lung process (e.g., infection) or a component of organizing pneumonia
      iv) May develop signs of fibrosis (traction bronchiectasis and irregular reticulation) 1 to 3 weeks after initial insult (**Fig. E**), although these findings are often reversible
      v) Mild residual fibrosis often persists in anterior and subpleural lung (**Fig. F**)
   d) Differential diagnosis includes edema, infection and hemorrhage

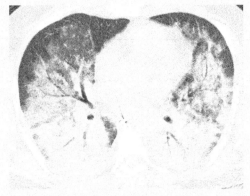

FIGURE D. Acute lung injury, 2 days after onset of symptoms: gradient of ground glass and consolidation from anterior to posterior

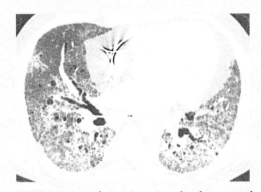

FIGURE E. Acute lung injury, 3 weeks after onset of symptoms: developing traction bronchiectasis and irregular reticulation

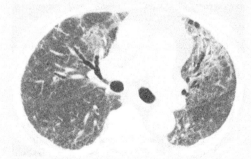

FIGURE F. Acute lung injury, 6 months after onset of symptoms: residual fibrosis in the anterior, subpleural lung

Chapter 9 Summary: The Interstitial Pneumonias

1) Key facts
   a) Histologic patterns of lung injury with characteristic features
   b) Each pattern has a HRCT correlate
   c) Each pattern may be idiopathic or associated with various diseases or exposures
2) Usual interstitial pneumonia (UIP)
   a) Common, 50% of interstitial pneumonia cases
   b) Most patients >50 years old
   c) Idiopathic UIP most common; termed idiopathic pulmonary fibrosis (IPF)
   d) Associated diseases
      i) Connective tissue disease (particularly rheumatoid arthritis)
      ii) Drug toxicity
      iii) Asbestosis (pleural plaques often present)
      iv) Hypersensitivity pneumonitis and sarcoidosis (usually have HRCT features that distinguish them from the other causes of UIP)
   e) Two classification schemes use HRCT findings and distribution to determine likelihood of UIP
      i) ATS/ERS/JRS/ALAT criteria
      ii) Fleischner society criteria
   f) HRCT features to make a confident diagnosis of UIP (biopsy not usually required) (**Fig. A**)
      i) Honeycombing
      ii) Other signs of fibrosis: irregular reticulation with or without traction bronchiectasis
      iii) Distribution: subpleural/basilar
      iv) Lack of features atypical for UIP (see h. below)
   g) HRCT features that are intermediate in likelihood for UIP (these cases often represent UIP) (**Fig. B**)
      i) Lack of honeycombing
      ii) Reticulation with or without traction bronchiectasis
      iii) Distribution: subpleural/basilar, variable, or diffuse
      iv) Atypical features may be seen but are present in nonsignificant amounts
   h) HRCT features that are atypical for UIP and suggestive of another diagnosis (only one of these needs to be present) (**Fig. C**)
      i) Distribution:
         (1) Mid-upper lung (craniocaudal)
         (2) Peribronchovascular distribution (axial)
      ii) Finding atypical for UIP is present (mosaic perfusion, air trapping, nodules, ground glass opacity, consolidation, cysts)

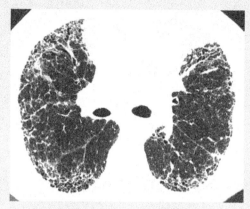

FIGURE A. High confidence in UIP: honeycombing and reticulation, peripheral distribution, no atypical features

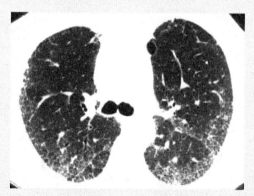

FIGURE B. Intermediate confidence in UIP: reticulation without honeycombing, peripheral distribution

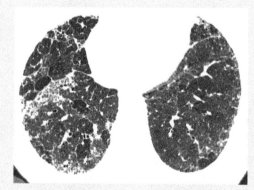

FIGURE C. Unlikely to represent UIP: patchy fibrosis with mosaic perfusion (geographic areas of dark lung) in at least three lobes

3) Nonspecific interstitial pneumonia (NSIP)
   a) Peak age range 40 to 50 years
   b) Less common than UIP
   c) Associated diseases
      i) Connective tissue disease
      ii) Hypersensitivity pneumonitis
      iii) Drug toxicity
      iv) Idiopathic NSIP
   d) HRCT features
      i) Cellular NSIP: ground glass opacity (**Fig. D**)
      ii) Fibrotic NSIP: reticulation and/or traction bronchiectasis (**Fig. E**)
      iii) Honeycombing very uncommon
      iv) Distribution: classically subpleural and basilar but may sometimes be peribronchovascular
      v) Subpleural sparing (very suggestive of NSIP)
   e) Biopsy often required for diagnosis except with connective tissue disease
4) Desquamative interstitial pneumonia
   a) Peak age: 30 to 40 years
   b) Most commonly associated with cigarette smoking
   c) HRCT features
      i) Ground glass opacity
      ii) Associated cystic lucencies
      iii) Subpleural/basilar distribution
      iv) Findings of fibrosis uncommon
5) Organizing pneumonia (OP)
   a) Subacute or chronic presentation
   b) May be seen in isolation or as a component of another diffuse lung disease (e.g., hypersensitivity pneumonitis, aspiration, vasculitis, etc.)
   c) Causes of OP: cryptogenic (COP; 50%), connective tissue disease, infection, drugs, toxic inhalations
   d) HRCT features (**Fig. F**)
      i) Consolidation > ground glass opacity
      ii) Focal, patchy, often nodular, or mass-like
      iii) Peribronchovascular and subpleural distribution
      iv) Atoll (or reversed halo) sign and perilobular sign are particularly suggestive
6) Lymphoid interstitial pneumonia (see Chapter 17)
7) Pleuroparenchymal fibroelastosis
   a) Newly described pattern of injury
   b) Apical distribution of fibrosis and pleural thickening
   c) HRCT features
      i) Apical/subpleural consolidation with architectural distortion, reticulation, traction bronchiectasis, and/or honeycombing
      ii) Pleural thickening (often fat attenuation)

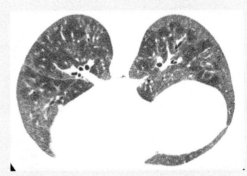

FIGURE D. Nonspecific interstitial pneumonia, cellular: isolated ground glass opacity, peripheral and peribronchovascular distribution, subpleural sparing

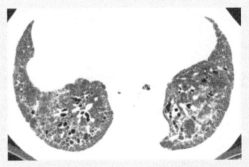

FIGURE E. Nonspecific interstitial pneumonia, fibrotic: reticulation and traction bronchiectasis, subpleural sparing

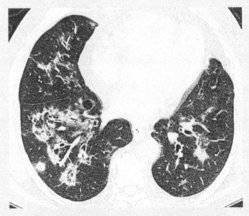

FIGURE F. Organizing pneumonia: peribronchovascular and subpleural consolidation with atolls

1) Role of HRCT in connective tissue disease (CTD)
   a) Diagnosis
      i) Made by clinical and serologic factors
      ii) Limited role of HRCT except in the setting of suspected, but not definite CTD
   b) Determine pattern of lung disease present
      i) Pathology generally not obtained in established CTD
      ii) HRCT is the primary method for determining pattern of injury present
      iii) Important for treatment and prognosis
   c) Follow up over time
      i) PFTs most helpful
      ii) HRCT useful with early disease or mixed disease (e.g., mixed interstitial and airways)
2) Patterns of injury in CTD
   a) Nonspecific interstitial pneumonia (NSIP)
      i) Most common pattern in CTD
      ii) Common with all CTDs except lupus
      iii) HRCT features (cellular and fibrotic types)
         (1) Ground glass opacity (GGO): cellular
         (2) Reticulation and/or traction bronchiectasis: fibrotic (honeycombing is rare)
         (3) Subpleural/basilar distribution most common
         (4) Subpleural sparing (particularly suggestive)
   b) Usual interstitial pneumonia (UIP)
      i) Most common with rheumatoid arthritis
      ii) Same HRCT features as with idiopathic pulmonary fibrosis
         (1) Honeycombing and reticulation
         (2) Subpleural/basilar distribution
         (3) Absence of features atypical for UIP
   c) Lymphoid interstitial pneumonia (LIP)
      i) Most common with Sjögren's disease and rheumatoid arthritis
      ii) HRCT features
         (1) GGO (nonspecific finding)
         (2) Nodules: centrilobular or perilymphatic
         (3) Cysts (in isolation or associated with the above findings)
   d) Organizing pneumonia (OP)
      i) Most common with myositis syndromes
      ii) HRCT features
         (1) Consolidation > GGO
         (2) Often nodular or mass-like
         (3) Peribronchovascular and subpleural distribution
         (4) Atoll or reversed halo sign (specific)

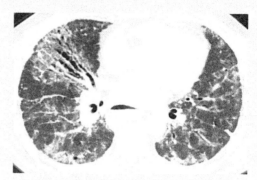

FIGURE A. Nonspecific interstitial pneumonia: scleroderma, irregular reticulation, traction bronchiectasis, subpleural sparing

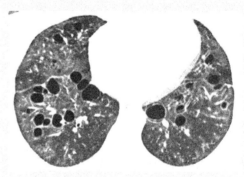

FIGURE B. Lymphoid interstitial pneumonia: rheumatoid, ground glass opacity, and cysts

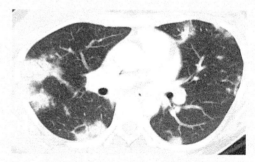

FIGURE C. Organizing pneumonia: systemic lupus erythematosus, focal patchy areas of consolidation

e) Pulmonary edema, hemorrhage, and diffuse alveolar damage (DAD)
   i) Acute presentation
   ii) Most common with lupus
   iii) HRCT features: bilateral GGO and consolidation
f) Airways disease (constrictive bronchiolitis or bronchiectasis)
   i) Most common with rheumatoid, lupus, and scleroderma
   ii) HRCT features
      (1) Mosaic perfusion and/or air trapping
      (2) Bronchial dilation and wall thickening
g) Other findings: pulmonary hypertension, serositis, esophageal dilation

3) Specific CTDs
a) Scleroderma
   i) Clinical: skin thickening, Raynaud's phenomenon, esophageal dysmotility
   ii) Lung disease is part of the criteria for diagnosis
   iii) Typical patterns
      (1) NSIP > UIP
      (2) Pulmonary hypertension (particularly with the CREST form)
b) Rheumatoid arthritis
   i) Clinical: arthritis predominant in hands, positive rheumatoid factor
   ii) Typical patterns
      (1) UIP and NSIP (most common)
      (2) LIP
      (3) Airways disease
c) Systemic lupus erythematosus
   i) Clinical: highly varied including rash, arthritis, serositis, renal, neurologic, hematologic
   ii) Typical patterns
      (1) Edema, hemorrhage, DAD
      (2) Airways disease
      (3) Serositis
d) Polymyositis and dermatomyositis
   i) Clinical: muscle weakness, arthritis, skin changes, Anti-Jo-1 antibodies
   ii) Typical patterns
      (1) NSIP
      (2) OP (often overlapping with NSIP)
e) Sjögren's disease
   i) Clinical: dry eyes and mouth, positive anti-SSA and anti-SSB
   ii) Typical patterns
      (1) NSIP
      (2) LIP (cysts often in isolation)
      (3) Airways disease

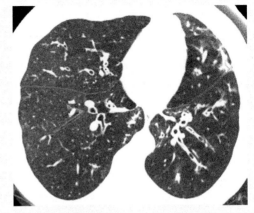

FIGURE D. Rheumatoid: airways disease, bronchiectasis, airway thickening and impaction, mosaic perfusion

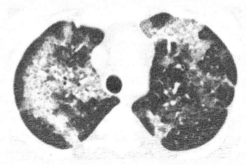

FIGURE E. Systemic lupus erythematosus: diffuse alveolar damage, bilateral ground glass opacity, and consolidation

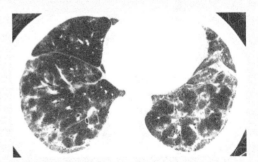

FIGURE F. Polymyositis: nonspecific interstitial pneumonia and organizing pneumonia overlap, subpleural ground glass opacity with subpleural sparing, peribronchovascular consolidation

Chapter 11 Summary: Smoking-Related Lung Disease

1) Respiratory bronchiolitis (RB) **(Fig. A)**
   a) Reaction to inhaled smoke around bronchioles
   b) Seen on pathology in all smokers
   c) Similar to, but less extensive than, desquamative interstitial pneumonia (DIP)
   d) Usually asymptomatic but when it causes symptoms is called RB-interstitial lung disease
   e) HRCT features (overlap with DIP, see below)
      i) Centrilobular ground glass nodules
      ii) Mild mosaic perfusion or air trapping
      iii) Distribution: upper lobes, central
   f) Differential diagnosis (other causes of centrilobular ground glass nodules)
      i) Hypersensitivity pneumonitis
      ii) Follicular bronchiolitis
      iii) Viral infection
      iv) Vascular diseases (e.g., hemorrhage)
2) Desquamative interstitial pneumonia (DIP) **(Fig. B)**
   a) More generalized reaction to inhaled smoke
   b) More commonly symptomatic than RB
   c) HRCT features (overlap with RB, see above)
      i) Ground glass opacity
      ii) Cystic lucencies (may resemble honeycombing but with thinner walls, irregular shapes, and often do not extend to subpleural lung)
      iii) Distribution: subpleural/basilar
      iv) Fibrosis develops in up to 25% **(Fig. C)**
   d) Differential diagnosis
      i) Significant overlap with appearance of NSIP from connective tissue disease, hypersensitivity pneumonitis, or drugs
      ii) IPF (cystic lucencies my resemble honeycombing)
3) Emphysema
   a) Lung destruction due to chronic inflammation
   b) Three types
      i) Centrilobular
         (1) Most common form seen in smokers
         (2) HRCT features: focal, air-density lucencies without a wall predominant in the central and upper lungs
      ii) Paraseptal
         (1) Idiopathic or associated with smoking
         (2) HRCT features: air-density cysts with a thin wall that are lined up in the subpleural lung in a single layer
      iii) Panlobular
         (1) Alpha-1 antitrypsin deficiency or associated with smoking
         (2) HRCT features: diffuse lung lucency and attenuated vessels with a lower lung predominance

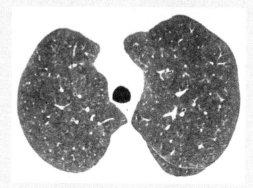

FIGURE A. Respiratory bronchiolitis: centrilobular ground glass nodules

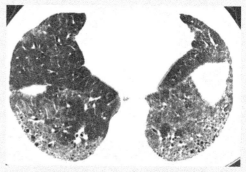

FIGURE B. Desquamative interstitial pneumonia: ground glass opacity associated with cystic lucencies

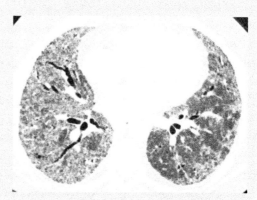

FIGURE C. Desquamative interstitial pneumonia: fibrosis with reticulation and traction bronchiectasis, significant ground glass opacity still present

4) Langerhans cell histiocytosis (**Fig. D**)
  a) Primarily smoking-related in adults
  b) Typical clinical symptoms
     i) Dyspnea
     ii) Pneumothorax
     iii) Incidental finding in asymptomatic patients
  c) HRCT features
     i) Nodules: soft tissue > ground glass attenuation, centrilobular distribution
     ii) Cavitation of nodules, thick or thin walled
     iii) Cysts (irregular shapes)
     iv) Distribution: spares lung bases
  d) Differential diagnosis
     i) Lymphangioleiomyomatosis (round cysts without sparing of the lung bases, nodules not usually present, associated pleural effusion)
     ii) Other causes of cystic lung disease (usually have fewer cysts): lymphoid interstitial pneumonia, pneumatoceles from prior infection, Birt–Hogg–Dubé, papillomatosis

5) Acute eosinophilic pneumonia
  a) Primarily a smoking-related lung disease
  b) Most patients have changed their smoking habits within a month of onset of symptoms
  c) Acute presentation
  d) Corticosteroid responsive
  e) HRCT features
     i) Ground glass opacity: diffuse or symmetric distribution
     ii) Smooth interlobular septal thickening

6) Smoking-related interstitial fibrosis and airspace enlargement with fibrosis
  a) Incidental finding of fibrosis on pathology seen in smokers
  b) Possibly the sequela of RB and DIP
  c) HRCT features
     i) Often normal
     ii) May show findings of RB and DIP
     iii) GGO often represents fibrosis in this setting

7) Combined pulmonary fibrosis and emphysema (**Fig. E**)
  a) Two components: emphysema and interstitial lung disease (most commonly idiopathic pulmonary fibrosis)
  b) Relatively normal lung volumes on pulmonary function tests
  c) Higher rate of pulmonary hypertension

8) Idiopathic pulmonary fibrosis
  a) 40% to 80% of IPF patients have a smoking history
  b) Emphysema and cystic lucencies of DIP (see above) complicate the diagnosis of fibrotic lung disease and may be mistaken for honeycombing (**Fig. F**)

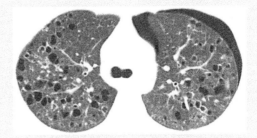

FIGURE D. Langerhans cell histiocytosis: solid nodules and irregular cysts, pneumothorax

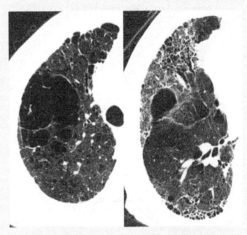

FIGURE E. Combined pulmonary fibrosis and emphysema: emphysema in the upper lung (left), fibrosis in a UIP pattern in the lower lung (right)

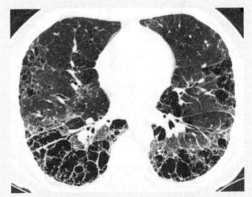

FIGURE F. Desquamative interstitial pneumonia: mimic of IPF, cystic lucencies with thin walls and irregular shapes, ground glass opacity with minimal fibrosis

Chapter 12 Summary: Sarcoidosis

1) General information
   a) Idiopathic systemic immune disorder
   b) Noncaseating granuloma deposition in one or more organs (thorax in ≥90%)
   c) Most common in patients <50 years old, although may also present in older patients
   d) Highest incidence in Scandinavians and African-Americans
   e) Relative low mortality (1% to 5%) compared with other diffuse lung diseases
2) Staging system
   a) Based on radiographic findings (not HRCT)
   b) May be helpful in predicting likelihood of spontaneous regression (60% to 90% in stage I but only 10% to 20% in stage III)
   c) Stages
      i) 0: normal
      ii) I: hilar lymphadenopathy (LAD) only
      iii) II: hilar LAD + parenchymal lung disease
      iv) III: parenchymal lung disease only
      v) IV: fibrosis
3) HRCT findings
   a) Perilymphatic nodules (Fig. A)
      i) Most typical locations
         (1) Parahilar, peribronchovascular interstitium
         (2) Subpleural interstitium
      ii) May also involve these locations, but usually to a lesser extent:
         (1) Centrilobular interstitium
         (2) Interlobular septa
      iii) Rarely nodules appear to represent a random distribution, but there are usually clues that the distribution is actually perilymphatic:
         (1) Inhomogeneous lung involvement
         (2) Proportionally too many nodules along fissures and/or peribronchovascular interstitium
   b) Consolidation and masses (Fig. B)
      i) Confluent granulomas
      ii) Distribution: upper lung and peribronchovascular
      iii) Satellite nodes around consolidation/masses (galaxy sign)
   c) Ground glass opacity (GGO) (Fig. C)
      i) Microscopic granulomas
      ii) Rare as an isolated abnormality
      iii) Even when GGO is present, nodules are also usually seen

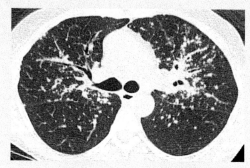

FIGURE A. **Sarcoidosis:** typical perilymphatic nodules, peribronchovascular and subpleural distribution

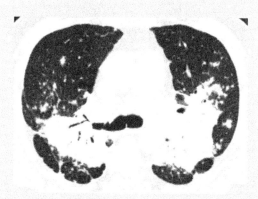

FIGURE B. **Sarcoidosis:** rounded and mass-like conglomerates of granulomas, smaller nodules at the peripheral, galaxy sign

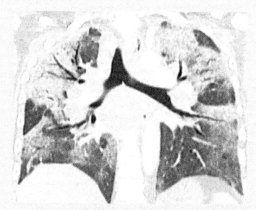

FIGURE C. **Sarcoidosis:** coronal image, patchy upper lobe predominant consolidation and ground glass opacity, chronic symptoms

d) Mosaic perfusion and/or air trapping (**Fig. D**)
   i) Reflection of granulomas obstructing central or distal airways
   ii) Lobular, segmental, or lobar distribution
   iii) Usually seen in association with nodules
   iv) May persist after nodules have been treated
e) Fibrosis (**Fig. E**)
   i) Occurs in 20% of patients
   ii) Associated with poor outcome
   iii) Key HRCT findings: irregular reticulation, traction bronchiectasis, and honeycombing
   iv) Distribution: upper lung and peribronchovascular
   v) Fibrosis may be mass-like, similar to progressive massive fibrosis
   vi) Associated findings: emphysema, cysts, and mycetoma
f) Lymphadenopathy (**Fig. F**)
   i) Hilar and mediastinal involvement
   ii) Symmetric distribution characteristic
   iii) Calcification of nodes is not uncommon
   iv) Necrosis of nodes is rare
4) Differential diagnosis: based on predominant finding seen in sarcoidosis
a) Perilymphatic nodules
   i) Lymphangitic spread of neoplasm (history of malignancy, usually interlobular septal thickening predominates)
   ii) Pneumoconioses (history of exposure, many centrilobular nodules)
   iii) Lymphoid interstitial pneumonia and amyloidosis (with an appropriate history)
b) Consolidation (chronic)
   i) Organizing pneumonia
   ii) Chronic eosinophilic pneumonia
   iii) Invasive mucinous adenocarcinoma
   iv) Lymphoma
   v) Lipoid pneumonia
c) Fibrosis (upper, peribronchovascular distribution)
   i) Pneumoconioses
   ii) Prior tuberculosis or fungal infection
   iii) Hypersensitivity pneumonitis (usually mid-lung)
d) Lymphadenopathy (symmetric hilar/mediastinal)
   i) Pneumoconioses
   ii) Amyloidosis
   iii) Castleman's disease
   iv) Metastatic disease (gastrointestinal and genitourinary tumors, lung cancer, breast cancer, leukemia)

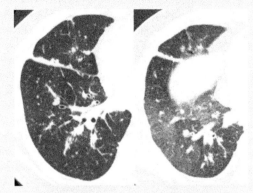

FIGURE D. Sarcoidosis: peribronchovascular and subpleural nodules on inspiratory CT (left) associated with air trapping on expiratory CT (right)

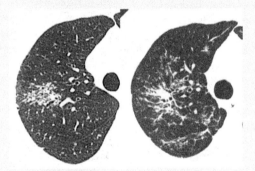

FIGURE E. Sarcoidosis: perilymphatic nodules on baseline CT (left); peribronchovascular fibrosis develops 4 years later (right)

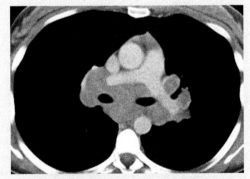

FIGURE F. Sarcoidosis: lymphadenopathy, symmetric, hilar and mediastinal

Chapter 13 Summary: Hypersensitivity Pneumonitis and Eosinophilic Lung Disease

1) Hypersensitivity pneumonitis (HP)
   a) An exaggerated immune response to inhaled organic antigens
      i) Most commonly related to birds or mold
      ii) Antigen identified in only 50% of patients
   b) Three categories
      i) Acute: rare, large antigen exposure, rapid onset of severe symptoms
      ii) Subacute: common, similar symptoms as acute HP; however, less severe; time course is weeks to months
      iii) Chronic: common, long-term exposure to low levels of antigen, presence of lung fibrosis
   c) HRCT findings
      i) Ground glass opacity (GGO)
         (1) May be seen in isolation in which case it is very nonspecific
         (2) Often associated with other abnormalities (nodules, mosaic perfusion, air trapping)
         (3) Patchy and bilateral distribution
         (4) Mid-lung predominance in some
      ii) Centrilobular nodules of GGO (**Fig. A**)
         (1) Distribution: symmetric and/or diffuse
         (2) Diagnostic of HP with history of exposure
         (3) Differential diagnosis
            (a) Respiratory bronchiolitis (smokers)
            (b) Follicular bronchiolitis (connective tissue disease)
            (c) Atypical infection
            (d) Vascular diseases (e.g., hemorrhage)
      iii) Mosaic perfusion and/or air trapping (**Fig. B**)
         (1) Seen in isolation or associated with other findings
         (2) HRCT: lobular areas of decreased lung attenuation with sharp margins
         (3) Differential diagnosis (when isolated)
            (a) Asthma
            (b) Constrictive bronchiolitis
      iv) The headcheese sign (**Fig. C**)
         (1) Reflects a mixed obstructive and infiltrative disorder
         (2) HRCT: three densities of lung present (all in significant amounts)
            (a) GGO
            (b) Mosaic perfusion/air trapping
            (c) Normal lung
         (3) Significance: HP represents the majority of cases with this pattern

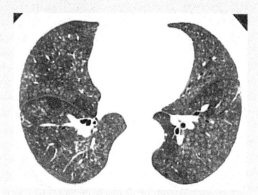

FIGURE A. **Hypersensitivity pneumonitis:** subacute, diffuse centrilobular nodules of GGO

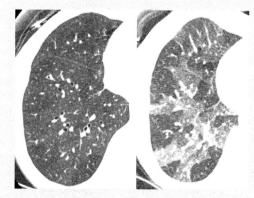

FIGURE B. **Hypersensitivity pneumonitis:** isolated mosaic perfusion on inspiration (left image) and air trapping on expiration (right image)

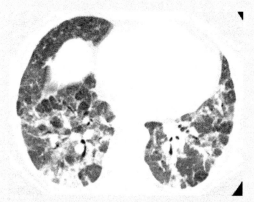

FIGURE C. **Hypersensitivity pneumonitis:** headcheese sign, geographic areas of ground glass opacity, mosaic perfusion and normal lung

v) Consolidation
   (1) Often represents organizing pneumonia associated with HP
   (2) Uncommon to be present in isolation in HP
   (3) Often present in small amounts and associated with other findings
vi) Fibrosis: chronic HP **(Fig. D)**
   (1) HRCT: irregular reticulation, traction bronchiectasis, and honeycombing
   (2) Often seen in association with other findings (nodules, ground glass opacity, mosaic perfusion, air trapping)
   (3) Distribution
      (a) Mid-lung, sparing costophrenic angles
      (b) Not subpleural predominant

d) Eosinophilic lung diseases (focusing on idiopathic disorders)
   i) Simple pulmonary eosinophilia (Loffler syndrome)
      (1) Acute presentation, mild symptoms, spontaneous regression within 1 months
      (2) Migratory, nonsegmental consolidation, often peripheral and in the upper lungs
   ii) Acute eosinophilia pneumonia
      (1) Acute presentation, does not recur
      (2) Most cases associated with smokers who change their smoking habits
      (3) Peripheral eosinophilia may be lacking
      (4) Highly steroid responsive
      (5) Extensive bilateral GGO and/or consolidation with smooth interlobular septal thickening (resembles edema)
   iii) Chronic eosinophilic pneumonia **(Fig. E)**
      (1) Chronic symptoms (several months)
      (2) Peripheral eosinophilia usually present
      (3) Highly steroid responsive
      (4) Consolidation most typical HRCT finding
      (5) Distribution: peripheral and upper lung most typical
   iv) Hypereosinophilic syndrome
      (1) >6 months clinical course
      (2) Systemic disorder: central nervous system (CNS) and cardiac involvement most common
      (3) HRCT
         (a) Pulmonary edema from cardiac disease
         (b) Nodules from eosinophilic infiltration
   v) Eosinophilic granulomatosis with polyangiitis (Churg–Strauss syndrome) **(Fig. F)**
      (1) Systemic vasculitis: lungs, CNS, skin
      (2) Seen in patients with asthma or allergy
      (3) HRCT: nonsegmental consolidation or GGO that is often peripheral and lobular

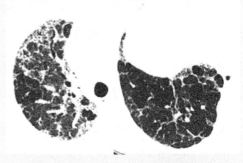

FIGURE D. Hypersensitivity pneumonitis: typical distribution, upper lobe (left image) predominance of fibrosis with sparing of the bases (right image)

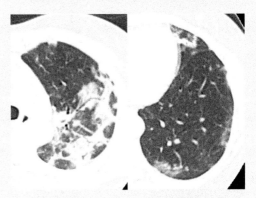

FIGURE E. Chronic eosinophilic pneumonia: patchy consolidation that is more severe in the upper lung (left image) compared with the lower lung (right image)

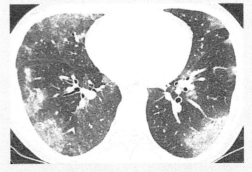

FIGURE F. Eosinophilic granulomatosis with polyangiitis: geographic and peripheral ground glass opacity and consolidation

1) Bacterial infection
    a) Lobar pneumonia
        i) Infection primarily within alveolar spaces
        ii) Most common organisms: *Streptococcus, Haemophilus influenzae, Klebsiella*, and *Moraxella catarrhalis*
        iii) HRCT findings
            (1) Consolidation marginated by fissures
            (2) Air bronchograms
            (3) Single or multiple lobes, nonsegmental
    b) Bronchopneumonia (**Fig. A**)
        i) Endobronchial spread of infection
        ii) Most common organisms: *S. aureus, P. aeruginosa, Klebsiella*, and *E. coli*
        iii) HRCT findings
            (1) Centrilobular nodules of soft tissue attenuation ± tree-in-bud opacities
            (2) Airway thickening, impaction and dilation
            (3) Consolidation
            (4) Patchy, lobular, or segmental distribution
    c) Septic emboli
        i) Embolization of infected thrombi to lungs
        ii) Most common sources: infective endocarditis and infected catheters
        iii) HRCT findings
            (1) Multiple, bilateral large nodules and masses
            (2) Cavitation common
            (3) Feeding vessel sign
2) Tuberculosis (TB)
    a) Primary TB: infection associated with initial exposure (**Fig. B**)
        i) Asymptomatic presentation (common)
            (1) Usually discovered as an incidental imaging finding
            (2) HRCT: small nodule, often calcified ± calcified lymph nodes
        ii) Symptomatic presentation (uncommon)
            (1) More frequently seen in children and immunosuppressed patients
            (2) HRCT: consolidation, nodule, and/or lymphadenopathy
    b) Reactivation TB (RTB): occurs after TB disseminates from the initial site of infection (**Fig. C**)
        i) Most common in upper lungs
        ii) Consolidation with cavitation, centrilobular nodules of soft tissue attenuation, and tree-in-bud opacities
        iii) Pleural effusions and/or thickening
        iv) Lung scarring
    c) Milliary TB: hematogenous spread of infection
        i) Diffuse small nodules
        ii) Random distribution on HRCT

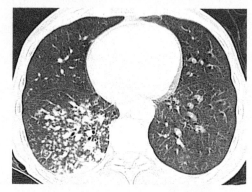

FIGURE A. Bacterial bronchopneumonia: clustered centrilobular nodules and consolidation in a segmental distribution

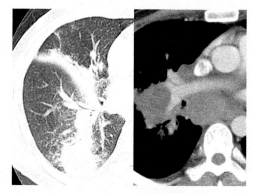

FIGURE B. Tuberculosis, primary: mid-lung consolidation associated with necrotic lymphadenopathy

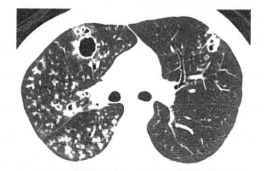

FIGURE C. Tuberculosis, reactivation: upper lobe cavities, centrilobular nodules, tree-in-bud opacities, asymmetric distribution

3) Nontuberculous mycobacterium (NTM)
   a) Multiple different organisms, *Mycobacterium avium-intracellulare* complex most common
   b) Most common form: airway-predominant disease
      i) Elderly women with normal immune status
      ii) HRCT findings
         (1) Bronchiectasis, airway thickening and impaction, centrilobular nodules, tree-in-bud opacities
         (2) Relative paucity of consolidation
         (3) Right middle lobe and lingular predominance
   c) Other forms of NTM include the following:
      i) Upper lobe cavitary consolidation resembling RTB (elderly immunocompromised men)
      ii) Nodular form (often asymptomatic): patchy, bilateral, large solid nodules resembling fungal infection or metastases
4) Fungal infection
   a) Two main categories of fungi that share similar HRCT features
      i) Endemic fungal infections: coccidioidomycosis, histoplasmosis, blastomycosis (most common in immunocompetent patients)
      ii) Other fungal infections: aspergillosis, mucormycosis, candidiasis, cryptococcosis (most common in immunocompromised patients)
   b) Primary HRCT patterns of fungal infection
      i) Upper lobe cavitary consolidation resembling RTB (most typical of endemic fungal infections or *Aspergillus*)
      ii) Solitary pulmonary nodule and/or lymphadenopathy (endemic infections or *Cryptococcus*)
      iii) Bronchopneumonia or lobar pneumonia (very nonspecific, can be seen with most infections)
      iv) Multifocal nodular or mass-like areas of consolidation ± halo sign (common with the nonendemic fungal infections and *Cryptococcus*) (**Fig. D**)
      v) Random distribution of small nodules (most typical of endemic fungal infections or candidiasis) (**Fig. E**)
5) Atypical infections including atypical bacterial infections, viral infections, and *Pneuomcystis jiroveci*
   a) Clinical features: less severe presentation, systemic symptoms more common
   b) HRCT features (**Fig. F**)
      i) Diffuse or symmetric distribution
      ii) Ground glass opacity ≫ consolidation
      iii) Centrilobular nodules and airways inflammation (particularly with viruses)
      iv) Cysts are particularly suggestive of *Pneumocystis* in HIV patients

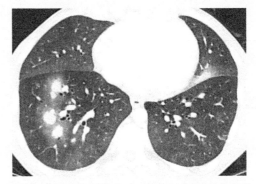

FIGURE D. Aspergillosis, multiple nodular regions of consolidation with halos of ground glass opacity

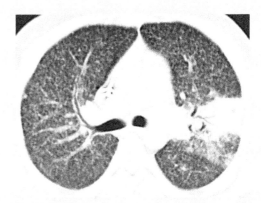

FIGURE E. Coccidioidomycosis: left upper lobe consolidation associated with a random distribution of small nodules

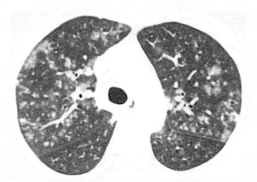

FIGURE F. Viral pneumonia: ground glass opacity, centrilobular nodules, symmetric distribution

1) Drug-induced lung disease
   a) General information
      i) Many possible patterns (listed below) that may be related to drugs or have other causes
      ii) History is critical for accurate diagnosis
      iii) Reference: https://www.pneumotox.com
      iv) Wide range of onset in symptoms in relation to start of drug; however, weeks to months most common
   b) Pulmonary edema
      i) HRCT: bilateral interlobular septal thickening, ground glass opacity, consolidation
      ii) Drugs: cocaine, aspirin, heroin, methotrexate, cyclophosphamide, carmustine
   c) Pulmonary hemorrhage
      i) HRCT: bilateral ground glass opacity and/or consolidation
      ii) Drugs: anticoagulants, cyclophosphamide, penicillamine
   d) Diffuse alveolar damage (**Fig. A**)
      i) HRCT: bilateral ground glass opacity and consolidation
      ii) Drugs: carmustine, busulfan, cyclophosphamide, bleomycin, amiodarone, methotrexate, aspirin, narcotics, cocaine
   e) Organizing pneumonia (**Fig. B**)
      i) HRCT: bilateral, patchy, nodular, or mass-like areas of consolidation, reversed halo sign
      ii) Drugs: carmustine, bleomycin, doxorubicin, cyclophosphamide, amiodarone, nitrofurantoin, cephalosporins, tetracycline, amphotericin B, gold salts, phenytoin, sulfasalazine, and cocaine
   f) Nonspecific interstitial pneumonia (**Fig. C**)
      i) HRCT: ground glass opacity or irregular reticulation and traction bronchiectasis in a peripheral and basilar distribution, subpleural sparing particularly suggestive
      ii) Drugs: bleomycin, busulfan, cyclophosphamide, methotrexate, amiodarone, nitrofurantoin, hydrochlorothiazide, statins, phenytoin, and gold
   g) Usual interstitial pneumonia
      i) HRCT: irregular reticulation, traction bronchiectasis, and honeycombing in a subpleural and basilar distribution
      ii) Drugs: cyclophosphamide, chlorambucil, nitrofurantoin, and pindolol

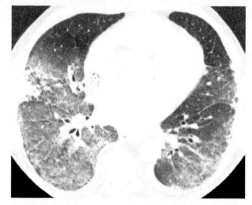

FIGURE A. Adriamycin: organizing diffuse alveolar damage, bilateral ground glass opacity, and focal areas of consolidation

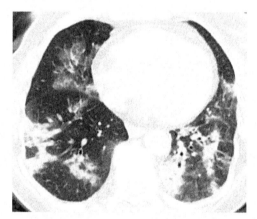

FIGURE B. Sirolimus: organizing pneumonia, patchy peribronchovascular and subpleural consolidation, reversed halo sign

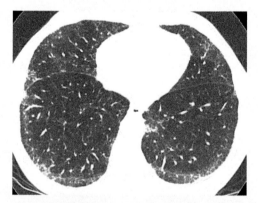

FIGURE C. Bleomycin: nonspecific interstitial pneumonia, peripheral irregular reticulation with subpleural sparing

h) Eosinophilic pneumonia
   i) HRCT: patchy bilateral consolidation that may be peripheral and upper lung in distribution
   ii) Drugs: bleomycin, amiodarone, nitrofurantoin, antidepressants, beta-blockers, hydrochlorothiazide, nonsteroidal anti-inflammatory drugs, phenytoin, sulfasalazine, and cocaine
i) Hypersensitivity pneumonitis (Fig. D)
   i) HRCT: ground glass opacity, centrilobular nodules, mosaic perfusion, air trapping, or fibrosis that spares the lung bases
   ii) Drugs: methotrexate, cyclophosphamide, mesalamine, fluoxetine, amitriptyline, and paclitaxel
j) Sarcoid-like reaction
   i) HRCT: perilymphatic nodules
   ii) Drug: interferon
k) Pulmonary vascultitis/hypertension
   i) HRCT: bilateral ground glass opacity, enlarged pulmonary arteries
   ii) Drugs: fenfluramine, busulfan, methylphenidate, and methadone
l) Constrictive bronchiolitis
   i) HRCT: mosaic perfusion, air trapping ± bronchiectasis
   ii) Drug: penicillamine

2) Radiotherapy (Rx) with lung injury
   a) Evolution over time
      i) Early: inflammation
      ii) Late: fibrosis (Fig. E)
   b) Typical distributions related to Rx
      i) Breast Rx: anterior subpleural lung
      ii) Axilla/supraclavicular Rx: lung apex
      iii) Neck Rx: biapical
      iv) Lymphoma/esophageal Rx: paramediastinal
   c) HRCT findings
      i) Inflammatory stage
         (1) Consolidation and ground glass opacity
         (2) Localized to the treated area
         (3) Often with sharp borders
      ii) Fibrotic stage
         (1) Volume loss and architectural distortion
         (2) Development of irregular reticulation and traction bronchiectasis
   d) May result in abnormalities outside the Rx field
      i) Resembles diffuse alveolar damage, organizing pneumonia, or eosinophilic pneumonia
      ii) HRCT (Fig. F)
         (1) Ground glass opacity and consolidation
         (2) Distribution is variable: patchy or diffuse

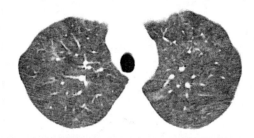

FIGURE D. Nitrofurantoin: hypersensitivity pneumonitis-like reaction, ground glass opacity, and centrilobular nodules

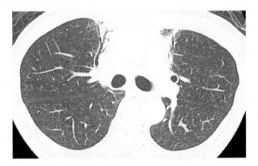

FIGURE E. Radiation fibrosis: paramediastinal fibrosis after radiation for thymic carcinoma

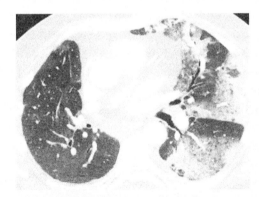

FIGURE F. Radiation pneumonitis: extensive left lung ground glass opacity and consolidation outside the radiation field

1) Lung disease resulting from environmental dust inhalation
   a) HRCT findings overlap with other diseases
   b) Exposure history is critical
   c) Key imaging findings
      i) Nodules
      ii) Fibrosis
      iii) Lymphadenopathy
   d) Several characteristic patterns (listed below) with an archetypal causative dust
2) Silicosis pattern
   a) Exposures: glass manufacturing, sandblasting, mining, stone cutting, quarrying
   b) Simple silicosis (**Fig. A**)
      i) Early stage with nodules but no fibrosis
      ii) HRCT
         (1) Perilymphatic nodules (often with many centrilobular nodules)
         (2) Nodules symmetric, soft tissue attenuation, may calcify
         (3) Hilar/mediastinal lymphadenopathy
   c) Complicated silicosis (**Fig. B**)
      i) Development of fibrosis
      ii) HRCT
         (1) Irregular reticulation and traction bronchiectasis
         (2) Upper lung and peribronchovascular distribution
         (3) Progressive massive fibrosis: consolidative masses of fibrosis
   d) Silicoproteinosis (**Fig. C**)
      i) Acute exposure to large amounts of silca dust
      ii) Closely resembles alveolar proteinosis
      iii) HRCT
         (1) Ground glass opacity often with interlobular septal thickening (e.g., crazy paving)
         (2) Symmetric bilateral distribution
   e) Differential diagnosis
      i) Other pneumoconiosis that may show this pattern: coal worker's pneumoconiosis, talcosis, berrylliosis
      ii) Sarcoidosis and other causes of perilymphatic nodules or upper lobe fibrosis
   f) Complications
      i) Tuberculosis (cavitation in a mass may be suggestive)
      ii) Primary bronchogenic carcinoma (PET may be helpful)

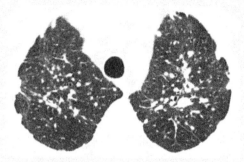

FIGURE A. Silicosis, simple: peribronchovascular and subpleural nodules, perilymphatic distribution

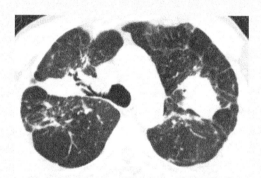

FIGURE B. Silicosis, complicated: rounded masses of fibrosis with volume loss, architectural distortion, and bronchiectasis

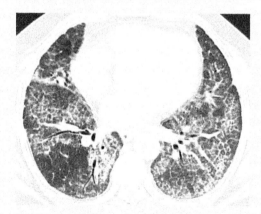

FIGURE C. Silicoproteinosis: bilateral crazy paving (ground glass and interlobular septal thickening)

3) Asbestosis pattern (**Fig. D**)
   a) Exposures: mining, shipbuilding, construction, textiles manufacturing, manufacture of brake lining, and exposure to insulation materials
   b) HRCT
      i) Pleural disease
         (1) Pleural effusion(s): exudative with pleural thickening and enhancement
         (2) Pleural plaques
      ii) Lung disease (asbestosis): typically a UIP pattern
         (1) Fibrosis with honeycombing
         (2) Subpleural/basilar distribution
         (3) Small centrilobular nodules (rare) may help to distinguish from idiopathic pulmonary fibrosis
   c) Differential diagnosis (other causes of a UIP pattern)
      i) Idiopathic pulmonary fibrosis (usually a more rapid rate of progression than asbestosis)
      ii) Connective tissue disease
      iii) Drugs
   d) Complications
      i) Primary bronchogenic carcinoma (should be distinguished from rounded atelectasis)
      ii) Mesothelioma

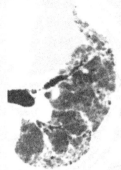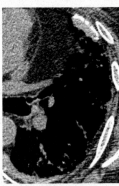

FIGURE D. Asbestosis: fibrosis with honeycombing (left image) associated with pleural plaques (right image)

4) Siderosis pattern (**Fig. E**)
   a) Exposure: primarily iron welding
   b) Deposition of iron oxide around airways
   c) Relative lack of immune reaction (fibrosis and lymphatic drainage not usually a feature)
   d) Mixed dusts that include iron oxide may result in mixed patterns
   e) HRCT
      i) Findings resemble subacute hypersensitivity pneumonitis
      ii) Ground glass opacity and/or centrilobular nodules of ground glass attenuation
      iii) Mosaic perfusion and/or air trapping (usually mild)
      iv) Fibrosis may occur, particularly in mixed dust exposures (often resembles nonspecific or usual interstitial pneumonia)
   f) Differential diagnosis
      i) Baritosis (barium) and stannosis (tin)
      ii) Hard metal pneumoconiosis: findings overlap with siderosis, fibrosis is more common (**Fig. F**)
      iii) Subacute hypersensitivity pneumonitis
   g) Complications are rare but include malignancy, particularly when mixed with silica

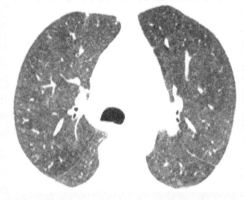

FIGURE E. Siderosis: bilateral ground glass opacity and centrilobular nodules of ground glass attenuation

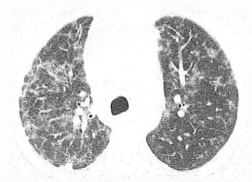

FIGURE F. Hard metal pneumoconiosis: ground glass opacity and centrilobular nodules of ground glass attenuation with irregular reticulation

Chapter 17 Summary: Neoplastic and Lymphoproliferative

1) Mechanisms of spread of malignancy
   a) Hematogenous: diffuse small nodules in a random distribution
   b) Intravascular: enlarged and nodular vessels
   c) Lymphangitic: smooth or nodular interlobular septal thickening
   d) Endobronchial: centrilobular nodules
2) Specific malignancies
   a) Invasive mucinous adenocarcinoma (**Fig. A**)
      i) Formerly called diffuse bronchioloalveolar carcinoma
      ii) Lepidic growth and endobronchial spread
      iii) Multifocal or diffuse lung involvement
      iv) HRCT features
         (1) Consolidation and/or ground glass opacity (resembling pneumonia)
         (2) Centrilobular nodules
         (3) Focal, patchy, or diffuse distribution
      v) Differential diagnosis includes other causes of chronic consolidation
   b) Kaposi sarcoma (**Fig. B**)
      i) Associated with herpes virus-8 infection
      ii) Most common in patients with human immunodeficiency virus (HIV)
      iii) HRCT features
         (1) Thickening of peribronchovascular interstitium
         (2) Large, irregular, "flame-shaped" nodules
         (3) Interlobular septal thickening
         (4) Pleural effusions and lymphadenopathy
   c) Pulmonary lymphoma
      i) Primary pulmonary lymphoma (**Fig. C**)
         (1) Isolated to lung without extrathoracic dissemination for 3 months after diagnosis
         (2) MALToma
            (a) Accounts for majority of primary pulmonary lymphomas
            (b) Risk factors: smoking, autoimmune disease, or infection
            (c) HRCT features
               (i) Solitary or multiple nodules or areas of consolidation
               (ii) Indolent course, slow growth
         (3) Diffuse large B-cell lymphoma: less common than MALToma
      ii) Secondary pulmonary lymphoma
         (1) More common than primary
         (2) Findings similar to primary lymphoma except that extrapulmonary findings are also present

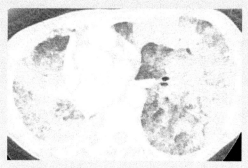

FIGURE A. Invasive mucinous adenocarcinoma: extensive bilateral consolidation and ground glass opacity, chronic symptoms

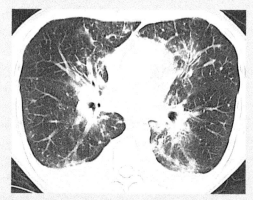

FIGURE B. Kaposi sarcoma: peribronchovascular interstitial thickening and small nodules

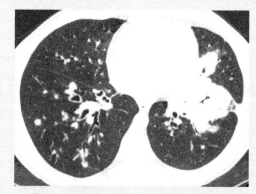

FIGURE C. Primary pulmonary lymphoma: peribronchovascular consolidation and nodules

Key Points, Differential Diagnosis and Classic Images

3) Lymphoproliferative diseases
   a) Focal nodular lymphoid hyperplasia (sometimes termed pseudolymphoma)
      i) Localized collection of nonneoplastic lymphocytes
      ii) Often associated with Sjogren's syndrome
      iii) HRCT features
         (1) Solitary, solid nodule (most common)
         (2) Consolidation or multiple nodules (uncommon)
   b) Lymphoid interstitial pneumonia (LIP) and follicular bronchiolitis (FB) (**Fig. D**)
      i) Polyclonal lymphocyte proliferation around small airways (FB) or in the interstitium (LIP)
      ii) Often associated with immunosuppression (HIV and common variable immunodeficiency) and connective tissue disease
      iii) HRCT features
         (1) Centrilobular nodules of ground glass attenuation (FB)
         (2) Mosaic perfusion or air trapping (mild)
         (3) Bilateral ground glass opacity and/or consolidation
         (4) Perilymphatic nodules (LIP)
         (5) Cysts
   c) IgG4-related disease (**Fig. E**)
      i) Systemic disorder
      ii) Lymphoplasmocytic infiltrates in various organs
      iii) HRCT: three main patterns of disease
         (1) One or more nodules or masses
         (2) Peribronchovascular and interlobular septal thickening
         (3) Findings of an interstitial pneumonia
   d) Lymphomatoid granulomatosis
      i) Angiocentric lymphoid infiltrate
      ii) Different grades depending on pathology
      iii) HRCT: bilateral, poorly defined nodules with or without cavitation
4) Posttransplant lymphoproliferative disorder (**Fig. F**)
   a) Solid organ or bone marrow transplantation
   b) Spectrum of disease from benign proliferation to malignant lymphoma
   c) HRCT (resembles lymphoma)
      i) Single or multiple pulmonary nodules/masses or consolidation
      ii) Lymphadenopathy commonly present
5) Leukemia: lung infiltration mainly shows peribronchovascular and interlobular septal thickening on HRCT

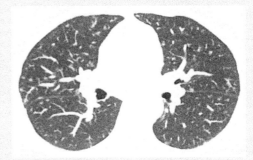

FIGURE D. Follicular bronchiolitis: centrilobular nodules of ground glass attenuation

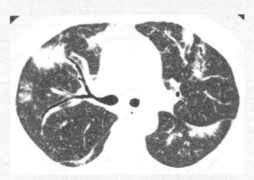

FIGURE E. IgG4-related disease: large, solid, peribronchovascular, and subpleural nodules

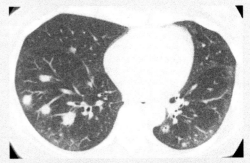

FIGURE F. Posttransplant lymphoproliferative disorder: scattered solid peribronchovascular nodules

1) Pulmonary alveolar proteinosis
   a) Accumulation of lipoprotein within alveoli
   b) Three forms
      i) Idiopathic (90% of cases): autoantibodies against granulocyte-macrophage colony-stimulating factor
      ii) Congenital
      iii) Secondary (associated with acute silicosis, infections, malignancy)
   c) HRCT
      i) Crazy paving (ground glass opacity and interlobular septal thickening)
      ii) Symmetric distribution, very geographic
2) Lipoid pneumonia
   a) Two forms
      i) Endogenous: distal to obstructed airway
      ii) Exogenous: aspiration of fat-containing substances
   b) HRCT (exogenous form)
      i) Consolidation with fat attenuation
      ii) Ground glass opacity ± crazy paving
      iii) Focal or patchy, bilateral distribution; often dependent
3) Amyloidosis
   a) Accumulation of extracellular protein in multiple organs (kidney, heart, nervous system, liver)
   b) Two subtypes
      i) Amyloid A: usually asymptomatic, associated with systemic inflammatory disorders
      ii) Amyloid light chain: accounts for most symptomatic cases, associated with myeloma
   c) Three HRCT manifestations in the lungs
      i) Focal parenchymal: single or multiple discreet lung nodules ± calcification
      ii) Diffuse parenchymal
         (1) Small nodules in a perilymphatic distribution, often calcified
         (2) Extensive involvement may result in high-density consolidation
      iii) Tracheobronchial
         (1) Involvement of trachea and central bronchi
         (2) Airway wall thickening and calcification
4) Light-chain deposition disease
   a) Accumulation of nonamyloid light chains in multiple organs
   b) Shares many features with amyloidosis
   c) Commonly associated with Waldenström's macroglobulinemia
   d) HRCT: single or multiple large solid nodules associated with cysts

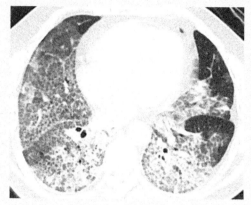

FIGURE A. Pulmonary alveolar proteinosis: geographic bilateral crazy paving and mild consolidation

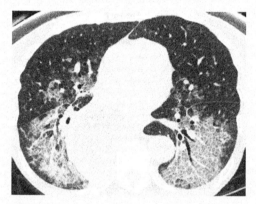

FIGURE B. Lipoid pneumonia: dependent bilateral crazy paving in a patient with achalasia

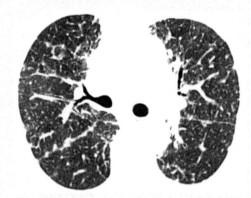

FIGURE C. Amyloidosis: subpleural nodules and peribronchovascular interstitial thickening

5) Pulmonary alveolar microlithiasis
   a) Accumulation of microliths in alveolar spaces
   b) Sporadic or familial
   c) HRCT
      i) Tiny, discreet, calcified nodules
      ii) Perilymphatic or centrilobular distribution
6) Erdheim–Chester disease
   a) Infilration of various organs by non-Langerhans histiocytes
   b) Organs: bones, nervous cysts, heart, kidneys, lymphatic system
   c) HRCT
      i) Smooth interlobular septal thickening
      ii) Small centrilobular or perilymphatic nodules
      iii) Hilar/mediastinal lymphadenopathy
7) Lymphangioleiomyomatosis
   a) Low-grade malignancy
   b) Proliferation of epithelioid cells
   c) Sporadic or related to tuberous sclerosis
   d) Presentation: dyspnea, pneumothorax, or as incidental finding
   e) HRCT
      i) Lung cysts: round regular shape
      ii) Distribution: uniform lung involvement
      iii) Nodules usually not present
      iv) Angiomyolipomas in the kidneys
8) Birt–Hogg–Dubé syndrome
   a) Genetic disorder
   b) Characteristics
      i) Skin fibrofolliculomas
      ii) Renal tumors
      iii) Lung cysts
   c) HRCT
      i) Lung cysts, thin-walled, variable size
      ii) Distribution: lung bases, subpleural, and directly adjacent to pulmonary arteries and veins
9) Hermansky–Pudlak syndrome
   a) Genetic disorder
   b) Characteristics: albinism, platelet dysfunction, and pulmonary fibrosis
   c) HRCT: nonspecific fibrosis, often peripheral
10) Minute pulmonary meningothelial-like nodules
   a) Usually an incidental finding
   b) HRCT: Small scattered nodules, well-defined borders, some of which contain cystic lucencies
11) Pulmonary ossification
   a) Often associated with interstitial lung disease but may also be idiopathic
   b) HRCT: multiple calcified nodules in the peripheral lung

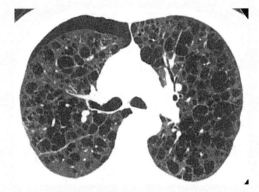

FIGURE D. Lymphangioleiomyomatosis: diffuse round cysts with a pneumothorax

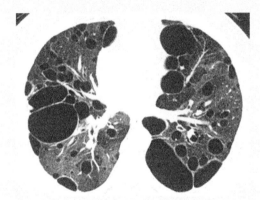

FIGURE E. Birt–Hogg–Dubé syndrome: subpleural and perivascular cysts at the lung bases

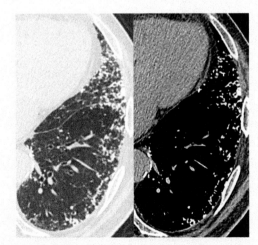

FIGURE F. Pulmonary ossification: subpleural-predominant calcified nodules seen in isolation

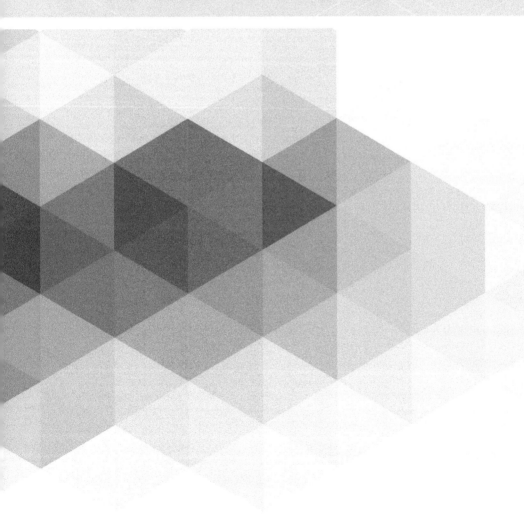

HRCT
FINDINGS

HRCT Indications, Technique, Radiation Dose, and Normal Anatomy

INTRODUCTION

High-resolution computed tomography (HRCT) is essential in the evaluation of diffuse lung disease. It is routinely obtained in all patients with diffuse lung disease and is a key component in the diagnosis and follow-up of these patients. The goal of this introductory chapter is to discuss the basics of HRCT, including indications, technique, and normal lung anatomy, as displayed using HRCT.

INDICATIONS FOR HRCT

HRCT has several indications in patients with, or suspected of having, diffuse lung disease (Table 1.1).

Detection of Diffuse Lung Disease

HRCT is more sensitive and specific than most other studies (including chest radiographs and pulmonary function tests [PFTs]) in the diagnosis of diffuse lung disease (Fig. 1.1A, B). HRCT may detect abnormalities in asymptomatic patients with an exposure or disease known to cause diffuse lung abnormalities (e.g., connective tissue disease), before PFTs become abnormal. Detecting abnormalities at an early stage by using HRCT may allow appropriate diagnosis and treatment, preventing progression of lung disease.

HRCT may also be used to exclude certain lung diseases as a cause of symptoms or abnormal PFT findings. For example, in patients with pulmonary hypertension, HRCT may be used to exclude emphysema and fibrotic lung disease as a cause.

Characterization of Diffuse Lung Disease

HRCT is of most value in identifying specific abnormal findings, allowing a characterization of the lung disease as interstitial, airways-related, or alveolar (airspace) (Figs. 1.2 and 1.3) and allowing a formulation of an appropriate differential diagnosis. The type of abnormality present and the specific distribution of lung abnormalities may be determined using HRCT. Both are very important in diagnosis (Fig. 1.3).

HRCT findings may have important implications for treatment and prognosis. When findings of fibrosis are present on HRCT, patients are less likely to respond to medications and, in general, have a poorer prognosis. Patients with HRCT findings suggestive of inflammatory disease are generally treated more aggressively because lung abnormalities may be reversible.

Differential Diagnosis and Guidance for Further Diagnostic Testing

HRCT is more specific than chest radiography, physical examination, and PFTs in the diagnosis and characterization of lung abnormalities in patients with diffuse lung disease (Fig. 1.4A, B). Although some HRCT findings suggest a particular disease, most require a differential diagnosis.

In general, the diagnosis of diffuse lung disease is based on a multidisciplinary approach, incorporating clinical information, HRCT findings, and sometimes pathology. Infrequently, one of these is sufficient to make

TABLE 1.1	Indications for HRCT

Detection of diffuse lung disease
- Detect abnormalities before other tests (e.g., chest radiograph) become abnormal
- Exclude certain diseases as a cause of symptoms

Characterization of diffuse lung disease
- Identification of specific abnormalities
- Formulation of a differential diagnosis
- Determine if reversible or irreversible abnormalities are likely present
- Help determine prognosis

Differential diagnosis and guidance for further testing
- HRCT findings (with clinical information) may be sufficiently diagnostic
- HRCT findings may suggest the appropriate study (transbronchial biopsy or VATS)

Sequential evaluation of abnormalities over time
- Response to treatment
- Assess patients with new symptoms

VATS, video-assisted thoracoscopic surgical.

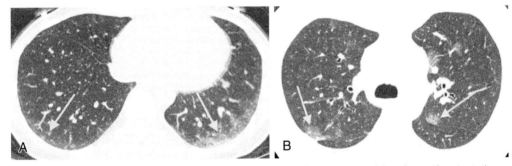

FIGURE 1.1 • **Detection of early lung disease.** HRCT may be more sensitive than other tests in detecting diffuse lung disease. **A.** Mild subpleural ground glass opacity (*arrows*) is seen in a patient with nonspecific interstitial pneumonia associated with scleroderma. This patient has a normal chest radiograph and pulmonary function tests. **B.** In a patient with acquired immune deficiency syndrome and a normal chest radiograph, patchy ground glass opacity (*arrows*) is visible on HRCT. Bronchoscopy confirmed *Pneumocystis jiroveci* infection.

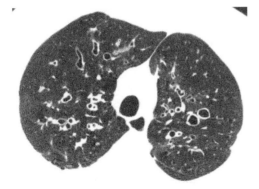

FIGURE 1.2 • **HRCT characterization of lung disease.** HRCT allows the diagnosis of airways disease in this patient with chronic symptoms. It provides an accurate assessment of both acute and chronic abnormalities in patients with airways disease. Bronchiectasis, airway wall thickening, and luminal impaction are present in this patient with cystic fibrosis.

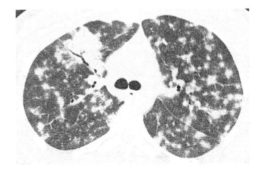

FIGURE 1.3 • **HRCT characterization of lung disease.** HRCT provides an accurate diagnosis of diffuse alveolar or airspace disease in a patient with patchy consolidation and an air bronchogram. In this example, patchy nodular areas of peribronchovascular and subpleural consolidation are present in a patient with organizing pneumonia.

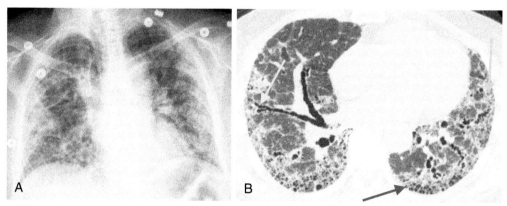

FIGURE 1.4 · Specificity of HRCT. A. Frontal chest radiograph in a patient with idiopathic pulmonary fibrosis (IPF) shows diffuse, nonspecific opacities. **B.** HRCT shows subpleural honeycombing (*red arrow*), traction bronchiectasis (*yellow arrow*), and reticulation (*blue arrow*) typical of usual interstitial pneumonia. In the absence of known diseases or exposures, these HRCT finding indicated the presence of fibrosis and are considered diagnostic of IPF.

TABLE 1.2	Clinical information that may be useful in the interpretation of HRCT abnormalities

Age
Acute or chronic symptoms
Cigarette smoking
Exposures (drugs, dusts, and organic antigens)
Immune status
Connective tissue disease
Family history of diffuse lung disease

a definitive diagnosis, but a combination of at least two is usually required to maintain a high degree of diagnostic accuracy and confidence. When HRCT is interpreted in conjunction with clinical information, the accuracy and specificity of diagnosis improve significantly (Table 1.2). Examples of clinical information useful in the diagnosis of diffuse lung abnormalities include patient age, duration of symptoms, a history of cigarette smoking, exposures (e.g., inhalational and environmental), immune status, drug treatment, known systemic disorders such as connective tissue disease, and a family history of diffuse lung disease.

In many cases, a combination of HRCT findings and clinical information may predict a single diagnosis with a high degree of accuracy (Fig. 1.5A, B). On the other hand, when the HRCT pattern is nonspecific, the

suggested differential diagnosis may help to guide additional tests, including lung biopsy (Fig. 1.6). Furthermore, because biopsy necessarily represents a small sample of the lung, the histologic diagnosis in some cases may not be representative of the overall lung abnormality present. HRCT, on the other hand, provides a global assessment of the lung disease present (Fig. 1.7).

Lung biopsy is often obtained in cases in which the combination of clinical information and HRCT is not considered sufficient for diagnosis. Histologic samples obtained at transbronchial biopsy have significant limitations, primarily because they represent very small samples of the lung; transbronchial biopsy is most useful in the diagnosis of sarcoidosis, lymphangitic tumor spread, infections, and a few other diseases that predominate in relation to airways (Fig. 1.6). Transbronchial lung cryobiopsy is a new technique that obtains larger samples than traditional transbronchial biopsies and could represent an alternative to surgical lung biopsies. Surgical lung biopsies still likely hold a significant advantage in terms of diagnostic yield; however, the precise indications for cryobiopsy have yet to be established.

Video-assisted thoracoscopic surgical (VATS) biopsies are generally the most accurate in the diagnosis of diffuse lung disease,

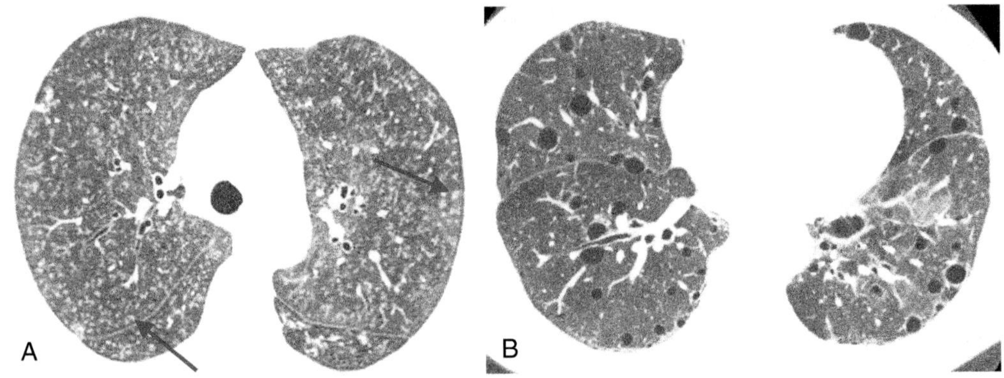

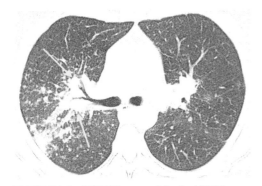

FIGURE 1.5 · **Correlation of HRCT findings with clinical information. A.** HRCT shows diffuse indistinct centrilobular nodules (*arrows*). There are several possible diagnoses based upon the HRCT pattern. This patient has chronic symptoms and a history of recurrent exposure to birds. This combination of HRCT findings and clinical information is highly suggestive of hypersensitivity pneumonitis, and biopsy is not usually needed. **B.** HRCT in a patient with Sjögren's syndrome shows scattered lung cysts. Although this finding is nonspecific, in a patient with a history of connective tissue disease, it is highly suggestive of lymphoid interstitial pneumonia.

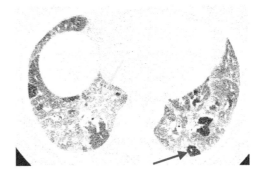

FIGURE 1.6 · **HRCT in sarcoidosis.** HRCT shows clusters of nodules in relation to the central bronchovascular bundles (*arrows*). This abnormality is typical of sarcoidosis but may also be seen with silicosis or other diseases. Given the proximity of the nodules to airways, bronchoscopy with transbronchial biopsy is the test of choice for making the diagnosis.

as they obtain relatively large samples from multiple sites within the lung. In patients with nonspecific fibrosis shown on HRCT, a VATS biopsy is usually required for diagnosis. HRCT may help guide the surgeon to the most appropriate regions for biopsy. It is important to recognize, however, that even if a VATS biopsy is obtained, it is often important to consider it in association with the HRCT findings (Fig. 1.7).

FIGURE 1.7 · **HRCT and biopsy in hypersensitivity pneumonitis.** HRCT provides a global assessment of anatomic abnormalities, whereas biopsy represents a small sampling of lung abnormalities. In some cases, biopsy of small areas of lung may not be representative of the overall pattern present. HRCT in this case shows a combination of ground glass opacity (*yellow arrow*) and air trapping (*red arrow*), highly suggestive of hypersensitivity pneumonitis. Pathology showed nonspecific interstitial pneumonia. In this case, the imaging is more suggestive of the correct diagnosis (hypersensitivity pneumonitis).

Sequential Evaluation of Lung Abnormalities Over Time

PFTs are generally the modality of choice for the serial evaluation of patients with diffuse lung disease. PFTs can accurately assess if a patient is responding to treatment or if his or her lung disease is worsening over time. HRCT is a complementary test that may provide information that PFTs do not.

HRCT is the primary method of following patients who have early lung disease that is undetectable using PFTs. Follow-up HRCT after treatment (Fig. 1.8A, B) is useful in determining the relative extent of inflammation and fibrosis and showing improvement, if present. Follow-up HRCT is particularly helpful in assessing the value of treatment in patients presenting with ground glass opacity; this finding may represent reversible inflammatory disease, irreversible fibrosis, or a combination of both. Also, PFTs may be difficult to interpret in patients with multicompartmental disease (e.g., airways, interstitial, vascular, and/or pleural disease). In these cases HRCT may be more accurate in discriminating the various components of disease and their changes over time.

New symptoms in a patient with diffuse lung disease may be due to worsening of the patient's established lung disease or a superimposed process. HRCT may be superior to PFTs in making this distinction. HRCT may be used to detect complications of diffuse lung disease, such as malignancy.

HRCT TECHNIQUES

Basic HRCT technique uses thin slices, scanning at full inspiration, and reconstruction with a sharp algorithm. To provide an accurate assessment of lung abnormalities, thin slices (≤1.25 mm) are required (Table 1.3). These are reconstructed using a sharp (edge-enhancing) algorithm to improve characterization of abnormal findings. Rapid gantry rotation is optimal in reducing motion artifacts. There are many CT protocols that may be used in obtaining high-resolution images for the purpose of diagnosing diffuse lung disease. No one protocol is the "correct" one, although several specific techniques are helpful. In nearly all patients, images are routinely obtained in the supine position, at full inspiration.

Axial versus Volumetric Imaging

Using single-slice scanners incapable of continuous (i.e., helical) image acquisition, HRCT was performed by obtaining single spaced axial images, at 1 or 2 cm intervals, during a breath-hold (Table 1.3). This method provided a sampling of lung anatomy (and pathology) and has been shown to be sufficient for diagnosis of diffuse lung diseases in most cases. This technique inherently results in a low radiation dose.

With multidetector, helical scanners, volumetric acquisition of thin sections through the entire thorax using a short breath-hold is possible. Volumetric imaging maximizes detection of all abnormalities present and allows for reconstruction of images in different planes, better depicting the distribution

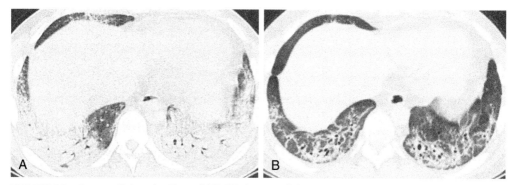

FIGURE 1.8 · Sequential evaluation of HRCT abnormalities over time. A. HRCT shows subpleural and basilar predominant consolidation. **B.** After treatment, the consolidation has resolved, but there has been interval development of irregular reticulation and traction bronchiectasis, indicative of fibrosis. HRCT is able to distinguish the reversible and nonreversible components after treatment.

of findings. Also, volumetric chest imaging is necessary if a quantification of lung abnormalities is desired. For these reasons, many centers use volumetric thin-section imaging rather than spaced axial imaging for HRCT studies (Table 1.3). Nonetheless, and although it is likely to provide some benefit, it has not been established that volumetric imaging provides improved diagnostic accuracy.

Disadvantages of volumetric HRCT include an increased radiation dose and images that are slightly fuzzier than axial images. As radiation reduction techniques, such as the use of modulated (variable or automatic) mA and iterative reconstruction, have become available, the radiation advantage of discontinuous scanning has become less pronounced. Additionally, some CT scanners allow for rapid, full-chest acquisition of true axial (nonhelical) images.

Prone Imaging

Prone imaging may be obtained routinely or in selected patients. Many interstitial lung diseases first present in the posterior subpleural lung regions. This is particularly common with usual interstitial pneumonia, nonspecific interstitial pneumonia, and desquamative interstitial pneumonia. In the supine position, normal patients may show increased opacity in the posterior subpleural region, reflecting dependent (gravitational) atelectasis.

Prone imaging is useful in distinguishing early interstitial lung disease from normal dependent opacity (Fig. 1.9A, B). When the patient is positioned prone, normal dependent opacity should disappear, whereas early interstitial lung disease persists. Prone imaging may also help in the identification of specific abnormalities in the dependent lung such as honeycombing. As full-chest imaging has

TABLE 1.3	HRCT scanning technique and examples of possible protocols

HRCT technique
  Full inspiration
  0.625- to 1.25-mm-thick sections
  Sharp (edge-enhancing) algorithm
  Fast gantry rotation speed
  Fixed mA or automatic mA adjustment
Axial (nonhelical) protocol
  Supine position
  No table motion
  Full inspiration
  Sections acquired at 1 cm intervals
  Prone scans at 1–2 cm intervals optional
Volumetric protocol
  Supine position
  Full inspiration
  Contiguous images throughout the chest
  Images reconstructed at 0.625–1.25 mm
  Prone scans at selected levels or with volumetric acquisition optional
Postexpiratory imaging (static)
  Supine position
  Suspended full expiration
  Levels of acquisition: aortic arch, tracheal carina, above diaphragm
Expiratory imaging (dynamic)
  Sequential images acquired during forced expiration
  Eight sequential images at 0.5 s intervals
  No table motion
  Levels of acquisition: aortic arch, tracheal carina, above diaphragm
  Fast gantry rotation speed
  mA = 100 or less

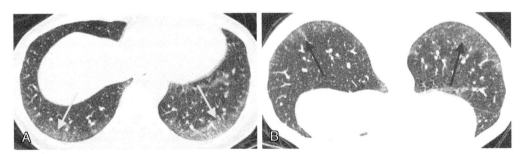

FIGURE 1.9 · **Use of prone HRCT. A.** Supine HRCT shows subtle ground glass opacity involving the posterior lung (*yellow arrows*). This could represent normal dependent density or early interstitial lung disease. **B.** Prone HRCT shows persistence of these abnormalities (*red arrows*). The prone scan confirms that this finding is due to early interstitial lung disease.

become more commonplace, prone imaging has largely been reserved for problem solving in selected patients with mild, posterior, subpleural lung abnormalities but should be routine in the initial evaluation of patients with suspected diffuse lung disease.

Expiratory Imaging

Expiratory images, obtained to detect air trapping, are important in the initial HRCT evaluation of most patients and in the follow-up of patients with airways disease or chronic obstructive lung disease. As an example, chronic hypersensitivity pneumonitis may mimic the appearance of usual interstitial pneumonia and idiopathic pulmonary fibrosis on inspiratory images, but air trapping on expiratory images may allow these diseases to be distinguished.

Expiratory images may be acquired using a static postexpiratory technique or a dynamic technique during forced expiration (Table 1.3). Static postexpiratory images are produced by obtaining single scans at selected levels at end expiration (i.e., "take a big breath, blow it out, and hold your breath"). Dynamic expiratory imaging (Fig. 1.10A–H) involves obtaining multiple (six to eight) sequential images (with a reduced mA setting) at the same anatomic location during forced expiration (i.e., "take a deep breath and blow it out as fast as you can"). The entire sequence may take 4 to 6 seconds. Dynamic imaging is more sensitive in the detection of air trapping than static postexpiratory techniques.

Expiratory images may be acquired at three anatomic levels: aortic arch, tracheal carina, and above the diaphragm. Sometimes five levels are chosen. Volumetric postexpiratory imaging through the entire chest is another option, but it requires a higher radiation dose.

HRCT AND RADIATION DOSE

We are all exposed to nonmedical radiation, primarily in the form of cosmic radiation. The yearly dose that an individual receives from cosmic radiation varies depending on a variety of factors, but on average, yearly exposure is approximately 2.5 milliSieverts (mSv).

For comparison, the dose from a posteroanterior chest radiograph is approximately 0.05 mSv. CT dose (Table 1.4) varies significantly among different patients, CT scanners, and HRCT protocols. Radiation dose is directly related to the mA used, which may range from 100 to 400 mA for most chest CTs. Decreased radiation dose is associated with increased image noise and decreased resolution, but images generally remain adequate for diagnosis.

HRCT using a variable mA of about 100, axial imaging, and 10 mm slice spacing results in a radiation dose of approximately 0.7 mSv. This dose is doubled if prone imaging is also used.

Volumetric multidetector HRCT results in a dose of 4 to 7 mSv if 300 mA is used, but volumetric HRCT with a reduced or modulated (automatic) mA (e.g., in the range of 100) produces adequate images with a dose of 1 to 2 mSv. Automatic tube current modulation uses a tube current that is adjusted for differences in body thickness and density at different locations. This technique attempts to produce images with similar noise levels throughout the anatomic locations being imaged. For a given dose, axial images are a little sharper than images obtained using helical technique. Some CT scanners allow for rapid, full-chest, true axial image acquisition.

Low-dose HRCT using spaced axial images may also be performed with 40 mA, although noise is increased and resolution is decreased. Dose using this technique may be as low as 0.02 mSv (with widely spaced images) to 0.2 mSv (with images at 2 cm intervals, supine and prone, and with dynamic expiratory images).

A variety of other dose reduction techniques are available. Alternative reconstruction algorithms, such as iterative reconstruction, have emerged as an alternative to filtered back projection (FBP). These techniques may result in up to 80% dose reduction or greater; however, image quality varies significantly compared with FBP; thus there is a possibility that interpretation might be affected.

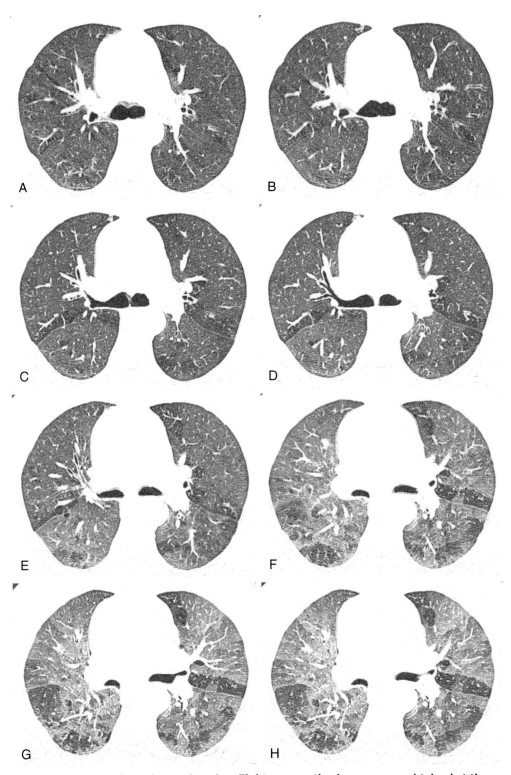

FIGURE 1.10 · **Dynamic expiratory imaging. Eight consecutive images were obtained at the level of the tracheal carina during forced expiration, using reduced mA.** Image **(A)** is obtained at the beginning of expiration and image **(H)** at the end. During expiration there are several regions of lung that do not change in attenuation and remain lucent. This represents air trapping in a patient with hypersensitivity pneumonitis.

TABLE 1.4	Comparison of radiation dose for chest imaging techniques

	Effective radiation dose (mSv)
Annual background radiation	2.5
Posteroanterior chest radiograph	0.05
Spaced axial HRCT supine (10 mm spacing)	0.7
Spaced axial HRCT supine (20 mm spacing)	0.35
Low-dose spaced axial HRCT	0.02–0.2
Volumetric helical HRCT supine (300 mA)	4–7
Volumetric helical HRCT supine (100 mA)	1–2

Modified from Mayo JR, Aldrich J, Muller NL. Radiation exposure at chest CT: a statement of the Fleischner Society. *Radiology*. 2003;228:15-21.

TABLE 1.5	Normal HRCT appearances

Large arteries and bronchi
  Outer walls of arteries and bronchi appear smooth and sharply marginated
  Bronchial walls measure 1/5th–1/10th of bronchial diameter
  Ratio of bronchial lumen to adjacent artery (bronchoarterial ratio) averages 0.7
  Bronchial walls similar in appearance in different lung regions
Secondary pulmonary lobule
  Usually 1–2.5 cm in diameter
  Interlobular septa uncommonly visible; very thin
  Centrilobular artery visible about 5 mm from pleural surface (dot or branching)
  Centrilobular bronchiole invisible
Pleural surfaces
  Smooth and sharply marginated; fissures thin
  A few linear or small nodular opacities are normal

In general, an adequate and appropriate diagnosis of diffuse lung disease may be obtained using a wide variety of CT techniques, and although using low radiation dose should be considered, obtaining representative and high-quality supine, prone, and expiratory imaging should be favored in an initial patient evaluation.

RECOMMENDATIONS FOR HRCT TECHNIQUE

Considering image quality, diagnostic accuracy, and radiation dose, our recommendations for HRCT in a patient with an undiagnosed diffuse lung disease, associated with significant but nonspecific symptoms, would consist of:

1. Volumetric imaging in the supine position, using dose reduction techniques, thin slices, and reconstruction using a high-resolution algorithm
2. Prone imaging, either with spaced axial images or volumentric imaging (optional)
3. Expiratory imaging

In patients being followed up for a known disease or abnormality, appropriate imaging could be modified.

NORMAL ANATOMY ON HRCT

The recognition of HRCT abnormalities is fundamentally based on an understanding of normal lung anatomy (Table 1.5). Understanding the *secondary pulmonary lobule* or simply *pulmonary lobule* is fundamental in HRCT interpretation. The secondary lobule is described in detail below, but first things first.

Large Bronchi and Arteries
Within the central lung, bronchi and pulmonary artery branches are closely associated and branch in parallel. Central pulmonary arteries imaged in cross section normally appear as rounded or elliptical opacities on HRCT, accompanied by uniformly thin-walled bronchi of similar size and shape. When imaged along their axis, bronchi and vessels should appear roughly cylindrical or show slight tapering as they branch, depending on the length of the segment that is visible; tapering of a vessel or bronchus is most easily seen when a long segment is visible.

The outer walls of pulmonary arteries form a smooth and sharply defined interface with the surrounding lung, whether they are seen in cross section or along their length. In normal subjects, the internal diameter of a bronchus (i.e., the bronchial lumen) averages about 0.7 of the diameter of the adjacent pulmonary artery. This measurement is termed the *bronchoarterial ratio*. A bronchoarterial ratio exceeding 1 generally indicates bronchial dilatation (i.e., bronchiectasis), although a ratio exceeding 1 may be seen in normal elderly patients or in people living at high altitudes (e.g., Denver).

The walls of large bronchi, outlined by lung on one side and air in the bronchial lumen on the other, should appear smooth and to be of uniform thickness. Generally speaking, the wall of a bronchus measures 1/5th to 1/10th of its outer diameter, and bronchial walls in different lung regions should appear similar in thickness. The lumen of a bronchus should be free of secretions.

Bronchi and pulmonary arteries are surrounded by the *peribronchovascular interstitium*, which extends from the pulmonary hila into the peripheral lung.

The Peribronchovascular Interstitium

The peribronchovascular interstitium, also known as the axial interstitium, accompanies pulmonary artery, bronchi, and lymphatics from the hilar regions into the lung periphery. It is invisible in normals.

The central or perihilar peribronchovascular interstitium is often affected by lymphatic diseases, such as sarcoidosis or lymphangitic spread of neoplasm, or infiltrative abnormalities, such as pulmonary edema. Such abnormalities may result in smooth, nodular, or irregular thickening of the peribronchovascular interstitium.

Pulmonary Lobule (Secondary Pulmonary Lobule)

The *secondary pulmonary lobule*, or simply *pulmonary lobule* (these are synonyms) (Fig. 1.11), is the smallest unit of the lung that is delineated by connective tissue septa, and many pathologic abnormalities occur in relation to specific components of the secondary lobule. Pulmonary lobules are generally polygonal in shape and measure from 1 to 2.5 cm.

Interlobular Septa

Pulmonary lobules are marginated by *interlobular septa* that contain pulmonary veins and lymphatics and form a web-like network throughout the lung. Only a few interlobular septa are seen on HRCT in normal subjects, and when visible, they are very thin and inconspicuous (Figs. 1.11 and 1.12). Certain processes, such as pulmonary edema, may result in interlobular septal thickening easily seen on HRCT (Fig. 1.13).

Centrilobular Structures

A pulmonary lobule is supplied by a single artery and bronchiole; these are located in the center of the lobule (i.e., the *centrilobular region*). The *lobular artery* is normally visible on HRCT as a dot-like or branching structure, 1 mm or more in diameter. The *lobular bronchiole*, although of similar size, is not normally visible because its wall is too thin to be resolved.

In the peripheral lung or adjacent to fissures, the centrilobular regions (i.e., the centers of pulmonary lobules), and thus, the centrilobular artery and bronchiole, are located approximately 0.5 cm from the pleural surface. The centrilobular artery is typically the most peripheral pulmonary vessel seen on HRCT. The centrilobular bronchiole and pulmonary artery, along with larger airways and arteries in the central lung, are invested by the distal continuation of the peribronchovascular interstitium. Thus, small airways diseases, vascular diseases, and some interstitial diseases often are manifested by abnormalities affecting the centrilobular region (Fig. 1.14).

The Pleural Surfaces, Fissures, and Subpleural Interstitium

In the peripheral lung, interlobular septa are contiguous with the *subpleural interstitium*, which lies beneath visceral pleura and adjacent to fissures. Fissures and the peripheral pleural surfaces should appear smooth in contour and sharply marginated, although a few linear opacities intersecting the pleura (interlobular septa) or nodular opacities (pulmonary veins or lymphoid aggregates) may

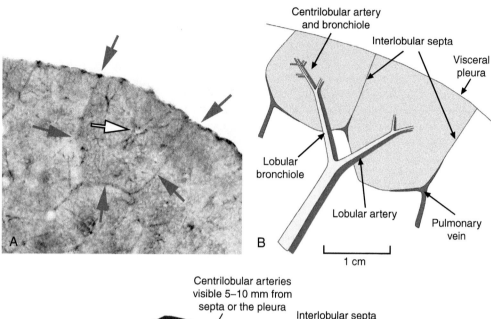

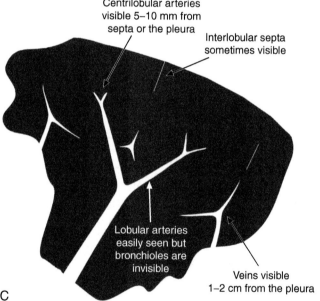

FIGURE 1.11 · **Normal (secondary) pulmonary lobules. A.** Histologic appearance of a normal pulmonary lobule at the pleural surface. Interlobular septa (*red arrows*) marginate a lobule in the lung periphery. The branching lobular bronchiole (*white arrow*) is visible in the centrilobular region, about 5 mm from the pleural surface. **B.** Anatomy of pulmonary lobules in the lung periphery. The lobules are delineated by interlobular septa, contiguous with the subpleural interstitium. The lobular bronchiole and artery are centrilobular in location. Veins are located within interlobular septa. **C.** HRCT visibility of lobular structures. The centrilobular artery and pulmonary vein branches can be seen. The centrilobular bronchiole is invisible. Interlobular septa are inconsipicuous and if visible, appear very thin.

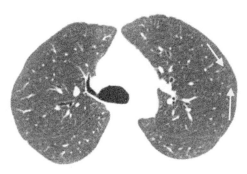

FIGURE 1.12 · **Normal interlobular septa.** HRCT in normal subjects may show a few interlobular septa (*yellow arrows*), but these are usually inconspicuous. Septa are easily seen only when they are thickened.

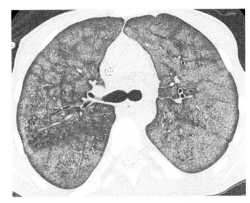

FIGURE 1.14 · **Disease affecting the centrilobular region.** Areas of ground glass opacity are present that have shapes resembling pulmonary lobules. The periphery of the lobule and interlobular septa are spared in this case. Diseases that are centrilobular in location are generally related to the centrilobular artery or bronchiole. This patient has metastatic calcification associated with renal failure.

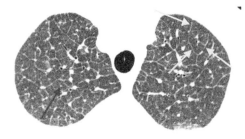

FIGURE 1.13 · **Interlobular septal thickening.** Thickening of interlobular septa (*yellow arrows*) is present in a patient with pulmonary edema. There is a web-like network of interconnecting lines outlining polygonal structures 1–2.5 cm in size, representing the pulmonary lobules. Note small dots at the center of some lobules (*red arrow*), representing the centrilobular arteries.

be seen. Thickening of interlobular septa is typically associated with subpleural interstitial thickening (and thickening of fissures). Nodules may also be located in relation to the interlobular septa. Abnormalities of the subpleural interstitium may result in the pleural surfaces or fissures having an irregular or nodular appearance.

The Intralobular Interstitium

A fine network of interstitial connective tissue fibers extends throughout the lung, within pulmonary lobules, bridging the space between the interlobular septa and the centrilobular peribronchovascular interstitium. This interstitial network has been termed

the *intralobular interstitium*. The intralobular interstitium is not normally visible, but it may become thickened in the presence of lung fibrosis or infiltration.

FURTHER READING

Arakawa H, Webb WR. Expiratory high-resolution CT scan. *Radiol Clin North Am.* 1998;36:189-209.

Austin JH, Müller NL, Friedman PJ, et al. Glossary of terms for CT of the lungs: recommendations of the Nomenclature Committee of the Fleischner Society. *Radiology.* 1996;200:327-331.

Elicker B, Pereira CA, Webb R, Leslie KO. High-resolution computed tomography patterns of diffuse interstitial lung disease with clinical and pathological correlation. *J Bras Pneumol.* 2008;34:715-744.

Gotway MB, Freemer MM, King TE Jr. Challenges in pulmonary fibrosis. 1: use of high resolution CT scanning of the lung for the evaluation of patients with idiopathic interstitial pneumonias. *Thorax.* 2007;62:546-553.

Gotway MB, Reddy GP, Webb WR, Elicker BM, Leung JW. High-resolution CT of the lung: patterns of disease and differential diagnoses. *Radiol Clin North Am.* 2005;43:513-542.

Griffin CB, Primack SL. High-resolution CT: normal anatomy, techniques, and pitfalls. *Radiol Clin North Am.* 2001;39:1073-1090.

Hansell DM, Bankier AA, MacMahon H, et al. Fleischner Society: glossary of terms for thoracic imaging. *Radiology.* 2008;246:697-722.

Klusmann M, Owens C. HRCT in paediatric diffuse interstitial lung disease—a review for 2009. *Pediatr Radiol.* 2009;39(suppl 3):471-481.

Mayo JR. CT evaluation of diffuse infiltrative lung disease: dose considerations and optimal technique. *J Thorac Imaging.* 2009;24:252-259.

Mayo JR, Aldrich J, Muller NL. Radiation exposure at chest CT: a statement of the Fleischner Society. *Radiology.* 2003;228:15-21.

Nishino M, Washko GR, Hatabu H. Volumetric expiratory HRCT of the lung: clinical applications. *Radiol Clin North Am.* 2010;48:177-183.

Quigley M, Hansell DM, Nicholson AG. Interstitial lung disease—the new synergy between radiology and pathology. *Histopathology.* 2006;49:334-342.

Sundaram B, Chughtai AR, Kazerooni EA. Multidetector high-resolution computed tomography of the lungs: protocols and applications. *J Thorac Imaging.* 2010;25:125-141.

Webb WR. High resolution lung computed tomography: normal anatomic and pathologic findings. *Radiol Clin North Am.* 1991;29:1051-1063.

Webb WR. Thin-section CT of the secondary pulmonary lobule: anatomy and the image—the 2004 Fleischner lecture. *Radiology.* 2006;239:322-338.

Reticular Opacities

Reticular opacities visible on high-resolution computed tomography (HRCT) in patients with diffuse lung disease indicate an interstitial abnormality and can be seen with infiltrative disorders, inflammatory disease, or lung fibrosis. Three specific patterns of reticulation can be seen. These are interlobular septal thickening (IST), honeycombing, and intralobular intersititial thickening.

INTERLOBULAR SEPTAL THICKENING

IST is easily recognized on HRCT and has a limited differential diagnosis.

HRCT Features

Interlobular septa variably marginate secondary pulmonary lobules (see Chapter 1). They consist of connective tissue and contain pulmonary veins and lymphatics. Interlobular septa are approximately 1 to 2 cm in length and are normally 1/10th of a millimeter in thickness. Only a few very thin interlobular septa are visible on HRCT in normal patients.

IST results in a web-like network of lines. These lines can usually be identified as thickened interlobular septa because they outline what can be recognized as pulmonary lobules because of their characteristic size (1 to 2.5 cm) and polygonal shape and because a centrilobular artery is usually visible as a dot-like or branching opacity in the center of the lobule (Fig. 2.1). IST is commonly associated with thickening of the subpleural interstitium, usually recognized as "thickening of the fissures,"

and thickening of the peribronchovascular interstitium, visible as "peribronchial cuffing," and mimicking the appearance of bronchial wall thickening.

When significant IST is present, the abnormal septa may appear smooth in contour (this is most common), nodular, or irregular. This appearance primarily determines the differential diagnosis (Figs. 2.1 and 2.2A–C, Table 2.1).

Smooth Interlobular Septal Thickening

Smooth IST is characterized by the presence of multiple thickened (and easily seen) septa, which are smooth in contour and otherwise normal in appearance (Figs. 2.1 and 2.2A). Smooth IST is almost always a manifestation of pulmonary edema or lymphangitic spread of a neoplasm, but rare causes of this pattern are occasionally seen (Table 2.1). Symmetric involvement of both lungs favors edema, while asymmetric, unilateral, or localized involvement favors lymphangitic spread of tumor. Furthermore, most patients with lymphangitic spread of tumor have a known malignancy or other findings to suggest this diagnosis. In different diseases, smooth septal thickening may reflect septal edema or septal infiltration (e.g., by tumor).

Nodular Interlobular Septal Thickening

A few small septal "nodules" can be seen in normal patients, reflecting the presence of pulmonary vein branches. Nodular IST is said to be present when multiple distinct nodules are visible within interlobular septa. Nodular IST is most common in patients with sarcoidosis or lymphangitic spread of tumor, reflecting, respectively, clusters of granulomas or tumor nodules in relation to lymphatics (Fig. 2.2B, Table 2.1). In sarcoidosis, nodules are almost always seen in other locations as well, including the peribronchovascular regions and the centrilobular and/or subpleural regions, with a

predominance of abnormalities in the upper lobes. In patients with lymphangitic spread of tumor, smooth IST is more common than nodular IST, but both appearances may be seen in combination. Nodular IST is part of a perilymphatic distribution of nodules, described in Chapter 3.

Irregular Interlobular Septal Thickening

Irregular IST usually reflects lung fibrosis. Architectural distortion associated with fibrosis causes the septa to appear jagged or angulated (i.e., irregular) (Fig. 2.2C, Table 2.1). Irregular septal thickening may be seen with any cause of fibrotic lung disease, but other findings, such as honeycombing and traction bronchiectasis, are more helpful in the formulation of a differential diagnosis.

Significance of Interlobular Septal Thickening

The presence of a few thickened interlobular septa can be seen in a wide variety of diffuse lung diseases and, in general, is a nonspecific finding. For the purposes of differential

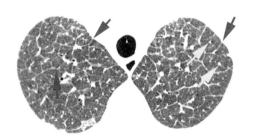

FIGURE 2.1 · **Smooth interlobular septal thickening in a patient with pulmonary edema.** Linear opacities, 1–2 cm long (*red arrows*), form a reticular network outlining polygonal pulmonary lobules. Dot-like opacities (*yellow arrows*) within the lobules represent centrilobular arteries. A few small nodular opacities in relation to the thickened septa represent pulmonary veins.

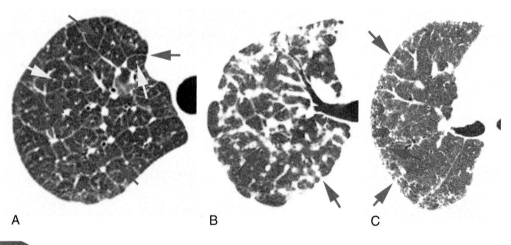

A   B   C

classic

FIGURE 2.2 · **Interlobular septal thickening (IST): Classic appearances.** When IST is the predominant abnormality seen on HRCT, the differential diagnosis depends on the morphology of the septal thickening. **A. Smooth IST.** The thickened septa are smooth in contour and uniform in thickness. This appearance is most likely pulmonary edema or lymphangitic carcinomatosis. This is interstitial pulmonary edema. **B. Nodular IST.** Multiple distinct nodules are visible within thickened septa (*red arrows*). Smooth septal thickening is also seen. This appearance is most likely sarcoidosis or lymphangitic carcinomatosis. This represents lymphangitis spread of tumor. **C. Irregular IST.** Septa are irregularly thickened (*red arrows*). This usually represents fibrotic lung disease. This represents idiopathic pulmonary fibrosis.

TABLE 2.1	Differential diagnosis of interlobular septal thickening as the predominant abnormality

Morphology of septal thickening	Differential diagnosis
Smooth	Pulmonary edema
	Lymphangitic carcinomatosis
	Lymphoproliferative disease
	Amyloidosis (rare)
	Pulmonary veno-occlusive disease (rare)
	Lymphangiomatosis (rare)
	Erdheim–Chester disease (rare)
Nodular	Sarcoidosis
	Lymphangitic carcinomatosis
	Lymphoproliferative disease
	Amyloidosis (rare)
Irregular	Fibrotic lung disease

TABLE 2.2	HRCT features of honeycombing

Cysts are subpleural in location
Cysts are usually 3–10 mm
Cysts have thick, easily seen walls
The cysts occur in a cluster or layer and share walls (multiple layers are seen in late disease)
Cysts are of air attenuation (i.e., black)
Cysts are empty; they contain no "anatomy"; they are black holes
The cysts do not branch
They are associated with other signs of fibrosis (traction bronchiectasis and reticulation)

diagnosis, thickened septa should be ignored unless they represent a predominant abnormality (Fig. 2.3A, B).

HONEYCOMBING

Pathologically, honeycombing represents interstitial lung fibrosis with destruction and dilatation of peripheral airspaces. It is relatively common and, in most cases, is easily recognized on HRCT.

HRCT Features

Honeycombing is a specific finding of lung fibrosis on HRCT; if clear-cut honeycombing is visible, you can be sure that fibrosis is present. However, in patients with early or minimal abnormalities, there can be significant disagreement, even among experts, as to the presence or absence of honeycombing. Thus, to make a confident diagnosis of honeycombing, a number of HRCT findings must be present (Table 2.2, Figs. 2.4 to 2.8):

1. *There must be black holes.* Honeycomb cysts are air-filled and should appear black on lung windows. They should have the same attenuation as air in bronchi.
2. *There should be no "anatomy" within the cysts.* Vessels, bronchi, or septations are not visible within honeycomb cysts. The cysts are empty black holes.

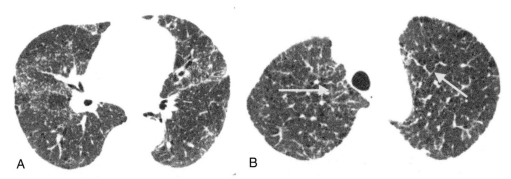

A   B

FIGURE 2.3 • **Interlobular septal thickening as an insignificant finding. A.** HRCT shows perilymphatic nodules with a patchy distribution and predominance along the fissures (*red arrow*) in a patient with amyloidosis. **B.** At a higher level, HRCT shows interlobular septal thickening (*yellow arrows*). Septal thickening should be ignored in terms of differential diagnosis unless it is the predominant finding.

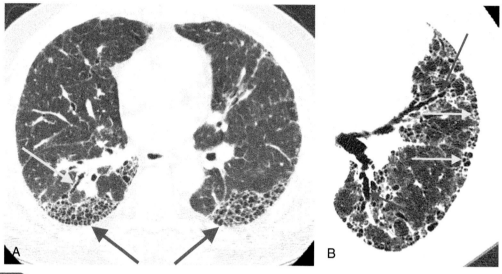

FIGURE 2.4 · **Honeycombing: Classic appearance in two patients with usual interstitial pneumonia and idiopathic pulmonary fibrosis. A.** HRCT shows advanced honeycombing. Note that cysts range from about 3 mm to less than 1 cm in diameter, are of air attenuation (i.e., black), have relatively thick walls, involve the subpleural lung, share walls, and are stacked in multiple layers (*red arrows*). There is associated traction bronchiectasis in the right lower lobe (*yellow arrow*). **B.** HRCT of a patient with idiopathic pulmonary fibrosis shows honeycombing (*yellow arrows*) and traction bronchiectasis (*red arrows*). The honeycomb cysts appear in clusters and layers in the subpleural lung.

3. *The cysts have a thick and easily recognizable wall.* The wall of honeycombing cysts should be easy to see. This finding helps in distinguishing honeycombing from emphysema or areas of subpleural air trapping.

4. *Most cysts are 3 to 10 mm in diameter.* Some may be larger or smaller.

5. *The subpleural lung must be involved.* Unless lucencies are visible in the immediate subpleural region, honeycombing cannot be diagnosed with certainty. Traction bronchiectasis and cystic lung disease may mimic its appearance more centrally.

6. *A layer or cluster of subpleural cysts should be visible.* Early honeycombing may be seen in only one layer beneath the pleural surface or as an isolated cluster of subpleural cysts. Adjacent cysts share walls, and the presence of three cysts in a row is often used as a minimum to diagnose honeycombing; a single subpleural cyst or a few scattered cysts are not sufficient. Keep in mind that subpleural honeycombing may be seen adjacent to fissures.

7. *Multiple layers of cysts* are typical of advanced cases, but this finding is not necessary for diagnosis of honeycombing. In patients with extensive disease, the stacked appearance of cysts, sharing walls with one another, is what gives this finding its name.

8. *The cysts of honeycombing do not branch.* Branching cystic structures, even in the subpleural lung, likely represent traction bronchiectasis (described below).

9. *Associated signs of fibrosis are present in the same lung regions.* These findings include traction bronchiectasis, irregular reticulation, and volume loss. If cysts are not associated with other findings of fibrosis, they may represent emphysema or cystic lung disease.

Significance of Honeycombing and the "UIP Pattern"

Honeycombing is often associated with the histologic pattern termed *usual interstitial pneumonia (UIP)*, and in some cases, honeycombing may be diagnostic of this pattern. However, there are a number of diseases that can show honeycombing on HRCT (Table 2.3).

The presence of honeycombing, by itself, is not sufficient to confidently diagnose what is termed a *UIP pattern* (i.e., a combination of HRCT abnormalities predicting the presence of UIP). In UIP, findings of fibrosis, including honeycombing, typically have a subpleural, posterior, and lower lobe predominance, and the posterior costophrenic

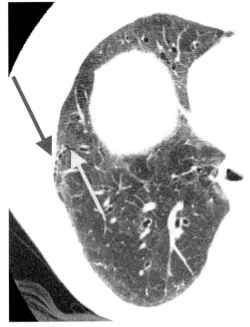

FIGURE 2.5 · **Early honeycombing in a single layer.** Early honeycombing is seen in a patient with mixed connective tissue disease. Note at least three adjacent subpleural, air-attenuation cysts with well-defined walls (*red arrow*) associated with mild traction bronchiectasis (*yellow arrow*).

angles are almost always involved (Fig. 2.7, Table 2.4). Also, features that would suggest an alternative diagnosis, such as isolated regions of ground glass opacity (seen in areas not showing findings of fibrosis), mosaic perfusion, air trapping, segmental or lobar consolidation, and small nodules, must be absent. The accurate HRCT diagnosis of UIP is particularly important in the diagnosis of patients with idiopathic pulmonary fibrosis (IPF; see Chapter 9). For a detailed review of this topic, refer to the paper by Raghu et al., listed at the end of this chapter.

When all of the features listed in Table 2.4 are present, a diagnosis of UIP can be made with a high degree of confidence (Figs. 2.6 and 2.7). In these classic cases, there is a close correlation between the HRCT and pathologic patterns, and lung biopsy is uncommonly performed. Remember that UIP is not a disease, but a histologic pattern with an HRCT correlate (i.e., the UIP pattern).

When a definite UIP pattern is present, the differential diagnosis of honeycombing is limited (Table 2.5) and generally includes four diseases or conditions: IPF, connective tissue disease, drug-related fibrosis, and asbestosis. IPF is the most common cause.

Think of IPF as idiopathic UIP. UIP associated with connective tissue disease, drug-related fibrosis, and asbestosis may be indistinguishable from IPF on HRCT (Fig. 2.8A–C), but there are often clinical clues that suggest the appropriate diagnosis. Patients with connective tissue disease may have joint

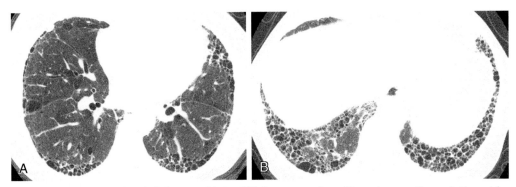

FIGURE 2.6 · **HRCT of a definite usual interstitial pneumonia pattern.** Images through the mid-lung **(A)** and lung bases **(B)** show subpleural and basilar fibrosis with significant honeycombing. No ground glass opacity, mosaic perfusion, or diffuse nodules are seen.

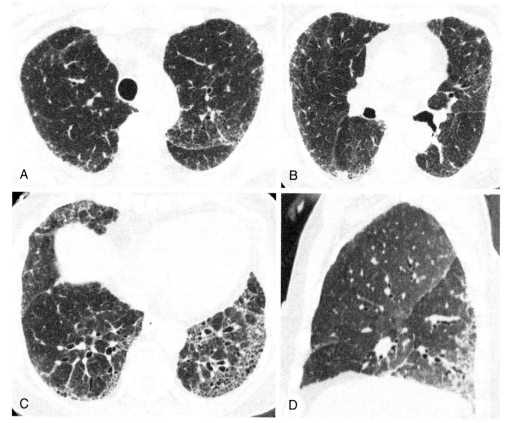

FIGURE 2.7 · **HRCT of a definite usual interstitial pneumonia pattern in a patient with idiopathic pulmonary fibrosis.** HRCT through the upper lungs **(A)** and mid-lung **(B)** shows reticulation and irregular interlobular septal thickening as the predominant abnormality. Scan through the lung bases **(C)** shows subpleural and basilar fibrosis with significant honeycombing. The abnormalities predominate at the lung bases. **D.** Sagittal reformation shows predominance of abnormalities at the bases and in the posterior lung, including the costophrenic angles.

symptoms, muscle weakness, rashes, or abnormal blood tests. Patients with drug fibrosis have a history of treatment with a drug that is a known offender such as cyclophosphamide, chlorambucil, nitrofurantoin, and pindolol. Patients with asbestosis usually have a clear exposure history and 90% or more have associated pleural thickening or plaques visible on HRCT.

If the patient has a classic HRCT appearance of a UIP pattern, and no appropriate history or clinical manifestations to suggest the later three diagnoses, a presumptive diagnosis of IPF will be made. As this diagnosis is based primarily on the HRCT appearance, it is very important to be conservative in labeling a patient as having a UIP pattern.

Significance of Honeycombing: Alternate Diagnoses

In patients with honeycombing visible on HRCT, the clinical history, the distribution of findings of fibrosis, and additional findings present may suggest that the diagnosis is not UIP.

Chronic hypersensitivity pneumonitis may be associated with a history of exposure to organic antigens in the environment (e.g., fungi, birds kept as pets), although as many as 50% of patients with hypersensitivity pneumonitis (HP) do not have a clear exposure. HP is classically mid- to lower lung predominant, with sparing of the inferior costophrenic angles but may predominate in the upper lobes. It often shows abnormalities that are diffuse or central in the axial plane, without the subpleural predominance typical of UIP

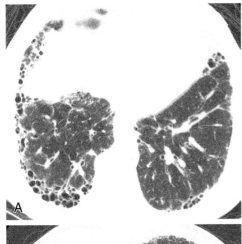
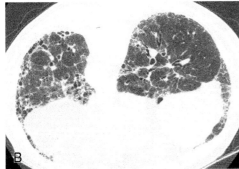
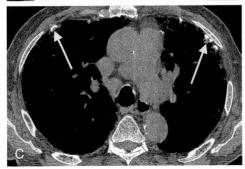

TABLE 2.3	Differential diagnosis of honeycombing on HRCT

Idiopathic pulmonary fibrosis
Connective tissue disease
Drug-related fibrosis
Asbestosis
Hypersensitivity pneumonitis
Sarcoidosis
Nonspecific interstitial pneumonia (mild honeycombing)
Pneumoconioses other than asbestosis
Post-acute respiratory distress syndrome fibrosis

TABLE 2.4	HRCT findings confidently predicting a usual interstitial pneumonia (UIP) pattern (all are necessary)

Honeycombing (in significant amounts)
Supportive signs of fibrosis (irregular reticulation and traction bronchiectasis)
Subpleural and basilar predominant distribution
Absence of upper or mid-lung or peribronchovascular predominance
Absence of extensive ground glass opacity
Absence of segmental or lobar consolidation
Absence of discrete bilateral cysts (away from honeycombing)
Absence of significant mosaic perfusion or air trapping (bilateral ≥ 3 lobes)
Absence of profuse micronodules

TABLE 2.5	Differential diagnosis of common causes of a UIP pattern on HRCT

Idiopathic pulmonary fibrosis
Connective tissue disease (rheumatoid arthritis most common)
Drug fibrosis
Asbestosis

classic

FIGURE 2.8 · Differential diagnosis of a usual interstitial pneumonia pattern. A. A patient with rheumatoid arthritis–related interstitial lung disease shows a classic usual interstitial pneumonia pattern of subpleural and basilar predominant fibrosis with honeycombing. **B** and **C.** A patient with asbestosis shows a usual interstitial pneumonia pattern of lung disease that is indistinguishable from idiopathic pulmonary fibrosis. Note pleural plaques (**C**, *arrows*) in the patient with asbestosis.

(Fig. 2.9). In other words, chronic HP may result in a predominance of fibrosis in the peribronchovascular regions or may involve the entire cross section of the lung as seen on HRCT. Furthermore, the presence of ground glass opacity or centrilobular nodules outside of areas of fibrosis, or mosaic perfusion or air trapping (Fig. 2.10), also suggests HP. It is rare for UIP to present with ground glass opacity as an isolated abnormality, but ground glass opacity in UIP is often visible in areas of lung that also show findings of fibrosis (i.e., honeycombing, reticulation, and traction bronchiectasis).

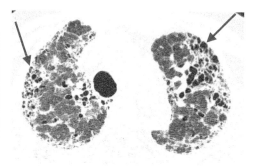

FIGURE 2.9 · **Honeycombing with patchy fibrosis in hypersensitivity pneumonitis.** While honeycombing is present (*red arrows*), the distribution of fibrosis is patchy and involves the central lung. It does not predominate in the subpleural lung, as would be typical of usual interstitial pneumonia, and involves the upper lobes, which is also atypical. This patient was diagnosed with hypersensitivity pneumonitis on lung biopsy.

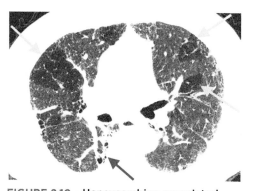

FIGURE 2.10 · **Honeycombing associated with mosaic perfusion in hypersensitivity pneumonitis.** Mild honeycombing is present in the right lower lobe (*red arrow*), but with significant associated mosaic perfusion (*yellow arrows*). This combination of findings is strongly suggestive of hypersensitivity pneumonitis.

Nonspecific interstitial pneumonia (NSIP), idiopathic or associated with connective tissue disease or drug treatment, may show findings of fibrosis with a distribution similar to that of UIP, being peripheral and basal predominant. Although honeycombing is present in a few percent of patients with fibrotic NSIP, it is often minimal in extent and other findings of fibrosis, such as reticulation and traction bronchiectasis, predominate (Fig. 2.11). Furthermore, NSIP often shows

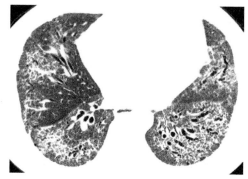

FIGURE 2.11 · **Severe fibrosis in nonspecific interstitial pneumonia.** Extensive reticulation, intralobular lines, and traction bronchiectasis are present at the lung bases, with only minimal honeycombing. Although it is possible that this represents idiopathic pulmonary fibrosis, the relative lack of honeycombing and relative sparing of the subpleural lung favor nonspecific interstitial pneumonia.

areas of isolated ground glass opacity and relative sparing of the immediate subpleural lung; these findings are atypical of UIP.

Sarcoidosis typically has an upper lobe and central peribronchovascular predominant distribution of fibrosis. Honeycombing is occasionally seen. Sarcoidosis often presents in a younger age distribution than IPF.

Pneumoconioses, such as silicosis, may show a distribution similar to sarcoidosis, being upper lobe and peribronchovascular predominant. Large mass-like areas of fibrosis, so-called progressive massive fibrosis, are common in pneumoconioses, but not typical of UIP. From a clinical perspective, these patients usually have a clear, identifiable exposure.

Post–acute respiratory distress syndrome (ARDS) fibrosis involves the subpleural lung but usually has an anterior and mid-lung predominance. A history of a severe, acute illness should be present, although this may also be seen in an acute exacerbation of IPF.

Keep in mind that IPF may present with atypical imaging findings, so even if the HRCT does not meet strict criteria for a definite UIP pattern, IPF is often included in the differential diagnosis (Fig. 2.12A, B). Although biopsy is commonly obtained in patients with imaging findings that are atypical for UIP, it also has limitations in diagnosis. Because of the

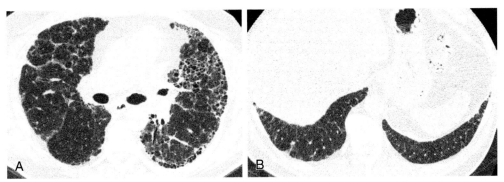

FIGURE 2.12 • **Atypical distribution of usual interstitial pneumonia (UIP) in idiopathic pulmonary fibrosis (IPF).** HRCT of a patient with IPF presenting with atypical HRCT findings not diagnostic of a UIP pattern. **A.** Honeycombing is present but the disease is patchy, asymmetrical, and not strongly subpleural predominant. **B.** Sparing of the posterior costophrenic angles, present in this case, is also atypical for IPF. Even with an atypical HRCT appearance, IPF is often still included in the differential diagnosis.

potential for sampling errors, pathology is not always representative of the disease present. A biopsy sample demonstrating findings of UIP may not be due to IPF or the other causes of a UIP pattern when a nonrepresentative region of lung is sampled (Table 2.6).

Honeycombing Pitfalls

Paraseptal emphysema (PSE) may resemble honeycombing because it occurs in a subpleural location, but there are several distinguishing features (Table 2.7, Fig. 2.13). PSE always occurs in one layer and is often associated with centrilobular emphysema; honeycombing may occur in multiple layers. Lucencies in PSE are usually larger than honeycomb cysts, ranging up to several centimeters in diameter, and may be associated with large bullae. Honeycombing is typically associated with other signs of fibrosis such as traction bronchiectasis, irregular reticulation, and volume loss, while PSE is not. Honeycombing is usually lower lobe predominant, whereas PSE is usually seen in the upper lobes. Keep in mind, however, that paraseptal emphysema and honeycombing may coexist. In such cases, bubbly lucencies may be seen from the lung apex to the base.

Reticulation in the subpleural lung may appear to outline rounded cysts that resemble honeycombing; however, the density of the central portion of these lucencies is not of air attenuation (i.e., it is not black) and may contain visible vessels (Fig. 2.14).

TABLE 2.6	Features atypical for UIP in patients with honeycombing
HRCT feature	**Likely alternative diagnoses**
Ground glass opacity outside areas of fibrosis	Nonspecific interstitial pneumonia (NSIP), hypersensitivity pneumonitis
Mosaic perfusion/air trapping	Hypersensitivity pneumonitis
Centrilobular nodules	Hypersensitivity pneumonitis
Perilymphatic nodules	Sarcoidosis, pneumoconioses
Subpleural fibrosis with only minimal honeycombing, subpleural sparing	NSIP
Upper lobe distribution of abnormalities	Sarcoidosis, pneumoconioses, hypersensitivity pneumonitis
Parahilar peribronchovascular predominance	NSIP, hypersensitivity pneumonitis, sarcoidosis, pneumoconioses
Lower lobe distribution of findings, not subpleural predominant	Hypersensitivity pneumonitis

Honeycombing must involve the subpleural lung if a confident diagnosis is to be made. If a cystic abnormality does not involve the subpleural lung, it likely represents another finding such as emphysema, bronchiectasis, traction bronchiectasis (Fig. 2.15), or cystic lung disease.

TABLE 2.7	Comparison of the features of paraseptal emphysema and honeycombing	
	Paraseptal emphysema	**Honeycombing**
Layers	Always one layer	One or more layers
Wall thickness	Very thin	Thick
Associated findings	±centrilobular emphysema	Traction bronchiectasis, irregular reticulation
Distribution	Upper lobes	Lower lobes
Size	Large	Small
Overall lung volume	Increased	Decreased
Associated reticulation or traction bronchiectasis	Absent	Present

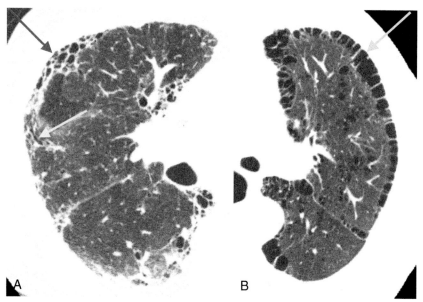

FIGURE 2.13 · **Paraseptal emphysema versus honeycombing.** Comparison of honeycombing **(A)** and paraseptal emphysema **(B)**. Both abnormalities are subpleural. Honeycomb cysts **(A**, *yellow arrow*) are clustered and stacked in multiple layers, have relatively thick walls, and are associated with reticulation and traction bronchiectasis **(A**, *red arrow*). Paraseptal emphysema **(B**, *blue arrow*) occurs in one layer, results in larger cysts, has very thin walls, and is associated with centrilobular emphysema, rather than signs of fibrosis.

Rarely primary cystic lung diseases, specifically lymphoid interstitial pneumonia (LIP), have a subpleural predominance (Fig. 2.16). In such cases, the cysts closely resemble honeycombing. Patients with LIP usually have a known history of connective tissue disease or immunosuppression (e.g., common variable immunodeficiency). Also, the lack of other signs of fibrosis in the same regions as the cysts may be a clue that honeycombing is not present.

INTRALOBULAR INTERSTITIAL THICKENING

Intralobular interstitial thickening (IIT) (i.e., thickening of the interstitial fiber network within pulmonary lobules) may be seen in isolation or in combination with IST or honeycombing.

IIT results in a network of opacities within pulmonary lobules, resulting in a reticular pattern with the lines (termed *intralobular*

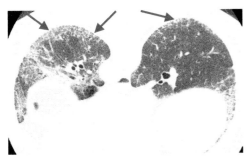

FIGURE 2.14 · Subpleural reticulation mimicking honeycombing. Reticular opacities (intralobular lines) are visible in the subpleural lung in a patient with nonspecific interstitial pneumonia. The areas of reticulation seem to outline several rounded structures (*arrows*). However, these are distinguished from honeycombing by the fact that they are not of air attenuation (i.e., they are not black).

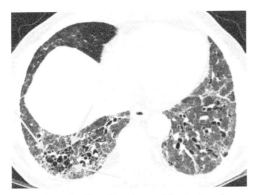

FIGURE 2.15 · Traction bronchiectasis mimicking honeycombing. Clusters of rounded air-density structures are seen at the lung bases (*arrows*), resembling honeycombing. However, they do not involve the subpleural lung. These represent areas of traction bronchiectasis in a patient with nonspecific interstitial pneumonia.

lines) separated by a few millimeters. IIT may be seen with infiltrative diseases such as pulmonary edema (Fig. 2.17), inflammatory diseases that cause interstitial thickening (such as NSIP), or in the presence of lung fibrosis (Figs. 2.10, 2.11, 2.14, 2.18, and 2.19A).

HRCT Features

Intralobular lines can be thick or thin, fine or coarse, and may or may not be associated with distortion of the underlying lung architecture.

If IIT is associated with honeycombing, it can be assumed to reflect fibrosis. In this case, it is the presence of honeycombing that is most important in the differential diagnosis. Another finding termed *traction bronchiectasis* is also helpful in suggesting that fibrosis is present when IIT is visible (Figs. 2.11, 2.18, and 2.19A). On the other hand, if IIT is associated with ground glass opacity (Fig. 2.17) and traction bronchiectasis is absent, consider an infiltrative or inflammatory disease as most likely.

Intralobular Interstitial Thickening with Traction Bronchiectasis

Traction bronchiectasis is a finding that is specific for fibrosis. The bronchi themselves are not intrinsically abnormal but are dilated secondary to traction on their walls from adjacent lung fibrosis. In traction bronchiectasis, bronchi appear irregular and distorted and "cork-screwed" in appearance (Figs. 2.11, 2.18, and 2.19A). Traction bronchiectasis may be distinguished from inflammatory bronchiectasis by a lack of mucous impaction and wall thickening, and by its association with IIT (Fig. 2.19A, B). When traction bronchiectasis is visible, a close inspection for the presence of honeycombing should be undertaken. If honeycombing is also present, then it should be used to formulate the differential diagnosis.

Traction bronchiectasis may be seen in association with any fibrotic lung disease and is less specific than honeycombing with respect to differential diagnosis. When significant traction bronchiectasis is unassociated with honeycombing, UIP is less likely as a diagnosis than when honeycombing is present, and other abnormalities, such as sarcoidosis, hypersensitivity pneumonitis, and NSIP, should be considered (Figs. 2.11, 2.18, and 2.19A). If reticulation with traction bronchiectasis is the predominant abnormality in a patient with known connective tissue disease, a diagnosis of connective tissue–related interstitial lung disease should generally be made. Otherwise, a biopsy is usually performed for diagnosis.

2

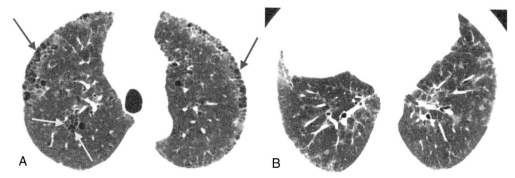

A   B

FIGURE 2.16 · Subpleural cystic lung disease mimicking honeycombing. A. HRCT of a patient with rheumatoid arthritis and lymphoid interstitial pneumonia shows subpleural cysts (*red arrows*) that closely resemble honeycombing. These are distinguished from honeycombing by the lack of other signs of fibrosis and by the presence of cysts in the more central lung regions (*yellow arrows*). **B.** Image through the lung bases shows ground glass opacity without evidence of fibrosis.

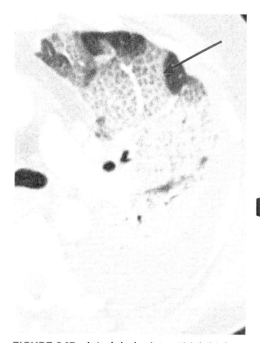

FIGURE 2.17 · Intralobular interstitial thickening. HRCT in a patient with pulmonary edema. A fine network of lines (*arrow*) represent intralobular interstitial thickening (i.e., intralobular lines) within areas of ground glass opacity.

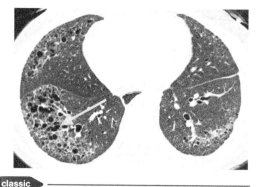

classic

FIGURE 2.18 · Intralobular interstitial thickening (intralobular lines): Classic appearance. In this patient with scleroderma, HRCT shows a peripheral distribution of fine reticulation (intralobular lines) in association with traction bronchiectasis (*arrow*). There is relative subpleural sparing and honeycombing is absent. This appearance is most typical of nonspecific interstitial pneumonia.

Intralobular Interstitial Thickening with Ground Glass Opacity

Often it is best to approach the differential diagnosis of this pattern by considering the differential diagnosis of ground glass opacity and associated symptoms (see Chapter 4).

Acute symptoms in the presence of ground glass opacity and IIT suggest pulmonary edema (Fig. 2.17), infection, diffuse alveolar damage, or hemorrhage. Chronic symptoms are most suggestive of hypersensitivity pneumonitis or NSIP. A biopsy is usually required for diagnosis in patients with chronic symptoms, unless the patient has a history of connective tissue disease.

Rarely UIP is associated with IIT and ground glass opacity as the predominant

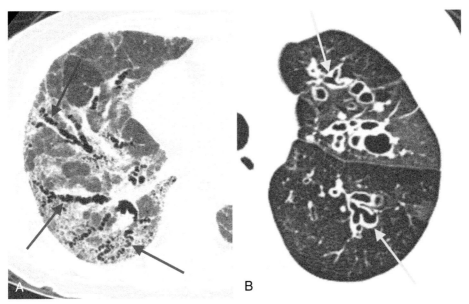

FIGURE 2.19 · **Traction bronchiectasis versus inflammatory bronchiectasis. A.** A fine reticular pattern represents intralobular interstitial thickening (i.e., intralobular lines) due to lung fibrosis. Traction bronchiectasis is present, with the bronchi appearing irregular and cork-screwed (*red arrows*). Associated lung disease is present. **B.** Inflammatory bronchiectasis (i.e., airways disease) shows extensive airway wall thickening, dilatation (*yellow arrows*), and mucoid impaction without signs of fibrosis.

findings, without honeycombing or traction bronchiectasis being visible. In this setting, these changes represent fibrosis below the resolution of HRCT.

Intralobular Interstitial Thickening as an Isolated Abnormality

When irregular reticulation is the predominant finding, and no significant honeycombing, traction bronchiectasis, or ground glass opacity is present, the appearance is nonspecific. It may reflect UIP and IPF (Fig. 2.20), NSIP, hypersensitivity pneumonitis, sarcoidosis, or other fibrotic, infiltrative, or inflammatory diseases. Biopsy may be pursued in such cases.

NONSPECIFIC OR IRREGULAR RETICULATION

Generally speaking, if reticular opacities cannot be characterized as representing IST, honeycombing, or intralobular interstitial thickening (intralobular lines), the nonspecific terms "reticulation," "irregular reticulation," or "reticular

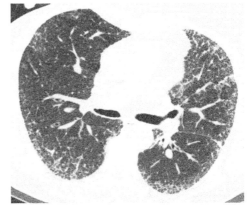

FIGURE 2.20 · **Intralobular lines as the predominant finding.** Mild subpleural reticulation is present without other signs of fibrosis. This abnormality is nonspecific with respect to diagnosis, but the subpleural distribution suggests one of the interstitial pneumonias. Lung biopsy yielded a diagnosis of usual interstitial pneumonia due to idiopathic pulmonary fibrosis.

pattern" can be used to describe the abnormality present. Although often associated with lung fibrosis, nonspecific reticulation can also be seen in the presence of various inflammatory diseases.

The differential diagnosis should be approached in a similar fashion to that of IIT and based on the presence or absence of traction bronchiectasis or ground glass opacity (Figs. 2.21 and 2.22).

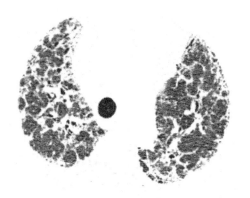

FIGURE 2.21 · Reticulation as the predominant finding. There is reticulation with irregular interlobular septal thickening, associated with mild traction bronchiectasis. This patient was diagnosed with hypersensitivity pneumonitis. It would be unusual for usual interstitial pneumonia to have such extensive abnormalities without honeycombing.

A GENERAL APPROACH TO THE DIAGNOSIS OF POSSIBLE FIBROTIC LUNG DISEASE

In the evaluation of HRCT in a patient with diffuse lung disease, a close inspection of findings of fibrosis is an important first step. The presence of fibrosis has significant implications in terms of diagnosis, prognosis, and potential response to treatment. Certain diseases, such as IPF, tend to be predominantly fibrotic, whereas others, such as desquamative interstitial pneumonia (DIP), typically have little to no fibrosis present. Regardless of the specific diagnosis, patients with significant fibrosis on HRCT tend to have a poorer prognosis than those who do not and are less likely to improve with treatment.

Several considerations are important in determining the differential diagnosis of fibrotic lung disease on HRCT, including the presence of honeycombing, the distribution of abnormalities, and presence of associated findings such as air trapping.

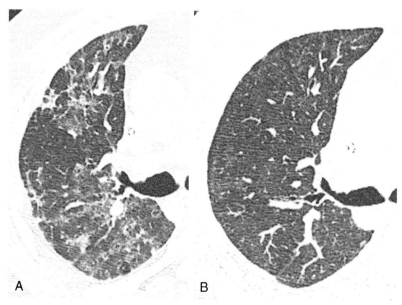

FIGURE 2.22 · Reticulation associated with ground glass opacity. HRCT at the same anatomic level is shown, performed 3 months apart. **A.** The initial HRCT shows irregular reticulation and ground glass opacity in a patient with bleomycin-induced pulmonary toxicity. **B.** Follow-up HRCT after treatment shows near-complete resolution of the previous abnormalities. Although irregular reticulation often represents fibrosis, it may in some cases represent inflammation particularly when associated honeycombing and traction bronchiectasis are absent.

HRCT Findings of Fibrosis

There are several HRCT findings that may indicate the presence of fibrosis. The most important of these are honeycombing, traction bronchiectasis, irregular IST, and IIT (Fig. 2.23A–C). Honeycombing is the most specific finding, and if present, one can be very confident about the presence of fibrosis (Fig. 2.4). Traction bronchiectasis usually indicates that fibrosis is present, particularly when associated with reticulation (Fig. 2.11). However, in some patients with ground glass opacity, traction bronchiectasis may be transient, resolving with treatment. Irregular septal thickening and IIT are moderately specific for the presence of fibrosis, but in some cases may represent infiltration or inflammation and can

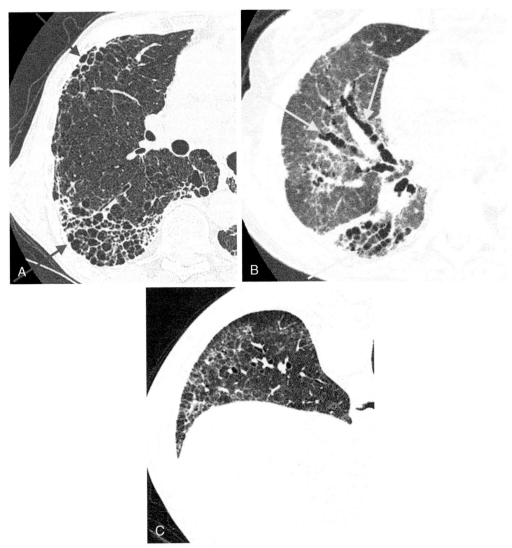

FIGURE 2.23 **HRCT signs of fibrosis. A. Honeycombing.** This is manifested by stacked subpleural cysts with relatively thick walls (*red arrows*). This finding is highly specific for fibrosis and is often seen in association with other findings such as traction bronchiectasis. **B. Traction bronchiectasis.** Bronchial dilatation associated with fibrosis is irregular and cork-screw shaped (*yellow arrows*), and findings of airway inflammation such as bronchial wall thickening are absent. This finding is also highly specific for fibrosis. **C. Reticulation.** Intralobular lines (seen in this example) suggest fibrosis but can be a manifestation of inflammatory or infiltrative disease, particularly in nonspecific interstitial pneumonia.

improve or resolve with treatment. Ground glass opacity is a nonspecific finding that reflects the presence of abnormalities below the resolution of HRCT and may occasionally be a manifestation of fibrotic lung disease.

Step-by-Step Analysis: A Checklist
Step 1: Is Fibrosis Present?

First, ask yourself this question. The presence of fibrosis is important in terms of diagnosis, prognosis, and possible response to treatment. Carefully search for any signs of fibrosis, specifically honeycombing, traction bronchiectasis, and reticulation (Figs. 2.23 and 2.24A, B).

Step 2: Is Honeycombing Present?

A careful inspection of scans for honeycombing should be undertaken (Fig. 2.25). It is highly specific for fibrosis and is often associated with a pattern of UIP and IPF. If present, determine if a "UIP pattern" is present.

Step 3: What Is the Craniocaudal Distribution of Abnormalities?

There are many ways to classify the distribution of a diffuse lung disease. Certain diseases tend to affect the upper lobes and others predominate in the mid- or lower lung (Table 2.8). An upper lobe predominance of disease is typical of sarcoidosis, prior granulomatous infection such as tuberculosis, pneumoconioses, radiation fibrosis, pleuroparenchymal fibroelastosis, and ankylosing spondylitis. A lower lobe predominance of disease is typical of IPF, connective tissue disease, asbestosis, and chronic aspiration. Chronic hypersensitivity pneumonitis and drug-related fibrosis may predominate in upper, mid-, or lower lung zones or may be diffuse.

Pay particular attention to the costophrenic angles. In general, the idiopathic interstitial pneumonias, including UIP, NSIP, and DIP, involve the posterior costophrenic angles. Fibrosis resulting from ARDS is often subpleural and anterior in distribution. Most other diseases will show sparing

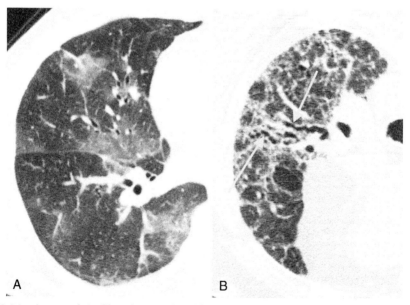

A   B

FIGURE 2.24 · **Approach to fibrosis, step 1: Is fibrosis present? A. Ground glass opacity only, no fibrosis present.** HRCT in a patient with subacute hypersensitivity pneumonitis shows ground glass opacity and no evidence of fibrosis. These changes represented inflammation and resolved after treatment. **B. Severe fibrosis present.** Prone HRCT in a patient with chronic hypersensitivity pneumonitis shows traction bronchiectasis (*arrows*) and reticulation. These findings represent fibrosis and were unresponsive to treatment.

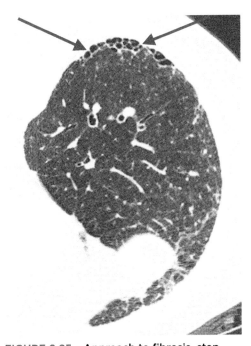

FIGURE 2.25 · **Approach to fibrosis, step 2: Is honeycombing present? Prone HRCT shows subpleural honeycombing (*arrows*) in a patient with idiopathic pulmonary fibrosis.** Although this finding may be found with several different diseases, its presence favors a pattern of usual interstitial pneumonia and represents irreversible fibrosis.

TABLE 2.8	Differential diagnosis of fibrosis based upon craniocaudal distribution of findings on HRCT

Upper lobe predominant	Lower lobe predominant
Sarcoidosis	Idiopathic pulmonary fibrosis
Prior tuberculosis	Connective tissue disease
Prior fungal infection	Drug fibrosis
Radiation fibrosis (e.g., head and neck cancer treatment)	Asbestosis
Pneumoconioses (silicosis, coal worker's, beryllium, talc)	Hypersensitivity pneumonitis
Pleuroparenchymal fibroelastosis	
Ankylosing spondylitis	Chronic aspiration

of the inferior-most costophrenic angles (Fig. 2.26A–C). This is particularly helpful in distinguishing chronic hypersensitivity pneumonitis from the interstitial pneumonias, as

hypersensitivity pneumonitis is often mid–lower lung predominant and yet spares the costophrenic angles.

Step 4: What Is the Axial (Cross-sectional) Distribution of Abnormalities?

The cross-sectional distribution of abnormalities (Fig. 2.27A, B) may also be helpful (Table 2.9). Whether a disease is strongly peripheral or involves the more central or peribronchovascular lung regions can serve to focus the differential diagnosis. The interstitial pneumonias tend to be strongly peripheral in distribution. Keep in mind that the subpleural region includes the interstitium just deep to the fissures. Other diseases tend to show a central or diffuse distribution. NSIP often spares the immediate subpleural lung.

Step 5: Are There Significant Associated Findings That Help in Diagnosis?

Ancillary findings may be important in diagnosis. The most important of these include mosaic perfusion, air trapping, and nodules. The combination of fibrosis and significant mosaic perfusion and/or air trapping suggests hypersensitivity pneumonitis (Fig. 2.28A, B). A patient with perilymphatic nodules and fibrosis likely has sarcoidosis. Note that these additional findings need to be significant in extent to be used for diagnosis. For instance, it is not uncommon for someone with IPF to have a small amount of air trapping (Fig. 2.29A, B). It is only when the presence of air trapping is moderate to severe that it should be considered helpful in diagnosing hypersensitivity pneumonitis.

Step 6: If Fibrosis Is Present, Is It the Predominant Abnormality?

If fibrosis is present, it is important to determine if the lung abnormality is predominantly fibrotic (Fig. 2.30). For example, IPF is predominantly a fibrotic disease. If there are areas of isolated ground glass opacity, consolidation, or nodules, findings that generally do not indicate fibrosis, then there may be

2

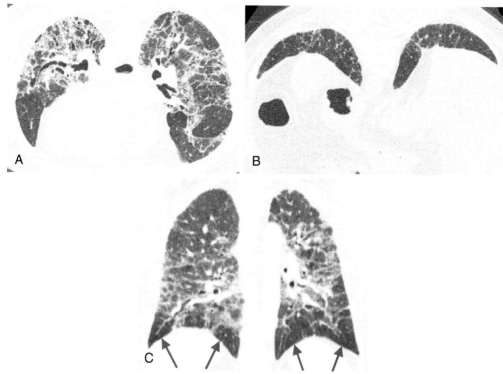

FIGURE 2.26 Approach to fibrosis, step 3: What is the craniocaudal distribution? Prone HRCT through the mid-lower lung (A), inferior costophrenic angles (B), and a coronal reformation(C) in a patient with hypersensitivity pneumonitis shows a mid-lower lung predominance with sparing of the costophrenic angles (C, *arrows*). This sparing of the costophrenic angle is very atypical for usual and nonspecific interstitial pneumonia and suggests an alternative cause of fibrosis.

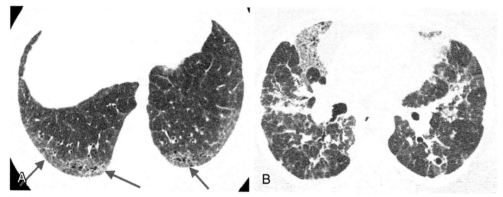

FIGURE 2.27 Approach to fibrosis, step 4: What is the axial distribution? **A. Peripheral distribution in nonspecific interstitial pneumonia.** HRCT shows a strong peripheral distribution (*arrows*) of ground glass opacity, irregular reticulation, and traction bronchiectasis. This distribution of findings strongly suggests an interstitial pneumonia, namely usual interstitial pneumonia, nonspecific interstitial pneumonia, or desquamative interstitial pneumonia. **B. Diffuse distribution of hypersensitivity pneumonitis.** In contrast to usual interstitial, nonspecific, and desquamative interstitial pneumonia, other fibrotic lung diseases tend to show a central or diffuse distribution of findings. This patient with hypersensitivity pneumonitis shows both peripheral and central areas of fibrosis.

TABLE 2.9	Differential diagnosis based on axial distribution of findings

Subpleural predominant	Diffuse or central distribution
Idiopathic pulmonary fibrosis	Sarcoidosis
Connective tissue disease	Pneumoconioses
Drug fibrosis	Hypersensitivity pneumonitis
Asbestosis	Chronic aspiration
Post-acute respiratory distress syndrome fibrosis	Prior tuberculosis or fungal infection

active inflammation present and the patient likely warrants more aggressive diagnosis or treatment.

Step 7: Is Useful Clinical Information Available?

Basic clinical information is vital in placing HRCT findings in context (Table 2.10). Age has an impact on which disease is most likely. For instance, IPF is rare in patients younger than 50 years, but in patients older than 50 years, it is one of the most common causes of lung fibrosis. Drug toxicity, asbestosis, and

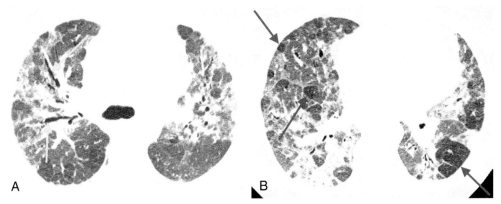

FIGURE 2.28 · Approach to fibrosis, step 5: Are there associated findings? Other findings associated with fibrosis may be useful in diagnosis. The combination of fibrosis and significant mosaic perfusion/air trapping is very suggestive of hypersensitivity pneumonitis. Note the patchy irregular reticulation and traction bronchiectasis (**A**, *yellow arrows*) associated with significant areas of air trapping on expiratory images (**B**, *red arrows*).

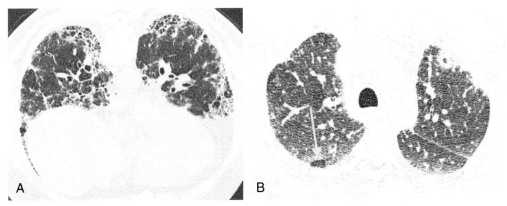

FIGURE 2.29 · Approach to fibrosis, step 5: Are there associated findings? A patient with idiopathic pulmonary fibrosis shows minimal air trapping. To be useful in diagnosis, additional findings associated with fibrosis need to be a significant part of the picture. This patient with idiopathic pulmonary fibrosis shows peripheral fibrosis with honeycombing in the lower lobes typical for a usual interstitial pneumonia pattern. The minimal air trapping in the right upper lobe (**B**, *arrow*) should be ignored as it is not a significant abnormality.

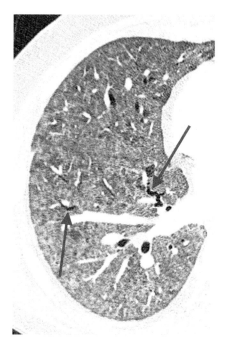

FIGURE 2.30 · **Approach to fibrosis, step 6: Is fibrosis the predominant abnormality? HRCT showing extensive ground glass opacity and minimal traction bronchiectasis (*red arrows*).** While fibrosis is present, it is a very small component to the disease. Most of the abnormality is likely inflammatory and reversible.

TABLE 2.10	Clinical information and the most likely associated diagnoses presenting with fibrosis
Age >50 y	Idiopathic pulmonary fibrosis, drug toxicity, asbestosis, pneumoconioses, hypersensitivity pneumonitis
Age <50 y	Sarcoidosis, collagen vascular disease, hypersensitivity pneumonitis
Cigarette smoking	Idiopathic pulmonary fibrosis, desquamative interstitial pneumonia
Exposures to dust	Silicosis, coal worker's pneumoconiosis, talcosis, and other pneumoconioses
Exposures to organic antigens	Hypersensitivity pneumonitis
Connective tissue disease	Nonspecific interstitial pneumonia and usual interstitial pneumonia

other pneumoconioses are also most common in patients older than 50 years. Sarcoidosis and collagen vascular disease typically present in patients younger than 50 years. Hypersensitivity pneumonitis has a wide age range at presentation.

Fibrosis in a cigarette smoker is most commonly due to UIP or DIP. Exposures to dust or organic antigens are associated with pneumoconiosis or hypersensitivity pneumonitis, respectively. Connective tissue disease is most commonly associated with NSIP, but a UIP pattern may also be seen in these patients. Drug-induced fibrosis will be seen in patients with an appropriate medication history. The most common categories of drugs to produce fibrosis are the chemotherapeutic agents, cardiac medications, and antibiotics.

FURTHER READING

Andreu J, Hidalgo A, Pallisa E, Majo J, Martinez-Rodriguez M, Caceres J. Septal thickening: HRCT findings and differential diagnosis. *Curr Probl Diagn Radiol*. 2004;33:226-237.

Austin JH, Müller NL, Friedman PJ, et al. Glossary of terms for CT of the lungs: recommendations of the Nomenclature Committee of the Fleischner Society. *Radiology*. 1996;200:327-331.

Collins J. CT signs and patterns of lung disease. *Radiol Clin North Am*. 2001;39:1115-1135.

Elicker B, Pereira CA, Webb R, Leslie KO. High-resolution computed tomography patterns of diffuse interstitial lung disease with clinical and pathological correlation. *J Bras Pneumol*. 2008;34:715-744.

Gotway MB, Freemer MM, KingJr TE. Challenges in pulmonary fibrosis. 1: use of high resolution CT scanning of the lung for the evaluation of patients with idiopathic interstitial pneumonias. *Thorax*. 2007;62:546-553.

Gotway MB, Reddy GP, Webb WR, Elicker BM, Leung JW. High-resolution CT of the lung: patterns of disease and differential diagnoses. *Radiol Clin North Am*. 2005;43:513-542.

Hansell DM, Bankier AA, MacMahon H, et al. Fleischner Society: glossary of terms for thoracic imaging. *Radiology*. 2008;246:697-722.

Kang EY, Grenier P, Laurent F, Müller NL. Interlobular septal thickening: patterns at high-resolution computed tomography. *J Thorac Imaging*. 1996;11:260-264.

Lynch DA, Travis WD, Muller NL, et al. Idiopathic interstitial pneumonias: CT features. *Radiology*. 2005;236:10-21.

Müller NL, Miller RR. Computed tomography of chronic diffuse infiltrative lung disease: part 1. *Am Rev Respir Dis*. 1990;142:1206-1215.

Müller NL, Miller RR. Computed tomography of chronic diffuse infiltrative lung disease: part 2. *Am Rev Respir Dis.* 1990;142:1440-1448.

Primack SL, Hartman TE, Hansell DM, Müller NL. End-stage lung disease: CT findings in 61 patients. *Radiology.* 1993;189:681-686.

Raghu G, Collard HR, Egan JJ, et al. An official ATS/ERS/JRS/ALAT statement: idiopathic pulmonary fibrosisAn official ATS/ERS/JRS/ALAT statement:: An official ATS/ERS/JRS/ALAT statement:evidence-based guidelines for diagnosis and management. *Am J Respir Crit Care Med.* 2011;183:788-824.

Souza CA, Müller NL, Flint J, Wright JL, Churg A. Idiopathic pulmonary fibrosis: spectrum of high-resolution CT findings. *AJR Am J Roentgenol.* 2005;185:1531-1539.

Suh RD, Goldin JG. High-resolution computed tomography of interstitial pulmonary fibrosis. *Semin Respir Crit Care Med.* 2006;27:623-633.

Webb WR. High resolution lung computed tomography: normal anatomic and pathologic findings. *Radiol Clin North Am.* 1991;29:1051-1063.

Webb WR. Thin-section CT of the secondary pulmonary lobule: anatomy and the image—the 2004 Fleischner lecture. *Radiology.* 2006;239:322-338.

Woodhead F, Wells AU, Desai SR. Pulmonary complications of connective tissue diseases. *Clin Chest Med.* 2008;29:149-164.

2

Nodular Lung Disease

INTRODUCTION

Diffuse lung diseases presenting with small nodules (less than 1 cm in diameter) represent a wide variety of entities in many different disease categories. High-resolution computed tomography (HRCT) is generally used to suggest a focused differential diagnosis and guide further diagnostic evaluation. In some cases, HRCT may be diagnostic of a single disease.

The HRCT evaluation of a patient with nodular lung disease is based on several findings and patterns. These include (1) the craniocaudal distribution of nodules, (2) the appearance and attenuation of the nodules, and (3) the specific distribution of the nodules relative to lung structures.

CRANIOCAUDAL DISTRIBUTION OF NODULES

The craniocaudal distribution of nodules is helpful in the differential diagnosis of nodular lung disease (Table 3.1). Certain diseases, such as sarcoidosis and other granulomatous diseases, tend to predominate in the upper lobes (Fig. 3.1A–C), whereas others, such as hematogenous metastases, tend to be lower lobe–predominant (Fig. 3.2A, B). However, on its own, the craniocaudal distribution of nodules is insufficient for diagnosis and should be used in combination with other findings. There is overlap between the distributions of different diseases and variability among patients with the same disease.

APPEARANCE AND ATTENUATION OF NODULES

The appearance of nodules may help to determine whether they are interstitial or alveolar (airspace) in origin (Table 3.2; Fig. 3.3A, B).

Interstitial nodules commonly have well-defined borders and are of soft tissue attenuation. Hematogenous metastases are an example; even small nodules in patients with metastases tend to be sharply marginated. *Alveolar (or airspace) nodules* typically have ill-defined borders. For instance, endobronchial spread of infection (bronchopneumonia) results from airway infection, and as the infection spreads outward from the airway to involve the adjacent alveoli, the leading edge of the resulting nodular opacity will be indistinct because of heterogeneous alveolar involvement. Alveolar nodules may be of soft tissue attenuation or of ground glass opacity (GGO). Soft tissue airspace nodules are typical of bacterial infection, whereas GGO nodules may be due to atypical infections or inflammatory disease.

Using the appearance of nodules to determine their differential diagnosis, without considering other findings, is of limited accuracy; there are many exceptions to the rule. For instance, hypersensitivity pneumonitis (HP) is predominantly an interstitial lung disease (ILD) but is characterized by very indistinct nodules. Also, many diseases have both interstitial and alveolar components.

DISTRIBUTION OF NODULES RELATIVE TO LUNG STRUCTURES

The preferred method by which to evaluate diffuse nodular lung disease on HRCT is to determine the specific distribution of nodules with respect to lung structures. This approach allows a limited differential diagnosis and also gives some insight into the pathophysiology of disease spread. When used in conjunction

TABLE 3.1	Differential diagnosis of nodules based on craniocaudal distribution	
Upper lobe predominant nodules	**Lower lobe predominant nodules**	**Variable (upper or lower lobe predominant nodules)**
Sarcoidosis	Hematogenous metastases	Lymphangitic carcinomatosis
Pneumoconioses (e.g., silicosis, coal worker's pneumoconiosis, berylliosis)		Hypersensitivity pneumonitis
Langerhans cell histiocytosis		Endobronchial spread of infection
Respiratory bronchiolitis		Invasive mucinous adenocarcinoma
Miliary tuberculosis		Miliary tuberculosis
		Miliary fungal infection
		Follicular bronchiolitis

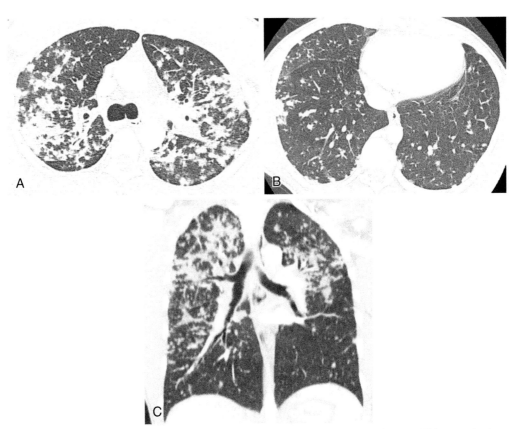

FIGURE 3.1 · **Upper lobe predominance of nodules in sarcoidosis. A** and **B.** HRCT in a patient with sarcoidosis shows nodules to be more numerous and larger in the upper **(A)** rather than in the lower **(B)** lungs. **C.** The marked upper lobe predominance of sarcoidosis is clearly demonstrated on a coronal reformation.

with clinical information, the craniocaudal distribution of nodules, and their appearance, it may be diagnostic of a single disease. When it is not diagnostic, the differential diagnosis is usually limited and HRCT can be helpful in guiding further tests.

There are three specific distributions of small nodules that can be distinguished on HRCT: (1) perilymphatic; (2) random; and (3) centrilobular. Recognizing one of these three distributions is fundamental to HRCT interpretation in patients with nodular lung

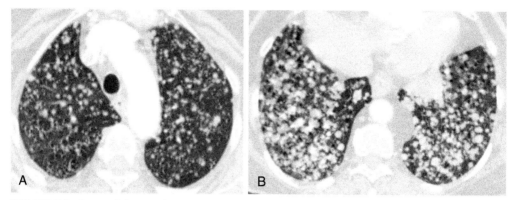

FIGURE 3.2 **Lower lobe predominance of nodules in metastatic neoplasm. A** and **B.** HRCT in a patient with hematogenous spread of thyroid cancer to the lungs. Note the marked lower lobe predominance in the size and number of nodules **(B)**, as compared with a scan through the upper lobes **(A)**. This reflects the differences in blood flow to the lower and upper lobes.

TABLE 3.2	Differential diagnosis of nodules based on appearance

Well-defined borders	Ill-defined borders	Either well-defined or ill-defined borders
Sarcoidosis	Hypersensitivity pneumonitis	Langerhans cell histiocytosis
Metastases	Respiratory bronchiolitis	Lymphoid interstitial pneumonia
Miliary infections	Follicular bronchiolitis	Pneumoconioses
Amyloidosis	Infections	
	Invasive mucinous adenocarcinoma (bronchioloalveolar carcinoma)	
	Aspiration	
	Pulmonary edema	
	Pulmonary hemorrhage	
	Pulmonary arterial hypertension	
	Metastatic calcification	

disease. HRCT is 90 to 95% accurate in determining the pattern present and the correct differential diagnosis.

Perilymphatic Nodules

Diseases with a perilymphatic distribution of nodules are characterized by involvement of, or spread through, pulmonary lymphatics. For example, sarcoidosis is characterized by clusters of granulomas occurring in relation to lymphatics. Also, silicosis and coal worker's pneumoconiosis (CWP) result from inhalation of dusts, which are cleared via lymphatic channels.

Pulmonary lymphatics predominate in four specific locations: (1) the parahilar peribronchovascular interstitium, (2) the subpleural interstitium, (3) the interlobular septa, and (4) the centrilobular peribronchovascular interstitium.

On HRCT, perilymphatic diseases typically show nodules predominating in, or limited to, one or more of these four locations (Fig. 3.4).

Peribronchovascular nodules are seen adjacent to large bronchi and vessels in the central lung regions (Fig. 3.4A, green dots). They can give the walls of bronchi and arteries a nodular appearance or may appear as clusters of nodules adjacent to bronchi. *Subpleural nodules*, or groups of nodules forming "plaques" or masses, are seen immediately beneath the pleural surfaces and adjacent to the interlobar fissures (Fig. 3.4A, yellow dots). *Interlobular septal nodules* give the septa a "beaded" appearance, as in nodular interlobular septal thickening (Fig. 3.4A, red dots), described in Chapter 2. *Centrilobular peribronchovascular nodules* are seen in relation to small airways and vessels in

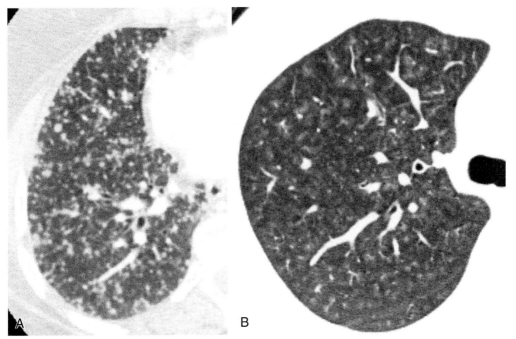

A   B

FIGURE 3.3 · **Appearances of different types of nodules.** Different HRCT appearances of interstitial and airspace nodules. **A.** Hematogenous metastases involving the lung interstitium are sharply defined. **B.** Ground glass opacity nodules associated with viral pneumonia, with variable involvement of alveoli, are indistinct with poorly marginated borders.

the centers of pulmonary lobules. They give the centrilobular artery a knobby appearance or result in a centrilobular cluster of small nodules (Fig. 3.4A, blue dots).

At the level of individual pulmonary lobules, perilymphatic diseases may show both centrilobular and interlobular septal nodules.

Each of these regions need not be involved in patients having a perilymphatic pattern. The combination of two of the four possible sites is usually sufficient for diagnosis. Globally, because the nodules occur only in relation to these specific locations, a perilymphatic distribution of nodules often appears patchy, with some lung regions appearing abnormal and some lung regions appearing normal (Fig. 3.4A).

The most common diseases that result in a perilymphatic distribution of nodules are (1) sarcoidosis (Figs. 3.4B, C and 3.5A–D), (2) lymphangitic spread of neoplasm, and (3) several pneumoconioses, such as silicosis, CWP, berylliosis, talcosis, and rare earth pneumoconiosis (Table 3.3). Rare causes include lymphoid interstitial pneumonia (LIP) and amyloidosis.

There is some variation in the specific distribution of nodules, and the predominant regions involved, among the different diseases associated with this pattern and in different patients with the same disease. These variations are discussed below.

HRCT findings, considered in conjunction with clinical information, may help distinguish among the several causes of perilymphatic nodules.

Sarcoidosis

Sarcoidosis is, by far, the most common disease in this category (see Chapter 12). On HRCT, nodules tend to predominate in the parahilar peribronchovascular and subpleural regions (Figs. 3.4B, C and 3.5A–D). Individual nodules are usually sharply marginated and of soft tissue attenuation and are easily seen when only a few millimeters in diameter.

HRCT may show a few peribronchovascular nodules, clusters of nodules, or large parahilar masses made up of multiple confluent nodules (Fig. 3.5C). Air-filled bronchi (air

3

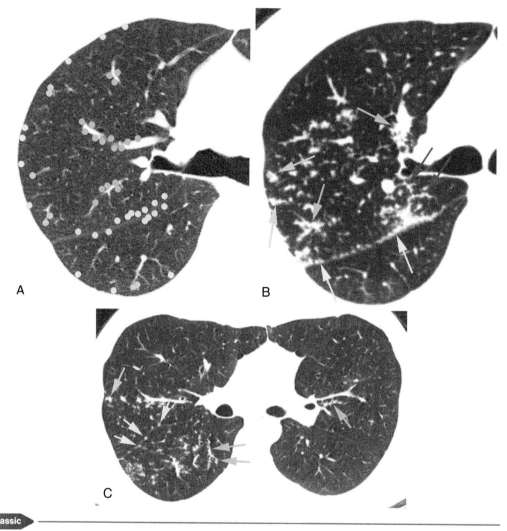

classic

FIGURE 3.4 · **Perilymphatic nodules: Classic appearances. A.** In a perilymphatic pattern, the nodules predominate in relation to the peribronchovascular interstitium (*green dots*), subpleural interstitium (*yellow dots*), centrilobular regions (*blue dots*), and interlobular septa (*red dots*). In patients with a perilymphatic pattern, the distribution of nodules is often patchy. The specific distribution of perilymphatic nodules varies in different diseases and in different patients. **B** and **C.** Perilymphatic nodules in two patients with sarcoidosis. As in **(A)**, nodules are seen involving peribronchovascular (*green arrows*), subpleural (*yellow arrows*), centrilobular (*blue arrows*), and interlobular septal (*red arrows*) interstitium. The overall appearance is that of patchy lung involvement, with some lung regions appearing abnormal and some appearing normal.

bronchograms) may be visible within large masses. Individual small nodules are usually visible adjacent to the large masses; these are termed *satellite nodules*, and the appearance of a large mass with satellite nodules has been termed *the galaxy sign* of sarcoidosis (Fig. 3.5C). Subpleural nodules are also common, being seen in the lung periphery or adjacent to fissures. They may appear as individual

nodules or as clusters or subpleural plaques or masses. Interlobular septal nodules and centrilobular peribronchovascular nodules are less common (Fig. 3.5B, D) but occasionally are a predominant feature (Fig. 3.5D). Mediastinal and hilar lymph node enlargement may be associated but need not be present to suggest the diagnosis when lung abnormalities are typical.

3

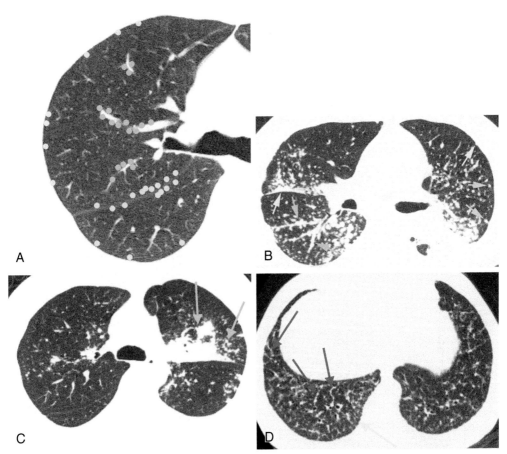

FIGURE 3.5 · **Perilymphatic nodules in sarcoidosis. A.** A typical perilymphatic distribution in sarcoidosis. In sarcoidosis, nodules typically predominate in relation to the peribronchovascular interstitium (*green dots*) and the subpleural interstitium (*yellow dots*), but centrilobular and septal nodules may also be seen. **B.** A classic perilymphatic pattern in a patient with sarcoidosis shows patchy, clustered nodules that predominate in relation to the central bronchovascular bundles (*green arrows*) and subpleural regions (*yellow arrows*). Note that some centrilobular peribronchovascular nodules (*blue arrows*) and septal nodules (*red arrow*) are also present. Conglomeration of nodules is visible in the left lung. **C.** CT "galaxy sign" in sarcoidosis. In a different patient, HRCT shows a parahilar mass-like conglomerate of confluent nodules in the left upper lobe. The mass reflects profuse peribronchovascular nodules. Smaller "satellite" nodules are visible at the periphery (*arrows*) of the confluent mass. This appearance is most common in the parahilar regions and has been termed the "galaxy sign." The galaxy sign may be seen in other diseases, such as silicosis and talcosis. Asymmetry, as seen in this case, may be seen in sarcoidosis. **D.** Interlobular septal nodules in sarcoidosis. A patient with sarcoidosis shows numerous nodules in relation to interlobular septa (*yellow arrow*). Numerous subpleural nodules (*red arrows*) are also present.

TABLE 3.3	Differential diagnosis of perilymphatic nodules

Sarcoidosis (common)
Lymphangitic carcinomatosis or lymphoma/ leukemia
Some pneumoconioses (e.g., silicosis, coal worker's pneumoconiosis, berylliosis, talc, rare earths)
Lymphoid interstitial pneumonia (rare)
Amyloidosis (rare)

Sarcoidosis usually shows an upper lobe predominance of nodules, but this is not always the case. Bilateral abnormalities are typical, but asymmetry is not uncommon.

Sarcoidosis is more frequently seen in younger patients than the other causes of perilymphatic nodules.

Often, patients with extensive nodules are relatively asymptomatic, so there

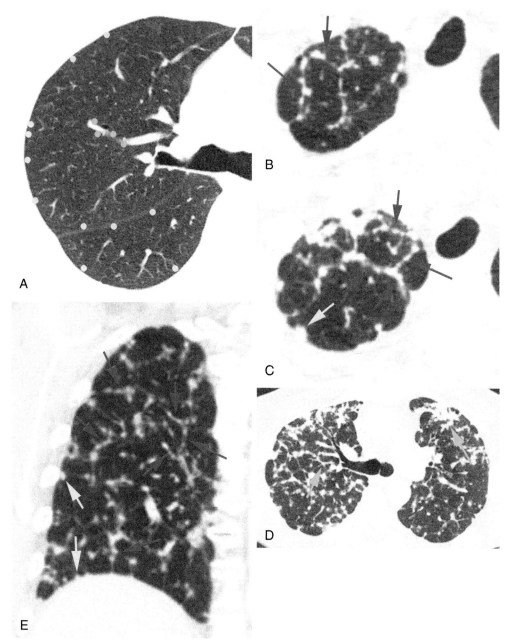

FIGURE 3.6 · **Perilymphatic nodules in lymphangitic spread of neoplasm. A.** In lymphangitic spread of neoplasm, perilymphatic nodules tend to predominate in relation to the interlobular septa (*red dots*), the parahilar peribronchovascular interstitium (*green dots*), and the subpleural regions (*yellow dots*). The abnormality may be diffuse or patchy. **B–D.** Colon cancer with lymphangitic carcinomatosis. Extensive nodular interlobular septal thickening (*red arrows*) is seen throughout both lungs. A few subpleural nodules are also present (*yellow arrow*, **C**). Although lymphangitic carcinomatosis often predominates in relation to interlobular septa, it may also involve the peribronchovascular lymphatics (*green arrows*, **D**). **E.** Coronal reconstruction in the same patient as in **(B)–(D)** shows nodular interlobular septal thickening (*red arrows*) and subpleural nodules (*yellow arrows*).

may be a discrepancy between the HRCT appearance and the severity of the patient's symptoms. There is a geographic variability in the incidence of sarcoidosis; sarcoidosis is much less common in countries close to the equator and in Asia than in the United States.

If sarcoidosis is suspected on HRCT, transbronchial biopsy is often the next diagnostic test. As the nodules are often located within the peribronchovascular interstitium, transbronchial biopsy has a high yield. Biopsy of mediastinal or hilar lymph nodes using endobronchial ultrasound guidance is another option with a high diagnostic yield.

Lymphangitic Spread of Neoplasm

On HRCT, lymphangitic spread of neoplasm, either carcinoma or lymphoma, most frequently results in smooth thickening of the interstitium, including the interlobular septa, peribronchovascular interstitium, and the subpleural interstitium (see Chapters 2 and 17). When nodules are present, which occurs in a minority of cases, they also tend to predominate in relation to the interlobular septa (Fig. 3.6A–E), the parahilar peribronchovascular interstitium, and the subpleural regions. A combination of smooth interstitial thickening and nodules may be seen; this appearance is not common in sarcoidosis. Mediastinal and hilar lymph node enlargement may be associated. Pleural effusion, rare in sarcoidosis, may be seen.

In lymphangitic spread of neoplasm, nodules are sharply marginated and of soft tissue attenuation. The overall distribution is variable. An upper or lower lobe predominance may be present, and nodules may be unilateral or bilateral.

Patients with lymphangitic spread of tumor usually have a history of malignancy and are older and more symptomatic (i.e., dyspneic) than patients with sarcoidosis. As with sarcoidosis, lymphangitic spread of neoplasm can often be diagnosed using transbronchial biopsy or endobronchial ultrasound-guided biopsy of lymph nodes.

Silicosis and CWP

History is important in suggesting silicosis or CWP in a patient with nodules (see Chapter 16). Patients with silicosis or CWP have a significant history of long-term exposure in professions such as mining, quarrying, stone cutting, or sand blasting. On HRCT, silicosis and CWP have a similar appearance despite the fact that different dusts are involved, and the histology is different.

Silicosis and CWP are frequently associated with centrilobular nodules (reflecting deposition of dust and fibrosis around small airways and involving lymphatics) and interlobular septal or subpleural nodules because of lymphatic clearance of the dust (Fig. 3.7A, B). Centrilobular nodules are more frequent in these pneumoconioses than with the other causes of perilymphatic nodules.

Large masses in the parahilar regions may be seen, usually representing central conglomeration of nodules in CWP or masses made up of confluent nodules and fibrosis (*progressive massive fibrosis*) in silicosis (Fig. 3.7B). As these masses develop, the number of lung nodules often appears to decrease. Satellite nodules are common, and areas of emphysema may be seen in the peripheral lung.

A distinct upper lobe predominance is typical in both silicosis and CWP, and nodules are often most numerous in the posterior lung. Abnormalities are usually symmetrical. Nodules are usually a few millimeters in diameter, of soft tissue attenuation, and more sharply marginated in silicosis than in CWP.

Rare Diseases

There is significant overlap in the HRCT findings of the various causes of perilymphatic nodules. History is most important in suggesting one of the rare causes of nodules in this distribution. *LIP* should be considered in patients with connective tissue disease or immunosuppression (e.g., human immunodeficiency virus infection and common variable immunodeficiency; see Chapters 9 and 17). The HRCT appearance

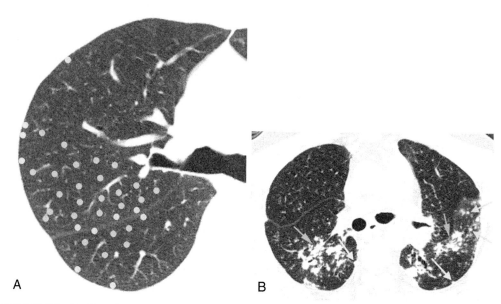

A

B

FIGURE 3.7 · **Perilymphatic nodules in silicosis. A.** In silicosis, nodules usually predominate in the centrilobular (*blue dots*) and subpleural regions (*yellow dots*). A posterior lung predominance is common. **B.** HRCT in a patient with silicosis shows nodules in the subpleural regions (*yellow arrows*) and centrilobular regions (*blue arrows*). Peribronchovascular nodules are also visible (*green arrows*).

of LIP is variable, but some combination of subpleural, interlobular septal, and centrilobular nodules is usually seen (Fig. 3.8). *Amyloidosis* may occur in patients with multiple myeloma or may be idiopathic (see Chapter 18). Subpleural and septal nodules are most typical.

Random Nodules

Random nodules have no particular distribution with respect to lung structures or pulmonary lobules (Fig. 3.9). They typically show a diffuse, uniform, and homogeneous distribution; they occur anywhere and everywhere. They are not clustered or concentrated adjacent to any specific lung structures.

As in patients with a perilymphatic pattern, subpleural nodules are present in patients with a random distribution, but there is no predominance of nodules in this location, as there often is with perilymphatic diseases. Overall, random nodules are diffuse and uniform in distribution, whereas perilymphatic nodules usually appear patchy. Random nodules are usually of soft tissue attenuation, sharply marginated, and easily

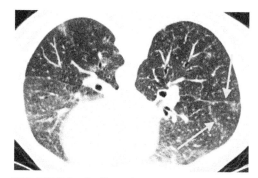

FIGURE 3.8 · **Perilymphatic nodules in lymphoid interstitial pneumonia.** Prone HRCT of a patient with human immunodeficiency virus infection shows small nodules with a patchy distribution. Note the predominance of nodules in the subpleural interstitium (*arrows*) reflecting a perilymphatic distribution of disease.

visible when only a few millimeters in size. At diagnosis, they may be smaller (1 to 2 mm) than nodules in patients with sarcoidosis.

A random pattern is most common with diseases that spread in a hematogenous fashion (Fig. 3.10A, B). As pulmonary blood flow is relatively homogeneous, but with greater blood flow in the lung bases, it stands to reason that processes that spread in this manner appear diffuse in distribution or show a basilar predominance in nodule size and number. An exception is miliary tuberculosis (TB); in some patients miliary TB predominates in the upper lobes because the TB bacillus grows best in the presence of high oxygen tension (which is present in the upper lobes).

The differential diagnosis (Table 3.4) of random nodules primarily includes miliary infection by TB or other mycobacteria, miliary fungal infection (e.g., histoplasmosis and coccidioidomycosis; see Chapter 14), and hematogenous spread of malignancy.

Occasionally, diseases that typically produce a perilymphatic pattern (e.g., sarcoidosis) appear random in distribution when the nodules are very numerous. However, there are usually clues to the correct diagnosis. For example, close inspection may show proportionally too many nodules along the fissures or within the peribronchovascular interstitium (Fig. 3.11). Also, in some patients with metastases, HRCT may show features of both random and perilymphatic patterns, likely because both types of spread are actually present.

The size of nodules may be helpful in determining the most likely diagnosis. Tiny nodules, a few millimeters in diameter, are most commonly due to miliary TB, whereas larger nodules are more commonly due to malignancy. However, there is considerable overlap in the size of nodules that each of these diseases produces. Miliary TB can result in nodules larger than 5 mm.

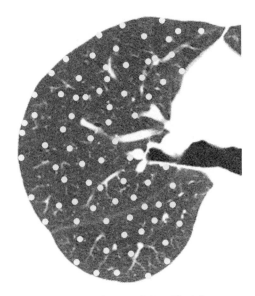

FIGURE 3.9 · **Random nodules. Nodules are diffuse and show a homogeneous distribution.** Note that subpleural nodules (dots) are present, but there is no preponderance of nodules in this location.

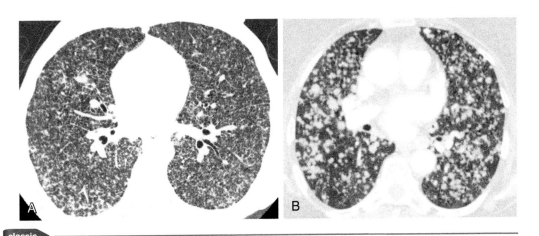

classic

FIGURE 3.10 · **Random nodules: Classic appearances. A and B.** Two examples of a random distribution of pulmonary nodules in patients with miliary tuberculosis **(A)** and hematogenous spread of metastases **(B).** Notice the diffuse and uniform distribution of nodules with involvement of the pleural surfaces.

TABLE 3.4	Differential diagnosis of random nodules

Miliary tuberculosis
Miliary fungal infection
Hematogenous metastases
Perilymphatic processes (occasionally appear random)

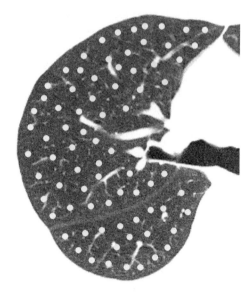

FIGURE 3.12 · **Centrilobular nodules. Nodules involve the centrilobular regions, and the most peripheral nodules are separated from the pleural surfaces by 5-10 mm; no subpleural nodules are present. Nodules also appear evenly spaced.** In patients with centrilobular nodules (*dots*), the overall distribution may be diffuse (as in this illustration) or patchy.

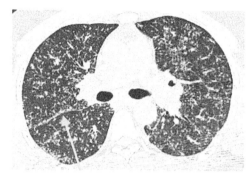

FIGURE 3.11 · **Perilymphatic nodules simulating a random distribution in sarcoidosis.** On initial inspection, the nodules in this case appear to have a diffuse random distribution. However, note the predominance of nodules along the major fissure (*arrow*), a finding that suggests a perilymphatic distribution in this patient.

History is also important in the differential diagnosis of this pattern. If the patient has a known diagnosis of malignancy, this pattern is usually diagnostic of hematogenous spread of tumor. If signs of infection are present (fever and increased white blood cell count), miliary TB or fungal infection is likely. One caveat: miliary TB may be associated with very few symptoms in elderly or debilitated patients. Transbronchial biopsy is often positive in patients with miliary infection or neoplasm.

Centrilobular Nodules

Centrilobular nodules occur in diseases that primarily involve the centrilobular bronchiole, artery, or lymphatics. The differential diagnosis of centrilobular nodules is quite broad and encompasses a wide variety of different etiologies and categories of disease. However, small airways disease is the most common cause of centrilobular nodules.

Centrilobular nodules demonstrate several HRCT findings that distinguish them from the other patterns. These include (1) sparing of the subpleural interstitium and (2) a similar spacing between adjacent nodules (Fig. 3.12).

As the centers of the most peripheral pulmonary lobules are about 5 to 10 mm from pleural surfaces, the most peripheral nodules seen with this pattern are generally 5 mm from the pleural surface or fissures. Subpleural nodules are characteristically absent with a centrilobular distribution (Fig. 3.13), although a large centrilobular nodule may reach the pleural surface, or the disease process may involve the entire lobule (Fig. 3.14). At a lobular level, centrilobular nodules (or a cluster of nodules) may be seen to surround the centrilobular artery but do not involve the interlobular septa.

As pulmonary lobules are all about the same size, the centers of the pulmonary lobules (and any centrilobular nodules present) are about the same distance from one another. In other words, centrilobular nodules appear evenly spaced on HRCT and because of this may superficially resemble a random pattern.

The differential diagnosis of centrilobular nodules varies depending on several additional findings, including (1) their attenuation (whether they are of GGO or homogeneous soft tissue attenuation), (2) their overall distribution (i.e., diffuse, symmetrical, or patchy), and (3) their association with the finding of tree-in-bud (TIB).

GGO Centrilobular Nodules

Centrilobular nodules of GGO may be the result of airways disease or vascular disease (Table 3.5). Airways disease is more likely. Centrilobular nodules with this appearance typically reflect processes that produce peribronchiolar inflammation, infiltration, or fibrosis without dense consolidation or obliteration of alveoli. The most common causes of GGO centrilobular nodules include HP, respiratory bronchiolitis (RB) and infection (particularly from viral organisms). Less common causes include follicular bronchiolitis, pneumoconioses (e.g., siderosis), and vascular diseases (edema, hemorrhage, pulmonary hypertension, metastatic calcification).

HP represents an allergic reaction to inhaled organic antigens, resulting in peribronchiolar inflammation and ill-defined granulomas (see Chapter 13). HP is one of the most common diseases to produce

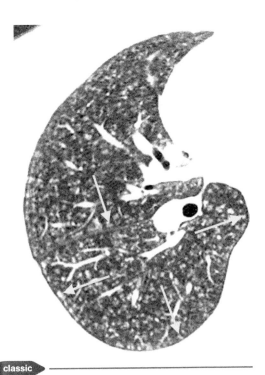

classic

FIGURE 3.13 · Centrilobular nodules: Classic appearance. Diffuse nodules are present in patient with subacute hypersensitivity pneumonitis. Note sparing of the subpleural interstitium in the peripheral lung and along the fissure; most peripheral nodules are about 5 mm from the pleural surface (*arrows*). No nodules arise at the pleural surface. The nodules appear evenly spaced.

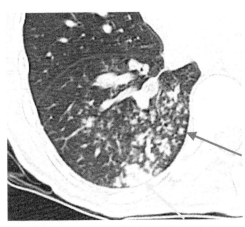

FIGURE 3.14 · Centrilobular nodules in bacterial bronchopneumonia. Centrilobular nodules are visible in the right lower lobe. Their centers are about 5 mm from the pleural surface (*red arrow*). In areas that are more severely affected, the entire pulmonary lobule is involved (*yellow arrow*).

TABLE 3.5	Differential diagnosis of ground glass opacity centrilobular nodules
Airways diseases	Hypersensitivity pneumonitis
	Respiratory bronchiolitis (RB or RB-ILD)
	Atypical/viral infection
	Follicular bronchiolitis
	Langerhans cell histiocytosis
	Pneumoconioses (e.g., coal worker's pneumoconiosis, siderosis)
	Infection (most commonly atypical/viral pneumonia)
Vascular diseases	Pulmonary edema
	Pulmonary hemorrhage
	Pulmonary arterial hypertension
	Metastatic calcification

RB-ILD, respiratory bronchiolitis interstitial lung disease.

centrilobular nodules of GGO (Fig. 3.15). Clinical history is extremely important in the diagnosis of a patient with diffuse GGO nodules. The combination of an identifiable exposure to an organic antigen and a HRCT showing diffuse centrilobular GGO nodules is usually considered diagnostic of HP and biopsy is not typically necessary. Bronchoalveolar lavage is sometimes used to further increase confidence in the diagnosis of HP by demonstrating an increased number of lymphocytes. In the absence of such an exposure, additional diagnostic workup is likely indicated. In patients with HP, symptoms are usually subacute or chronic.

RB or *RB-ILD* is the most likely diagnosis when diffuse GGO nodules are visible in a patient with a history of cigarette smoking (Fig. 3.16; see Chapter 11). RB represents an inflammatory bronchiolitis present histologically in almost all smokers. RB-ILD is said to be present when RB is associated with symptoms, such as dyspnea. Langerhans cell histiocytosis in a smoker may occasionally present with GGO nodules. Symptoms in each of these smoking-related diseases are usually subacute or chronic.

Infection: Acute infection may result in a bronchiolitis and peribronchiolar inflammation that manifests with diffuse GGO nodules on HRCT. Nodules of this attenuation are most frequently seen with viral organisms. Bacterial, mycobacterial, and fungal may also demonstrate GGO nodules; however, soft tissue attenuation nodules are more typical. Acute symptoms are typical of viral infection, whereas most other causes of GGO nodules will present with subacute or chronic symptoms. Nodules may be diffuse in viral infection or patchy and asymmetrical in bacterial, mycobacterial, and fungal infection.

Follicular bronchiolitis, an inflammatory bronchiolitis associated with lymphoid follicles, may present with diffuse GGO nodules (Fig. 3.17; see Chapters 10 and 17). Patients usually have a history of connective tissue disease or immunosuppression. Follicular bronchiolitis is the sole manifestation of LIP in some patients.

Pneumoconioses can show centrilobular GGO nodules that indicate peribronchiolar deposition of the inhaled dust or mild peribronchiolar fibrosis (see Chapter 16). The pneumoconioses typically showing ground glass nodules as the predominant abnormality tend to be those that are not highly fibrogenic, such as CWP and siderosis. Obviously, in these cases, an exposure history is important.

Vascular abnormalities and diseases affecting centrilobular vessels may produce

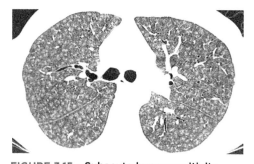

FIGURE 3.15 · **Subacute hypersensitivity pneumonitis (HP) with ground glass opacity centrilobular nodules.** Diffuse centrilobular nodules of ground glass opacity are visible. There is sparing of the subpleural interstitium in the lung periphery and adjacent to the fissures. In the presence of an identifiable exposure, such as birds kept as pets, this pattern is diagnostic of HP. Otherwise lung biopsy is typically required for diagnosis.

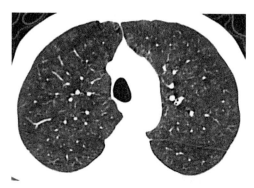

FIGURE 3.16 · **Respiratory bronchiolitis interstitial lung disease with ground glass opacity centrilobular nodules.** HRCT shows very indistinct centrilobular nodules of ground glass opacity with sparing of the subpleural interstitium. This patient was a smoker with mild dyspnea.

centrilobular GGO nodules; such diseases and abnormalities include pulmonary edema, pulmonary hemorrhage (Fig. 3.18), metastatic calcification (calcification occurring in relation to small vessels in patients with abnormal serum calcium and phosphate), and pulmonary arterial hypertension (see Chapter 7). The cause of

centrilobular nodules in association with pulmonary hypertension is not clear but is most likely due to perivascular edema or hemorrhage or their residua. These vascular causes should be considered in the appropriate clinical setting or when other supportive HRCT findings are present (e.g., interlobular septal thickening, pleural effusions, pulmonary artery dilation).

Invasive mucinous adenocarcinoma (IMA) of the lung (formerly termed diffuse bronchioloalveolar carcinoma; see Chapter 17) may result in GGO nodules, but the nodules are more commonly of soft tissue attenuation. Nodules are often patchy rather than diffuse, some nodules may be large, and a combination of GGO and soft tissue nodules may be present.

In a patient with chronic symptoms and diffuse GGO nodules, the most likely causes include HP, RB, and follicular bronchiolitis. In a patient with acute symptoms and diffuse GGO nodules, atypical (viral) pneumonia, pulmonary edema, and pulmonary hemorrhage are considerations (see Chapters 8 and 14). HP may occasionally present with acute symptoms.

Soft Tissue Attenuation Centrilobular Nodules

Centrilobular nodules of homogeneous soft tissue attenuation are characterized by inflammation or infiltration with consolidation of peribronchiolar alveoli or dense peribronchiolar fibrosis (Fig. 3.19). Bronchiolar filling or impaction may be present. As the disease progresses, the entire lobule may be involved.

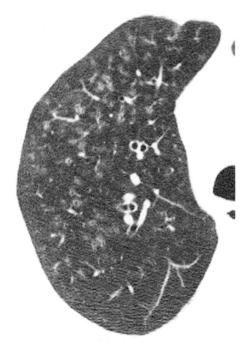

FIGURE 3.17 · Follicular bronchiolitis with centrilobular nodules. HRCT shows centrilobular nodules of ground glass opacity. Many of the nodules are associated with abnormal airways. Biopsy showed follicular bronchiolitis.

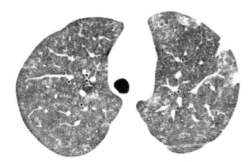

FIGURE 3.18 · Pulmonary hemorrhage in a patient with systemic lupus erythematosus and hemoptysis. HRCT shows symmetric, diffuse centrilobular nodules of ground glass opacity. While this pattern is nonspecific, it may be seen with vascular diseases resulting in hemorrhage or edema.

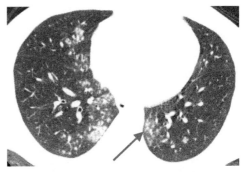

FIGURE 3.19 · Endobronchial spread of infection in bacterial bronchopneumonia. HRCT shows patchy, asymmetric soft tissue attenuation centrilobular nodules. Note that the nodules all spare the subpleural regions (*arrow*).

The differential diagnosis of centrilobular nodules of soft tissue attenuation includes processes that are associated with endobronchial spread, such as bronchopneumonia, aspiration, and tumor (IMA) (Table 3.6; Fig. 3.20).

Bronchopneumonia resulting from bacterial, mycobacterial (TB and atypical mycobacteria), fungal, or sometimes viral organisms is the most common cause of this abnormality (see Chapter 14). Symptoms are generally acute, and the nodules are focal, multifocal, or patchy in distribution, rather than diffuse.

IMA may result in multifocal or patchy nodules, sometimes associated with larger areas of consolidation or GGO. Multiple lobes and both lungs may be involved.

Langerhans cell histiocytosis may be associated with centrilobular nodules early in the course of the disease. The nodules represent peribronchiolar accumulation of Langerhans cells, other inflammatory cells, or peribronchiolar fibrosis (see Chapter 11). An upper lobe distribution of disease, cavitation within nodules, or the presence of cysts may suggest this diagnosis. In adults, this disease is predominantly related to cigarette smoking.

Vascular diseases may produce either GGO or soft tissue attenuation centrilobular nodules depending on the severity and confluence of alveolar involvement. Pulmonary edema and pulmonary hemorrhage are the most common vascular diseases to appear as soft tissue attenuation nodules.

Distribution of Centrilobular Nodules in Differential Diagnosis: Diffuse, Symmetrical, and Patchy

The overall distribution of centrilobular nodules should be used in conjunction with nodule attenuation in formulating a differential diagnosis (Table 3.7).

In general, a diffuse and symmetrical distribution of centrilobular nodules is seen

TABLE 3.6	Differential diagnosis of soft tissue attenuation centrilobular nodules

Endobronchial spread of infection (bacterial, mycobacterial, fungal, viral)
Endobronchial spread of tumor (invasive mucinous adenocarcinoma)
Aspiration
Langerhans cell histiocytosis
Pulmonary edema
Pulmonary hemorrhage

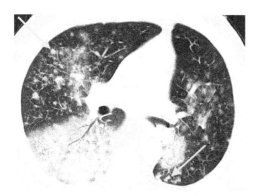

FIGURE 3.20 · Invasive mucinous pulmonary adenocarcinoma. Extensive patchy consolidation and soft tissue attenuation centrilobular nodules (*arrows*) are present. The nodules are evenly spaced and show striking sparing of the subpleural interstitium. This reflects endobronchial spread of tumor. Some ground glass opacity centrilobular nodules are also visible.

TABLE 3.7	Differential diagnosis of centrilobular nodules based upon overall distribution
Diffuse distribution	Hypersensitivity pneumonitis
	Respiratory bronchiolitis (RB or RB-ILD)
	Follicular bronchiolitis
	Atypical/viral infections
	Pneumoconioses
	Pulmonary edema
	Pulmonary hemorrhage
	Pulmonary arterial hypertension
Upper or mid-lung predominance	Hypersensitivity pneumonitis
	Respiratory bronchiolitis (RB or RB-ILD)
	Langerhans histiocytosis
	Pneumoconioses
	Metastatic calcification
Patchy distribution	Endobronchial infection (bacterial, mycobacterial, fungal)
	Invasive mucinous adenocarcinoma
	Aspiration
	Langerhans cell histiocytosis

RB-ILD, respiratory bronchiolitis interstitial lung disease.

in patients with HP, RB or RB-ILD, follicular bronchiolitis, atypical infections, pneumoconioses, pulmonary edema, and other vascular abnormalities.

A symmetrical distribution of nodules with an upper or mid-lung predominance may be seen in HP, RB, Langerhans histiocytosis, pneumoconioses (e.g., CWP, silicosis, and siderosis), and metastatic calcification.

Patchy or multifocal nodules are most frequent with endobronchial spread of infection (bacterial, mycobacterial, and fungal), IMA, aspiration, and Langerhans cell histiocytosis. Such nodules are often asymmetric.

Tree-in-Bud

TIB opacities, when present, are seen in a centrilobular location. They may be associated with centrilobular nodules (see Chapter 14). On HRCT, TIB is characterized by the presence of branching opacities, 1 to 2 mm in thickness and 1 to 2 cm in length, often associated with small nodules at the tips of the branches or along their length. The HRCT finding of TIB is usually due to dilatation and impaction of centrilobular bronchioles by pus or mucus (the branches), associated with small regions of peribronchiolar inflammation or fibrosis (the buds). TIB resembles a budding tree; its appearance is characteristic (Fig. 3.21A–E).

TIB is important because of its specificity; it is almost always due to infection or aspiration with involvement of the small peripheral airways (Table 3.8). In fact, in a patient with lung disease, it is only necessary to visualize one good example of TIB to be confident that infection or aspiration is present. TIB is not specific with regard to the type of infection, but bacterial and mycobacterial infections are most frequent. Depending on the cause or duration of infection, bronchiectasis or bronchial wall thickening may also be present (Figs. 3.21C–E and 3.22).

Because TIB is generally taken to mean that infection or aspiration is present, it is vital to describe this finding only when you are sure that it is present. Your goal should be not to overcall TIB.

There are several noninfectious causes of TIB associated with bronchiolar abnormalities, but these are relatively rare and findings are often atypical. These include endobronchial spread of IMA, follicular bronchiolitis (usually in patients with connective tissue disease), mucoid impaction in asthma and allergic bronchopulmonary aspergillosis, and panbronchiolitis.

On occasion, a centrilobular vascular abnormality can mimic the appearance of TIB. Examples include *talcosis* due to injection of crushed pills (Fig. 3.23) in which fibrosis occurs in relation to small vessels and *intravascular metastases* with nodules of tumor in small vessels.

Perilymphatic processes such as sarcoidosis are sometimes associated with small clusters of nodules in a centrilobular location. As the nodules are visible adjacent to the branching centrilobular artery, the appearance can mimic a TIB pattern. However, nodules in other locations, such as the parahilar peribronchovascular and subpleural regions, are often present, allowing a correct diagnosis to be made (Fig. 3.24).

HRCT may guide the next diagnostic test in patients with centrilobular nodules. In patients with patchy, soft tissue attenuation centrilobular nodules or the TIB pattern, sputum analysis or bronchoscopy with bronchoalveolar lavage often yields a diagnosis; infection is a very common cause of these appearances.

In patients with GGO nodules and acute symptoms, further evaluation is usually clinical. On occasion, bronchoscopy may be performed to diagnose a suspected infection. Sputum analysis in a patient with centrilobular nodules of GGO is not usually helpful. In patients with chronic symptoms and GGO nodules, a video-assisted thoracoscopic surgical biopsy is typically required for definitive diagnosis.

AN APPROACH TO DIAGNOSIS OF NODULAR LUNG DISEASE

Being able to differentiate the three patterns of nodules on HRCT will enable the formulation of an appropriate and focused differential diagnosis. A comparison of the characteristics of the three different distributions of nodules

3

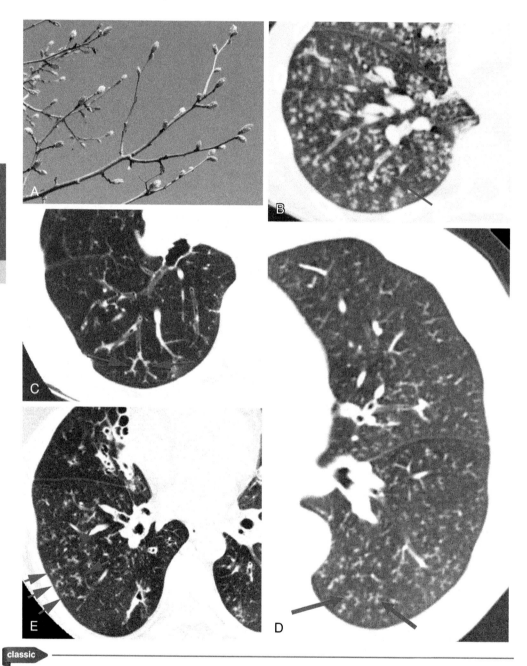

classic

FIGURE 3.21 · Tree-in-bud pattern: Classic appearances. A. Tree-in-bud resembles the branches of a tree as its buds begin to swell before opening. **B.** On CT, tree-in-bud results in the appearance of a centrilobular branching opacity with nodules at the tips of the branches. This appearance reflects the presence of dilatation and impaction of small distal airways (*arrows*) and is highly specific for endobronchial infection. As in this patient with pneumonia, it may be associated with centrilobular nodules. **C.** Tree-in-bud (*arrows*) in a patient with chronic airway infection. Note associated bronchial wall thickening. **D.** Multiple tree-in-bud opacities (*arrows*) in the dependent lung in aspiration. **E.** Tree-in-bud (*arrows*) associated with bronchiectasis and chronic infection.

TABLE 3.8	Differential diagnosis of the tree-in-bud pattern and its mimics
Infections	Bacterial infection
	Mycobacterial infection
	Fungal infection
	Viral infection
Infectious variants	Cystic fibrosis
	Ciliary disorders
	Immunodeficiency
	Panbronchiolitis
	Allergic bronchopulmonary aspergillosis
Noninfectious bronchiolar diseases	Invasive mucinous adenocarcinoma
	Follicular bronchiolitis
	Aspiration
Vascular abnormalities	Talcosis
	Intravascular metastases
Perilymphatic disease	Sarcoidosis

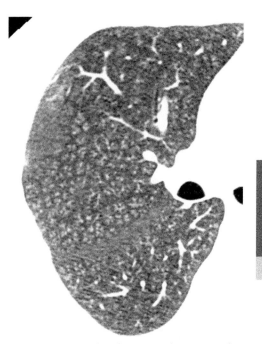

FIGURE 3.23 · **Talcosis, a vascular cause of centrilobular nodules.** HRCT of the right lung in a body builder who injected crushed steroid tablets shows branching opacities that resemble the tree-in-bud sign. The process is diffuse. This distribution would be very unusual for endobronchial infection. Note the sparing of the fissures and peripheral subpleural interstitium. Talcosis results in deposition of mineral and fibrosis in relation to small centrilobular arteries.

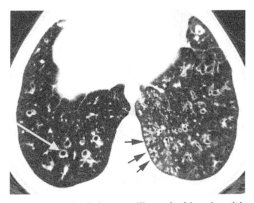

FIGURE 3.22 · **Primary ciliary dyskinesia with tree-in-bud.** Extensive large airways inflammation is present, manifested by bronchiectasis and bronchial wall thickening (*yellow arrow*). Chronic infection and mucostasis in the distal airways is manifested primarily by tree-in-bud opacities (*red arrows*).

is shown in Fig. 3.25A–D and Table 3.9. A simple algorithm for evaluating nodules on HRCT is shown in Fig. 3.26.

The following are a few important points to remember when attempting to identify the pattern of nodules:

1. Subpleural nodules are present in both perilymphatic and random patterns, but they should not be present in patients with centrilobular nodules. If the distribution

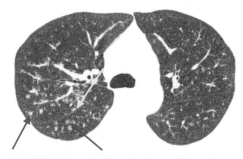

FIGURE 3.24 · **Perilymphatic nodules mimicking a centrilobular pattern.** Clusters of centrilobular peribronchovascular nodules (*red arrows*) in a patient with sarcoidosis resemble the tree-in-bud sign. However, perilymphatic diseases such as sarcoidosis also show nodules in other locations such as the subpleural (*yellow arrow*) and parahilar peribronchovascular interstitium.

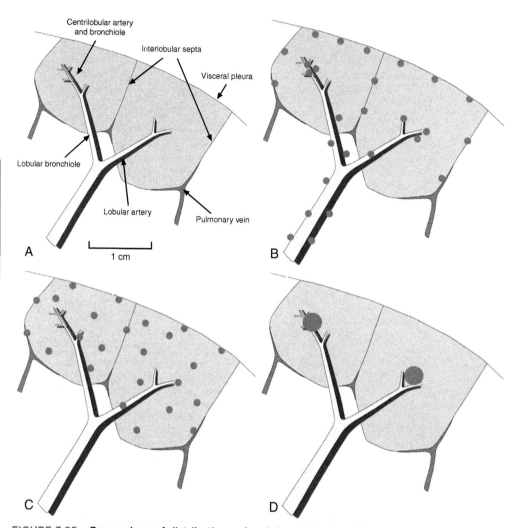

FIGURE 3.25 · **Comparison of distributions of nodules at the level of the secondary pulmonary lobule. A.** Normal anatomy of the secondary pulmonary lobule. **B.** Perilymphatic nodules involve the subpleural lobule, interlobular septa, and the centrilobular peribronchovascular region. **C.** Random nodules involve the septa and pleural surfaces but have no specific distribution with respect to the pulmonary lobule. **D.** Centrilobular nodules are found only at the center of the lobule.

is unclear, attention should be paid to the fissures and peripheral subpleural interstitium to determine if nodules are present in these locations.

2. A diffuse distribution is typical of a random pattern, whereas a patchy distribution is typical of perilymphatic nodules. Centrilobular nodules may be diffuse or patchy in distribution depending on the cause. For instance, HP is often diffuse and endobronchial spread of infection is typically patchy.

3. When centrilobular nodules are present, close inspection for the presence of TIB pattern should be made. When TIB is present, infection or aspiration is very likely. When not present, the differential depends on the attenuation and distribution of nodules. The symptoms present may also be helpful in diagnosis.

TABLE 3.9	Characteristics of nodules based on their distribution with respect to lung structures and the secondary pulmonary lobule		
Distribution	**Perilymphatic**	**Random**	**Centrilobular**
Pathophysiology	Primary lymphatic involvement or lymphatic drainage	Hematogenous spread	Bronchiolar, small vessel, or lymphatic disease
Nodule locations	Peribronchovascular, subpleural, interlobular septal, centrilobular	No specific distribution	Centrilobular only
Features	Patchy, clustered	Diffuse, uniform	Separated from pleura/fissures, evenly spaced, diffuse or patchy
Subpleural nodules present	Yes	Yes	No
Common diseases	Sarcoidosis, lymphangitic carcinomatosis	Miliary tuberculosis or fungal infection, metastases	Endobronchial infection or tumor, hypersensitivity pneumonitis, respiratory bronchiolitis, edema

3

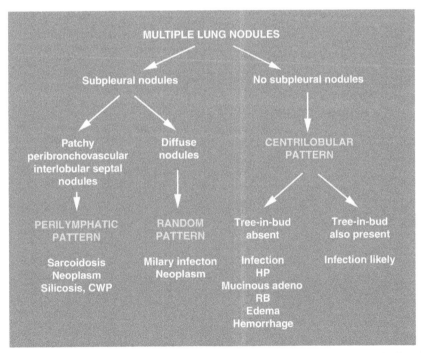

FIGURE 3.26 · **Algorithm for determining the distribution of small nodules on HRCT.** CWP, coal worker's pneumoconiosis; HP, hypersensitivity pneumonitis; Adeno, adenocarcinoma; RB, respiratory bronchiolitis.

FURTHER READING

Aquino SL, Gamsu G, Webb WR, Kee SL. Tree-in-bud pattern: frequency and significance on thin section CT. *J Comput Assist Tomogr*. 1996;20:594-599.

Bendeck SE, Leung AN, Berry GJ, Daniel D, Ruoss SJ. Cellulose granulomatosis presenting as centrilobular nodules: CT and histologic findings. *AJR Am J Roentgenol*. 2001;177:1151-1153.

Elicker B, Pereira CA, Webb R, Leslie KO. High-resolution computed tomography patterns of diffuse interstitial lung disease with clinical and pathological correlation. *J Bras Pneumol*. 2008;34:715-744.

Gruden JF, Webb WR, Warnock M. Centrilobular opacities in the lung on high-resolution CT: diagnostic considerations and pathologic correlation. *AJR Am J Roentgenol*. 1994;162:569-574.

Gruden JF, Webb WR, Naidich DP, McGuinness G. Multinodular disease: anatomic localization at thin-section CT-multireader evaluation of a simple algorithm. *Radiology*. 1999;210:711-720.

Hansell DM, Alexander AB, MacMahon H, et al. Fleischner Society: glossary of terms for thoracic imaging. *Radiology*. 2008;246:697-722.

Lee KS, Kim TS, Han J, et al. Diffuse micronodular lung disease: HRCT and pathologic findings. *J Comput Assist Tomogr*. 1999;23:99-106.

Müller NL, Miller RR. Diseases of the bronchioles: CT and histopathologic findings. *Radiology*. 1995;196:3-12.

Murata K, Itoh H, Todo G, et al. Centrilobular lesions of the lung: demonstration by high-resolution CT and pathologic correlation. *Radiology*. 1986;161:641-645.

Okada F, Ando Y, Yoshitake S, et al. Clinical/pathologic correlations in 553 patients with primary centrilobular findings on high-resolution CT scan of the thorax. *Chest*. 2007;132:1939-1948.

Webb WR. High resolution lung computed tomography: normal anatomic and pathologic findings. *Radiol Clin North Am*. 1991;29:1051-1063.

Webb WR. Thin-section CT of the secondary pulmonary lobule: anatomy and the image—the 2004 Fleischner lecture. *Radiology*. 2006;239:322-338.

3

Increased Lung Attenuation: Ground Glass Opacity and Consolidation

INTRODUCTION

Abnormalities characterized by increased lung opacity can be divided into two general categories based on their attenuation: ground glass opacity (GGO) and consolidation. Each of these findings tends to be nonspecific and has a long differential diagnosis. Clinical information, particularly the duration of symptoms, can limit the diagnosis when either of these findings is present.

GROUND GLASS OPACITY

On high-resolution computed tomography (HRCT), GGO is characterized by hazy regions of increased lung opacity (i.e., attenuation) within which vessels remain visible (Fig. 4.1). GGO represents the presence of abnormalities below the resolution of HRCT. It may reflect the presence of air space (alveolar) filling diseases, interstitial diseases with alveolar wall thickening, or a combination of both, and it may be a manifestation of lung infiltration, active inflammation, or fibrosis (Fig. 4.2). GGO may also result from atelectasis.

The differential diagnosis of GGO is broad and includes a variety of diseases in different disease categories. The duration of symptoms (i.e., acute or chronic) is important in limiting the initial differential diagnosis (Table 4.1). In general, the symptoms should be considered acute when they have been present for hours to less than a few weeks and chronic if they have been present for 6 weeks or more.

GGO with Acute Symptoms

In a patient with acute symptoms, the most common causes of GGO include infection, most notably atypical infections such as viral pneumonia, *Pneumocystis jiroveci*, and atypical bacterial infections (e.g., Legionella, *Mycoplasma pneumoniae*, and *Chlamydia pneumoniae*); pulmonary edema, either hydrostatic or increased permeability edema; acute lung injury (i.e., the clinical syndrome associated with patients who have diffuse alveolar damage on histopathology); pulmonary hemorrhage; and aspiration (Table 4.1). Additional causes include an acute presentation of hypersensitivity pneumonitis and acute eosinophilic pneumonia.

In the acute setting, the various causes of GGO are difficult to distinguish from one another based on their appearance. The specific distribution of GGO (diffuse, symmetric, patchy, nodular, or focal) is of limited use in narrowing the differential diagnosis (Fig. 4.3). Even processes such as pulmonary edema, which are commonly symmetric or diffuse, can produce patchy, focal, or nodular opacities in some patients (Fig. 4.4).

Suggesting a specific diagnosis in a patient with acute symptoms and GGO is greatly aided by history (e.g., immunosuppression or acquired immunodeficiency syndrome [AIDS], exposures, known cardiac disease) and the specific presenting symptoms (e.g., fever, sputum production, hemoptysis).

One HRCT finding that may be helpful in diagnosis is the presence of smooth

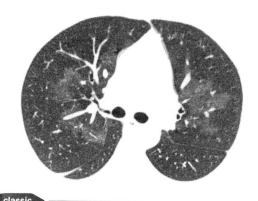

FIGURE 4.1 · Ground glass opacity (GGO): Classic appearance. Hazy regions of opacity are noted in the parahilar lung in this patient with acute pulmonary hemorrhage due to granulomatosis with polyangiitis. Vessels are well seen in the areas of opacity; this finding defines GGO.

interlobular septal thickening. When this finding is conspicuous and associated with GGO, pulmonary edema is the most likely diagnosis (Fig. 4.5). The presence of lung cysts associated with GGO suggests *Pneumocystis jiroveci* infection.

GGO with Chronic Symptoms

When GGO is associated with chronic symptoms, the differential diagnosis is not only different but also broad. Possible causes include hypersensitivity pneumonitis, nonspecific interstitial pneumonia (NSIP), desquamative interstitial pneumonia (DIP) and respiratory bronchiolitis (RB), lymphoid interstitial pneumonia (LIP) and follicular bronchiolitis, pulmonary invasive mucinous adenocarcinoma (IMA), organizing pneumonia (OP), eosinophilic pneumonia, sarcoidosis, lipoid

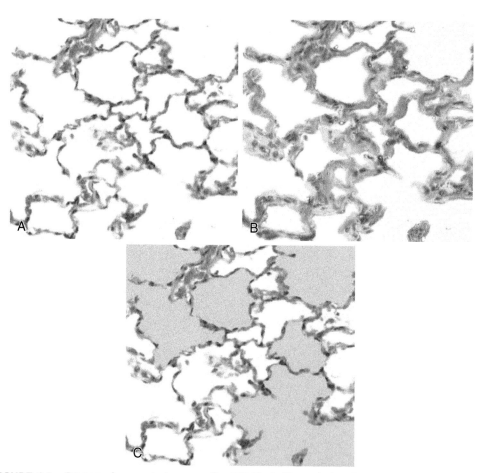

FIGURE 4.2 · Causes of ground glass opacity (GGO). A. Normal alveoli. **B.** Simulated alveolar wall thickening in interstitial disease. Increased tissue within the volume scanned results in GGO. **C.** Simulated alveolar disease, with some alveoli filled with fluid. This results in increased attenuation, but because some alveoli remain aerated, consolidation does not result.

TABLE 4.1	Differential diagnosis of GGO based on symptom duration

Acute	Chronic
Infection (usually atypical)	Hypersensitivity pneumonitis
Edema	Nonspecific interstitial pneumonia
Acute lung injury	Desquamative interstitial pneumonia/respiratory bronchiolitis
Hemorrhage	Lymphoid interstitial pneumonia/follicular bronchiolitis
Aspiration	Invasive mucinous adenocarcinoma
Hypersensitivity pneumonitis (acute)	Organizing pneumonia
Acute eosinophilic pneumonia	Eosinophilic pneumonia
	Sarcoidosis
	Lipoid pneumonia
	Alveolar proteinosis

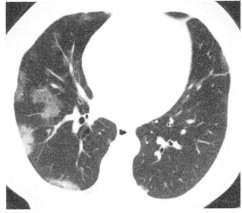

FIGURE 4.4 · **Acute pulmonary edema with patchy GGO.** The distribution of GGO in the setting of acute symptoms is not particularly helpful in diagnosis. Even processes that are classically diffuse or symmetric, such as pulmonary edema, may occasionally present with focal or patchy abnormalities.

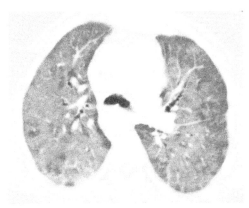

FIGURE 4.3 · **Acute drug reaction with pulmonary edema and diffuse ground glass opacity (GGO).** The differential diagnosis of GGO is broad. In a patient with acute symptoms, the distribution of GGO is of limited value in helping distinguish among the various possible causes. The diagnosis is often determined by the clinical history, as in this patient with drug toxicity resulting from treatment of lymphoma.

pneumonia, and alveolar proteinosis. Several findings may be helpful in limiting the differential diagnosis (Table 4.2).

Distribution of GGO

A peripheral distribution of GGO is typical of NSIP and DIP; however, eosinophilic pneumonia

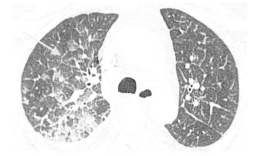

FIGURE 4.5 · **Pulmonary edema with a combination of ground glass opacity (GGO) and interlobular septal thickening.** GGO in the acute setting is nonspecific, but when interlobular septal thickening (*arrow*) is a significant associated finding, pulmonary edema is the most likely etiology.

and OP may also show this appearance (Fig. 4.6). Subpleural sparing associated with peripheral GGO is highly suggestive of NSIP (Fig. 4.7).

A patchy and geographic distribution of GGO with significant involvement of the central lung is suggestive of hypersensitivity pneumonitis (Fig. 4.8), RB, LIP and follicular bronchiolitis, OP, sarcoidosis, and alveolar proteinosis.

Most causes of chronic GGO are bilateral. A unilateral or highly asymmetric distribution of GGO may be seen with invasive pulmonary mucinous adenocarcinoma or lipoid pneumonia.

TABLE 4.2	Ground glass opacity with chronic symptoms. Use of associated findings to suggest a particular diagnosis(es)
Associated HRCT finding	**Likely diagnosis(es)**
Fibrosis (honeycombing, traction bronchiectasis, irregular reticulation)	Nonspecific interstitial pneumonia, hypersensitivity pneumonitis, usual interstitial pneumonia
Peripheral distribution	Nonspecific interstitial pneumonia, desquamative interstitial pneumonia
Peripheral distribution with sparing of the immediate subpleural interstitium	Nonspecific interstitial pneumonia
Patchy and geographic distribution	Hypersensitivity pneumonitis, nonspecific interstitial pneumonia
Significant mosaic perfusion and/or air trapping	Hypersensitivity pneumonitis
Centrilobular nodules	Hypersensitivity pneumonitis, respiratory bronchiolitis/desquamative interstitial pneumonia, follicular bronchiolitis/lymphoid interstitial pneumonia, invasive mucinous adenocarcinoma
Interlobular septal thickening	Alveolar proteinosis, invasive mucinous adenocarcinoma, lipoid pneumonia

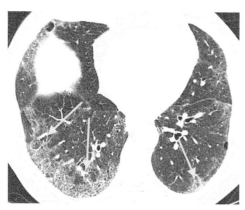

FIGURE 4.6 · Desquamative interstitial pneumonia (DIP) with a peripheral distribution of ground glass opacity (GGO). In the chronic setting, GGO with a peripheral distribution (*arrows*) is suggestive of an interstitial pneumonia or more specifically nonspecific interstitial pneumonia, DIP, or usual interstitial pneumonia. This patient is a smoker with DIP.

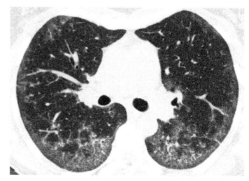

FIGURE 4.7 · Nonspecific interstitial pneumonia (NSIP) with a peripheral distribution of ground glass opacity (GGO) and subpleural sparing. In this patient with NSIP, GGO shows a peripheral predominance, but the immediate subpleural lung is relatively spared. This distribution is typical of NSIP.

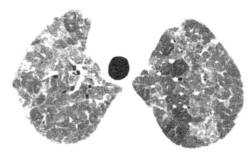

FIGURE 4.8 · Hypersensitivity pneumonitis (HP) with a patchy and geographic distribution of ground glass opacity (GGO). In this patient with HP, the areas of GGO lack a peripheral predominance. This appearance is typical of HP.

Associated Mosaic Perfusion and/or Air Trapping

If GGO is associated with significant mosaic perfusion and/or air trapping (involvement of multiple lobules in three or more lobes), the diagnosis of hypersensitivity pneumonitis is strongly favored (Fig. 4.9A, B). GGO associated with centrilobular nodules may be seen with hypersensitivity pneumonitis (Fig. 4.10), RB, follicular bronchiolitis, and invasive mucinous adenocarcinoma.

Crazy Paving

The combination of GGO and smooth interlobular septal thickening in the same lung

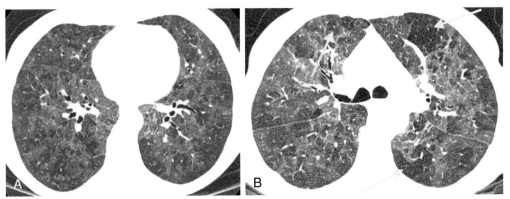

FIGURE 4.9 · **Hypersensitivity pneumonitis with patchy ground glass opacity (GGO) and air trapping.** HRCT **(A)** shows nonspecific patchy GGO in a patient with chronic symptoms. Expiratory image **(B)** shows patchy air trapping (*arrows*). This combination of findings is strongly suggestive of hypersensitivity pneumonitis.

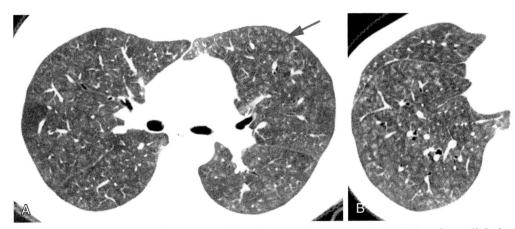

FIGURE 4.10 · **Hypersensitivity pneumonitis with ground glass opacity (GGO) and centrilobular nodules. A** and **B.** When chronic GGO is associated with centrilobular nodules (**A**, *arrow*), the differential diagnosis includes hypersensitivity pneumonitis, respiratory bronchiolitis, follicular bronchiolitis, or invasive mucinous adenocarcinoma. Numerous centrilobular nodules of GGO are visible in **(B)**.

regions is termed "crazy paving." This name refers to the appearance of irregularly shaped paving stones in an English garden.

Although originally described as a typical HRCT finding in pulmonary alveolar proteinosis (Fig. 4.11), this finding is nonspecific and may be seen in any disease resulting in GGO. In the acute setting, the differential diagnosis is identical to that of isolated GGO and includes edema, atypical infections (Fig. 4.12), diffuse alveolar damage, hemorrhage, acute hypersensitivity pneumonitis, and acute eosinophilic pneumonia. In a patient with chronic symptoms, the list of diagnostic possibilities is the same as for GGO, but alveolar proteinosis, which is otherwise quite rare, should be considered a distinct possibility (Fig. 4.11).

Associated Fibrosis

In the presence of chronic symptoms, GGO may reflect one of two very different processes, active inflammatory or infiltrative disease, or microscopic lung fibrosis. If GGO is unassociated with HRCT findings of fibrosis, such as traction bronchiectasis, irregular reticulation, or honeycombing, then it is likely that inflammatory or

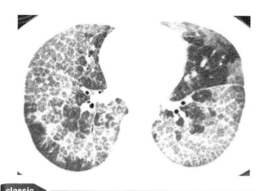

FIGURE 4.11 · Crazy paving: Classic appearance. In this patient with pulmonary alveolar proteinosis, the combination of ground glass opacity (GGO) and smooth interlobular septal thickening is termed "crazy paving." The differential diagnosis of crazy paving includes all causes of GGO, but in a patient with chronic symptoms, alveolar proteinosis, which is otherwise rare, becomes an important consideration.

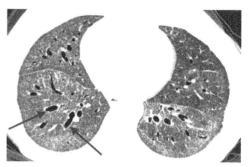

FIGURE 4.13 · Nonspecific interstitial pneumonia with ground glass opacity (GGO) and traction bronchiectasis. When GGO is associated with signs of fibrosis, such as traction bronchiectasis (*arrows*) and reticulation, it is likely related to a chronic interstitial lung disease such as fibrotic nonspecific interstitial pneumonia secondary to scleroderma.

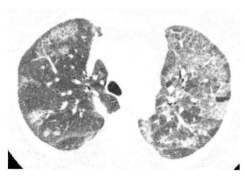

FIGURE 4.12 · *Pneumocystis jiroveci* infection with crazy paving. The differential diagnosis of crazy paving in the acute setting is identical to that of ground glass opacity and primarily includes edema, atypical infections, diffuse alveolar damage, and hemorrhage.

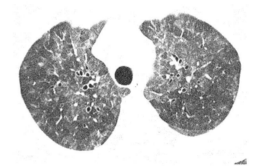

FIGURE 4.14 · Hypersensitivity pneumonitis with ground glass opacity and chronic symptoms. Patchy central and peripheral areas of ground glass opacity are present in a patient with chronic symptoms. The most common causes of ground glass opacity in the chronic setting include hypersensitivity pneumonitis, nonspecific interstitial pneumonia, and desquamative interstitial pneumonia.

infiltrative disease is present (Fig. 4.13). On the other hand, if GGO is associated with signs of fibrosis in the same lung regions, then it is likely that the GGO represents (microscopic) lung fibrosis. In some patients with GGO, both inflammatory disease and fibrosis coexist.

Hypersensitivity pneumonitis and NSIP, related to connective tissue disease or drug exposures, are the most common diffuse fibrotic lung diseases to show GGO on HRCT

(Fig. 4.14). Usual interstitial pneumonia and idiopathic pulmonary fibrosis may present with GGO as a significant finding, but in such patients, findings of fibrosis are generally visible in the same lung regions; isolated regions of GGO are distinctly unusual.

CONSOLIDATION

Consolidation is characterized on HRCT by homogeneous increased lung opacity, which results in obscuration of vessels (Fig. 4.15).

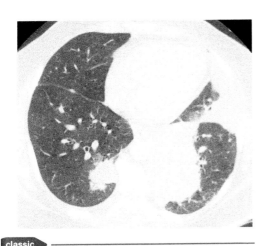

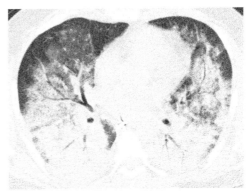

FIGURE 4.16 · Acute lung injury with diffuse consolidation. In the acute setting, diffuse consolidation is nonspecific and may be seen with infection, acute lung injury, edema, or hemorrhage. These entities are primarily distinguished clinically.

classic

FIGURE 4.15 · Consolidation: Classic appearance. Patchy bilateral consolidation is present in a patient with invasive mucinous adenocarcinoma. Note that the vessels are obscured in the regions of abnormality.

TABLE 4.3	Differential diagnosis of consolidation based on symptom duration

Acute	Chronic
Infections	Organizing pneumonia
Edema	Eosinophilic pneumonia
Acute lung injury	Invasive mucinous adenocarcinoma
Hemorrhage	Sarcoidosis
Aspiration	Lymphoma (usually recurrent)
Hypersensitivity pneumonitis	Lipoid pneumonia
Acute eosinophilic pneumonia	Hypersensitivity pneumonitis

Consolidation with Acute Symptoms

The differential diagnosis of consolidation in the acute setting is essentially the same as that of GGO with acute symptoms (Table 4.3), but acute consolidation is most commonly seen with bacterial pneumonia and aspiration. Other causes of acute consolidation include pulmonary edema, acute lung injury, and hemorrhage, but GGO is a more typical finding with these abnormalities.

Occasionally, lung diseases that are primarily interstitial may present with acute symptoms and consolidation. This is most commonly seen with hypersensitivity pneumonitis and acute eosinophilic pneumonia. GGO is a more common manifestation of these diseases.

Distribution

A diffuse distribution of consolidation is common with edema, acute lung injury (Fig. 4.16), certain infections, hemorrhage, and acute eosinophilic pneumonia. Of the infections, viral pneumonia, atypical bacterial (Legionella, *Mycoplasma pneumoniae*, and *Chlamydia pneumoniae*) pneumonia, and *Pneumocystis jiroveci* pneumonia are the most common to present with diffuse abnormalities, but these more commonly show GGO. Other types of infections (bacterial, fungal, or mycobacterial) tend to be focal or patchy

Air bronchograms are often seen in affected regions. As with GGO, the abnormality may be alveolar or interstitial in origin, although filling of alveoli is most commonly responsible. Interstitial abnormalities must be extensive to result in the appearance of consolidation; an example is sarcoidosis with confluent interstitial granulomas. As with GGO, the differential diagnosis is broad and depends primarily upon symptom duration (Table 4.3) and distribution. The differential diagnosis overlaps with that of GGO.

4

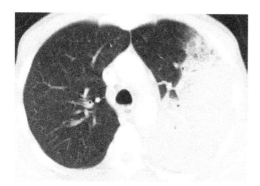

FIGURE 4.17 · Bacterial pneumonia with focal consolidation. A focal distribution of consolidation in the acute setting is typically associated with pneumonia, aspiration, and hemorrhage. While nonspecific with regard to the type of infection, this is most typical of bacterial, mycobacterial, and fungal infections.

TABLE 4.4	Causes of chronic consolidation based on distribution on HRCT
Distribution	**Causes of chronic consolidation**
Patchy	Any cause may show this pattern
Single, focal region	Invasive mucinous adenocarcinoma
	Lymphoma
	Lipoid pneumonia
	Organizing pneumonia
Diffuse consolidation	Invasive mucinous adenocarcinoma
	Organizing pneumonia
Peribronchovascular	Sarcoid
	Organizing pneumonia
	Chronic eosinophilic pneumonia
Peripheral	Chronic eosinophilic pneumonia
	Organizing pneumonia (polymyositis/dermatomyositis)

in distribution (Fig. 4.17). Aspiration may be focal or patchy and typically involves the lower lobes or posterior upper lobes.

Consolidation with Chronic Symptoms

In patients with chronic symptoms, the most frequent causes of consolidation are OP, chronic eosinophilic pneumonia, sarcoidosis, IMA, lymphoma, and lipoid pneumonia. The distribution of consolidation, and several other findings, may be helpful in narrowing the differential diagnosis.

Distribution

While distribution may be helpful in narrowing the list of possibilities (Table 4.4), it is unusual for distribution, by itself, to suggest a single diagnosis. All causes of chronic consolidation may present with a patchy, bilateral distribution of consolidation.

Extensive or diffuse chronic consolidation is most typical of IMA or, less likely, OP. A single, focal region of consolidation may be seen with IMA, lymphoma, lipoid pneumonia, or, rarely, OP. Lipoid pneumonia typically presents with patchy abnormalities in dependent regions of both lungs. A peribronchovascular distribution of consolidation may be seen with sarcoidosis, OP, or chronic eosinophilic

pneumonia. Peripheral consolidation is typical of chronic eosinophilic pneumonia or OP, particularly in patients with polymyositis/dermatomyositis.

The "Atoll" or "Reversed Halo" Sign and OP

The atoll sign is characterized by a ring of consolidation (sometimes incomplete) surrounding a central area of GGO or clearing (Fig. 4.18). It resembles a coral atoll, a circular coral reef with a sandy lagoon in its center. This sign has also been called the "reversed halo sign" because it is the opposite of the well-recognized "halo sign" (a dense nodule with a ring of GGO surrounding it). The atoll sign or reversed halo sign is suggestive of OP or one of its associated diseases (Table 4.5). The typical appearance results from active inflammation in the periphery of the abnormal lung, with healing or clearing in its center.

OP represents an organizing inflammatory reaction, typically associated with shortness of breath and fever of more than 6 weeks' duration (see Chapter 9). It may be idiopathic, in which case it is termed cryptogenic organizing pneumonia (COP), or may be associated with one of its many possible causes

4

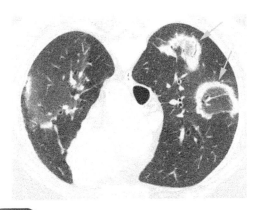

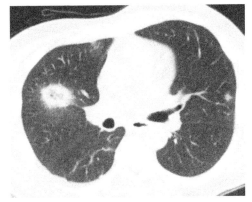

classic

FIGURE 4.18 • **The atoll or reversed halo sign: Classic appearance.** The atoll or reversed halo sign is characterized by a peripheral rim of consolidation (*arrows*) surrounding a central area of ground glass opacity or clearing. This finding is highly specific for organizing pneumonia. This patient has organizing pneumonia as a complication of chemotherapy.

FIGURE 4.19 • **Fungal infection with the atoll sign.** The atoll sign is present in invasive fungal infection. The history of neutropenia, in this case, suggests an alternative diagnosis to organizing pneumonia.

TABLE 4.5	Differential diagnosis of organizing pneumonia

Causes of organizing pneumonia	Diseases associated with organizing pneumonia
Cryptogenic organizing pneumonia	Chronic eosinophilic pneumonia
Drugs	Hypersensitivity pneumonitis
Connective tissue disease	Infections (e.g., fungal infection)
Toxic inhalations	GPA (Wegener's granulomatosis)
Immunodeficiencies	
Graft vs. host disease	

including drug treatment, connective tissue disease, toxic inhalations, immunodeficiency, and graft-versus-host disease.

There are a number of diseases that may be associated with a significant component of OP and thus can have an identical appearance on HRCT. These include chronic eosinophilic pneumonia, hypersensitivity pneumonitis, granulomatosis with polyangiitis (GPA; formerly Wegener's granulomatosis), and some infections (most commonly fungal and viral). Although the atoll sign generally indicates OP, its presence should not dissuade you from

making an otherwise obvious alternative diagnosis. Other reported causes of the atoll sign include pulmonary infarction, infection (e.g., paracoccidioidomycosis or invasive fungal infection), sarcoidosis, and GPA. Clinical or radiologic clues are usually present to suggest one of these alternative diagnoses. Pulmonary infarction may show one or a few atoll signs in the peripheral lung that have a wedge-shaped appearance. The atoll sign in association with perilymphatic nodules should suggest sarcoidosis. In the setting of neutropenia (Fig. 4.19), invasive fungal infection, particularly mucormycosis, should be considered.

OP classically shows patchy, bilateral focal regions of consolidation in a peripheral or peribronchovascular distribution. The atoll or reversed halo sign is visible in 20 to 40% of patients with OP.

The "Galaxy Sign" and Sarcoidosis

Sarcoidosis may present with consolidation that represents confluent granulomatous lesions; air bronchograms may be visible within the consolidated lung. The consolidation tends to appear as a focal, patchy area or mass-like. Although this appearance is sometimes called "alveolar sarcoidosis," this term is a misnomer.

In most cases, the diagnosis of sarcoidosis can be suggested when discrete, small nodules ("*satellite nodules*") are seen at the periphery of the areas of consolidation (Fig. 4.20). The combination of focal consolidation or mass with satellite nodules has been termed the *"galaxy sign."* It may also be seen in patients with other granulomatous diseases, infections, silicosis, and coal worker's pneumoconiosis.

Lipoid Pneumonia with Low-Attenuation Consolidation

Lipoid pneumonia is a rare cause of consolidation. This disease results from repeated aspiration of fat-containing liquids. Areas of consolidation are usually located in the posterior lung, are irregular in shape, and often contain areas of low (fat) attenuation, measuring less than −30 Hounsfield units (Fig. 4.21). This appearance is nearly diagnostic of lipoid pneumonia.

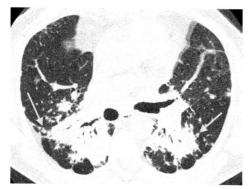

FIGURE 4.20 · **"Alveolar sarcoid." Mass-like areas of consolidation with air bronchograms, due to confluent interstitial granulomas, are seen in both upper lobes.** At the periphery of these areas, more discrete small pulmonary nodules are seen (*arrows*). The consolidation represents confluent interstitial granulomas.

DIFFERENTIAL DIAGNOSIS BASED ON WHETHER GGO OR CONSOLIDATION IS PRESENT

Although many of the diseases discussed in this chapter may show either GGO or consolidation, some more commonly present with GGO while others more commonly present with consolidation (Table 4.6).

Atypical/viral infections, hemorrhage (Fig. 4.22), edema, hypersensitivity pneumonitis, acute eosinophilic pneumonia, NSIP, DIP, and alveolar proteinosis typically present with GGO.

Bacterial, fungal, or mycobacterial pneumonia; aspiration; OP; chronic eosinophilic pneumonia; IMA; lymphoma (Fig. 4.23); and sarcoidosis more commonly present with consolidation.

Acute lung injury commonly presents with both GGO and consolidation with the predominant HRCT abnormality depending on the severity of the disease.

Nonetheless, despite these tendencies, it is important to recognize that overlap occurs. For instance, the majority of patients with OP present with consolidation, but occasionally GGO will be the major finding, particularly in patients with immunosuppression (Fig. 4.24). In contrast, hypersensitivity pneumonitis typically presents with GGO but may be manifest with patchy consolidation, particularly when associated OP is present pathologically (Fig. 4.25).

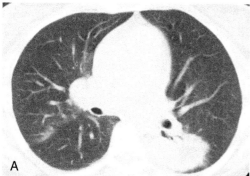

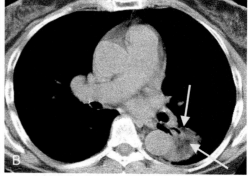

FIGURE 4.21 · **Lipoid pneumonia, fat attenuation consolidation.** Lung windows **(A)** show nonspecific consolidation in a patient with focal, chronic consolidation. Soft tissue windows **(B)** show areas of fat attenuation (*arrows*) in consolidation compatible with lipoid pneumonia.

TABLE 4.6	Differential diagnosis based on the predominant abnormality seen on HRCT: ground glass opacity or consolidation

Ground glass opacity	Consolidation
Viral, atypical, PCP infection	Bacterial, fungal, mycobacterial infection
Hemorrhage	Aspiration
Edema	Invasive mucinous adenocarcinoma
Hypersensitivity pneumonitis	Organizing pneumonia
Nonspecific interstitial pneumonia	Eosinophilic pneumonia
Desquamative interstitial pneumonia	Sarcoid
Alveolar proteinosis	Lymphoma
Acute eosinophilic pneumonia	

PCP, Pneumocystis carinii *pneumonia.*

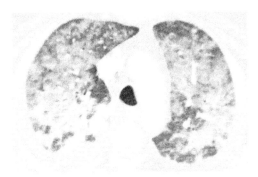

FIGURE 4.22 · **Pulmonary hemorrhage; diffuse ground glass opacity (GGO).** Although both GGO and consolidation are present, GGO is the predominant abnormality in this patient with diffuse pulmonary hemorrhage resulting from mitral stenosis.

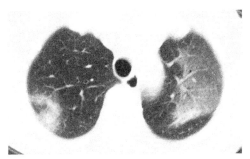

FIGURE 4.24 · **Organizing pneumonia with patchy ground glass opacity (GGO).** Organizing pneumonia usually presents with consolidation; however, it may occasionally present with GGO, particularly in the setting of immunosuppression.

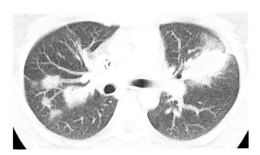

FIGURE 4.23 · **Recurrent non-Hodgkin's lymphoma with patchy consolidation.** The two malignancies that may present with chronic consolidation include invasive mucinous adenocarcinoma and lymphoma. When lymphoma presents with consolidation, it is most commonly recurring after initial treatment.

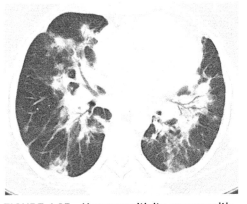

FIGURE 4.25 · **Hypersensitivity pneumonitis with patchy consolidation.** Hypersensitivity pneumonitis usually presents with ground glass opacity. It rarely may present with consolidation, particularly when pathologically there is significant associated organizing pneumonia.

FURTHER READING

Austin JH, Müller NL, Friedman PJ, et al. Glossary of terms for CT of the lungs: recommendations of the Nomenclature Committee of the Fleischner Society. *Radiology*. 1996;200:327-331.

Collins J. CT signs and patterns of lung disease. *Radiol Clin North Am*. 2001;39:1115-1135.

Elicker B, Pereira CA, Webb R, Leslie KO. High-resolution computed tomography patterns of diffuse interstitial lung disease with clinical and pathological correlation. *J Bras Pneumol*. 2008;34:715-744.

Engeler CE, Tashjian JH, Trenkner SW, Walsh JW. Ground-glass opacity of the lung parenchyma: a guide to analysis with high-resolution CT. *AJR Am J Roentgenol*. 1993;160:249-251.

Flaherty KR, Martinez FJ. Nonspecific interstitial pneumonia. *Semin Respir Crit Care Med*. 2006;27:652-658.

Hansell DM, Bankier AA, MacMahon H, et al. Fleischner Society: glossary of terms for thoracic imaging. *Radiology*. 2008;246:697-722.

Hewitt MG, Miller WT Jr, Reilly TJ, Simpson S. The relative frequencies of causes of widespread ground-glass opacity: a retrospective cohort. *Eur J Radiol*. 2014;10:1970-1976.

Lee KS, Kim EA. High-resolution CT of alveolar filling disorders. *Radiol Clin North Am*. 2001;39:1211-1230.

Leung AN, Miller RR, Müller NL. Parenchymal opacification in chronic infiltrative lung diseases: CT-pathologic correlation. *Radiology*. 1993;188:209-214.

Lynch DA, Travis WD, Muller NL, et al. Idiopathic interstitial pneumonias: CT features. *Radiology*. 2005;236:10-21.

Miller WT Jr, Shah RM. Isolated diffuse ground-glass opacity in thoracic CT: causes and clinical presentations. *AJR Am J Roentgenol*. 2005;184:613-622.

Nowers K, Rasband JD, Berges G, Gosselin M. Approach to ground-glass opacification of the lung. *Semin Ultrasound CT MR*. 2002;23:302-323.

Polverosi R, Maffesanti M, Dalpiaz G. Organizing pneumonia: typical and atypical HRCT patterns. *Radiol Med*. 2006;111:202-212.

Remy-Jardin M, Giraud F, Remy J, Copin MC, Gosselin B, Duhamel A. Importance of ground-glass attenuation in chronic diffuse infiltrative lung disease: pathologic-CT correlation. *Radiology*. 1993;189:693-698.

Travis WD, Brambilla E, Noguchi M, et al. International Association for the Study of Lung Cancer/American Thoracic Society/European Respiratory Society International Multidisciplinary Classification of lung adenocarcinoma. *J Thorac Oncol*. 2011;6:244-285.

Travis WD, Hunninghake G, King TE Jr, et al. Idiopathic nonspecific interstitial pneumonia. *Am J Respir Crit Care Med*. 2008;15(177):1338-1347.

Webb WR. High resolution lung computed tomography: normal anatomic and pathologic findings. *Radiol Clin North Am*. 1991;29:1051-1063.

4

Decreased Lung Attenuation: Emphysema, Mosaic Perfusion, and Cystic Lung Disease

INTRODUCTION

Multifocal, regional, or focal areas of decreased lung attenuation (i.e., increased lung lucency) are sometimes seen on high-resolution computed tomography (HRCT) as a manifestation of diffuse lung disease. Decreased lung attenuation can have several HRCT appearances and a variety of causes. These include lung destruction due to emphysema, decreased lung perfusion resulting from airway or vascular obstruction, cyst formation, and airway dilatation. Lucencies due to airway dilatation (i.e, bronchiectasis) are usually identifiable as such and will be discussed in the next chapter.

EMPHYSEMA

Emphysema represents lung destruction that may result from several different processes including cigarette smoking, enzyme deficiency, and drug abuse. Emphysema is categorized by the part of the secondary pulmonary lobule that is involved as centrilobular, panlobular, or paraseptal. Each of these has a different HRCT appearance and different possible causes (Table 5.1).

Centrilobular Emphysema

Centrilobular emphysema (CLE) is common and strongly associated with cigarette smoking; in general, the presence and severity of CLE correlate with the pack-years smoked. Tobacco smoke results in chronic inflammation in and around small centrilobular airways (so-called respiratory bronchiolitis),

which is associated with a cellular infiltrate and the release of several enzymes. Through a complex process, this is thought to result in centrilobular lung destruction (i.e., CLE). As lung destruction becomes more extensive, emphysema may involve entire pulmonary lobules.

On HRCT, CLE is visible as multiple, scattered, focal air-attenuation lucencies, which are a few millimeters to 1 cm in diameter, usually without a visible wall. The lucencies of CLE tend to predominate in the upper lobes and are most severe in the central lung regions. Small areas of CLE may be seen to surround the dot-like centrilobular artery (Fig. 5.1).

In a smoker, this appearance on HRCT is diagnostic of CLE and biopsy is not required. HRCT is able to detect very early stages of CLE and is often more sensitive than pulmonary function testing.

Panlobular Emphysema

Panlobular emphysema (PLE) is commonly associated with alpha-1-antitrypsin deficiency but may also be seen in association with cigarette smoking and intravenous injection of oral Ritalin. PLE involves the entire secondary pulmonary lobule. For this reason, it is generally unassociated with focal areas of lucency on HRCT, as is CLE. Instead, it shows generalized lung lucency with vessels that appear smaller than normal, and lung volume is increased. In other words, PLE results in a lung that is too big, too black, and contains vessels that are too small. PLE tends to be

TABLE 5.1	Comparison of the different types of emphysema		
	Centrilobular	**Panlobular**	**Paraseptal**
Distribution HRCT appearance	Upper lobes, central Focal lucencies without visible walls	Lower lobes, diffuse Generalized increase in lung lucency	Subpleural Focal, round, well-defined lucencies with thin walls, in a single layer
Causes	Cigarette smoking	Alpha-1-antitrypsin deficiency, cigarette smoking, intravenous injection of oral Ritalin	Cigarette smoking or idiopathic

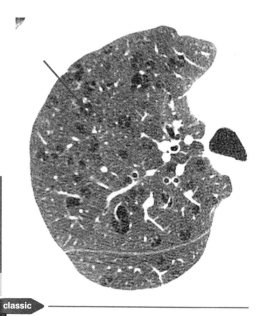

`classic`

FIGURE 5.1 · Centrilobular emphysema: Classic appearance. HRCT in a smoker shows focal, upper lobe, central, air-attenuation lucencies without a recognizable wall. Note the centrilobular artery at the center of some of these lucencies (*arrow*).

to 2 cm or more in diameter, occurring in a single layer in the subpleural lung (Fig. 5.3). It is also seen in the peripheral lung, adjacent to the mediastinum, and adjacent to fissures. The cysts of PSE are outlined by discrete, thin walls. These walls may correspond to interlobular septa. Given its association with smoking, there is often coexistent CLE.

PSE versus Honeycombing

As discussed in Chapter 2, PSE should not be confused with honeycombing, which may have a similar appearance. There are several distinguishing features:

PSE occurs in a single layer, while honeycomb cysts may occur in multiple layers. The walls of PSE are thinner than those of honeycombing, and the cystic spaces are usually larger. PSE is unassociated with signs of fibrosis such as traction bronchiectasis and irregular reticulation, which are typically seen with honeycombing. PSE is most severe in the upper lobes, while honeycombing usually predominates at the lung bases. One caveat: both PSE and honeycombing may be seen in the same patient if two diseases are present.

Bullous Emphysema

There is no specific pathologic type of emphysema termed "bullous emphysema," but this term is often used to refer to emphysema that is associated with large bullae. A bulla is defined as a sharply defined area of emphysema measuring more than 1 cm in diameter. Bulla walls are usually well seen on HRCT.

Bullae occur most commonly in patients with PSE or CLE. They are less frequent with PLE. Bullous emphysema is often asymmetrical.

diffuse or lower lobe predominant or diffuse in distribution (Fig. 5.2A, B). In cases of early PLE, the diagnosis may be difficult because focal abnormalities are not present.

Paraseptal Emphysema

Paraseptal emphysema (PSE) may be associated with cigarette smoking or may be idiopathic. On HRCT, PSE is characterized by air-attenuation cysts from a few millimeters

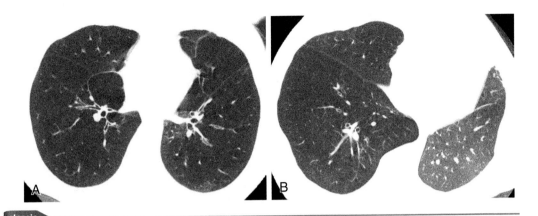

FIGURE 5.2 · Panlobular emphysema: Classic appearance. A. HRCT in a patient with alpha-1-antitrypsin deficiency shows basilar predominant, diffuse, increased lung lucency with small vessels. This appearance is typical of panlobular emphysema. **B.** In another patient with a left lung transplant for panlobular emphysema, the abnormal, markedly, hyperinflated and lucent native right lung can be contrasted with a normal-appearing transplanted left lung.

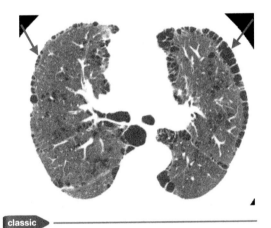

FIGURE 5.3 · Paraseptal emphysema: Classic appearance. PSE in a smoker. Subpleural, air-density cysts (*arrows*) are present in a single layer. Note a thin wall at the periphery of the areas of emphysema. There is associated centrilobular emphysema in the central lung.

MOSAIC PERFUSION

The term *mosaic perfusion* refers to the presence of geographic regions of varying lung attenuation owing to regional differences in lung perfusion. Approximately 50% of lung attenuation is derived from blood. Consequently, when blood flow is decreased to a specific region of lung, its attenuation appears decreased on HRCT. On HRCT, the attenuation of regions of mosaic (decreased) perfusion is intermediate between that of normal lung and room air.

Mosaic perfusion may result from either airways disease or vascular disease; airways disease is the most common cause. In cases of airways disease, stenosis or obstruction of the abnormal airways results in decreased ventilation and hypoxia in the downstream lung. This leads to reflex vasoconstriction and decreased lung perfusion. With vascular disease, such as chronic pulmonary embolism, decreased perfusion is due to stenosis or occlusion of pulmonary arterial branches, with decreased blood flow.

In patients with mosaic perfusion, the vessels in areas of relative lung lucency usually appear smaller on HRCT than those in normal, denser lung regions. This finding is key in making the diagnosis of mosaic perfusion as a cause of patchy lung attenuation.

Mosaic Perfusion versus Ground Glass Opacity

Mosaic attenuation is a term used to indicate that lung parenchyma shows patchy or geographic areas of heterogeneous lung attenuation, without implying what the nature of the abnormality is. When the lung shows mosaic attenuation, one must first determine if the relatively opaque or the relatively lucent lung regions are abnormal. If the opaque lung is abnormal, the abnormality represents ground

5

glass opacity. If the lucent lung is abnormal, the pattern represents mosaic perfusion. There are several features that suggest that the lucent lung is abnormal and mosaic perfusion is the predominant abnormality.

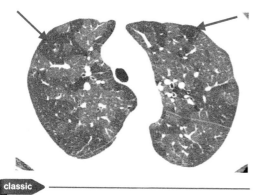

classic

FIGURE 5.4 · Mosaic perfusion: Classic appearance. Heterogeneous lung density with geographic areas of decreased lung attenuation (*arrows*) is present in a patient with constrictive bronchiolitis due to neuroendocrine hyperplasia. This sharp demarcation between opaque and lucent lung suggests that the lucent lung is abnormal. Vessels in lucent regions appear small in comparison with vessels in the denser regions.

Geographic Areas of Decreased Lung Attenuation

With mosaic perfusion, regions of heterogeneous attenuation tend to be geographic and sharply demarcated (Fig. 5.4). Usually there is a sharp border between the lung that is affected (relatively lucent) and the unaffected normal lung (relatively opaque), reflecting the geographic vascular supply. Ground glass opacity, on the other hand, usually has ill-defined borders because the responsible process results in variable involvement of the interstitium or alveoli (Fig. 5.5). When the lucent regions appear to represent pulmonary lobules, mosaic perfusion is the likely diagnosis. On the other hand, if some areas of increased opacity are centrilobular, ground glass opacity is present.

On occasion, however, ground glass opacity presents with geographic abnormalities. For instance, viral infections or alveolar proteinosis may present with geographic regions of ground glass opacity (Fig. 5.6). In these cases, there is usually a greater attenuation difference between opaque and lucent lung, whereas the difference is usually not as pronounced with mosaic perfusion.

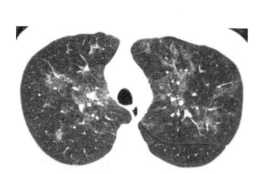

FIGURE 5.5 · "Mosaic" ground glass opacity. Patchy perihilar areas of increased lung attenuation are present in a patient with pneumocystis pneumonia. The edges of the regions of ground glass opacity are ill-defined rather than sharply demarcated. The vessels in regions of varying lung attenuation appear similar in size.

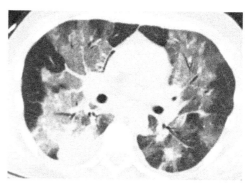

FIGURE 5.6 · Geographic ground glass opacity in viral infection. Although geographic areas of heterogeneous lung attenuation are usually due to mosaic perfusion, occasionally, ground glass opacity may have sharply demarcated borders. The marked difference in attenuation between affected and unaffected lung in this case would be unusual for mosaic perfusion, and frank consolidation is also visible.

5

Decreased Vessel Size in Lucent Lung Regions

As mosaic perfusion represents regional decreases in lung perfusion, the vessels in affected regions usually appear smaller than in areas of normal lung (Fig. 5.7). This finding is more commonly seen with vascular causes of mosaic perfusion and is accentuated in severe cases. The absence of a difference in vessel size does not exclude mosaic perfusion as a cause of geographic attenuation.

Air Trapping on Expiratory Imaging

When mosaic perfusion is due to airways disease, lucent lung regions usually show air trapping on expiratory imaging (Fig. 5.8A,

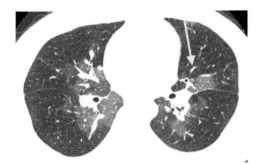

FIGURE 5.7 · **Mosaic perfusion due to chronic pulmonary embolism.** Note the geographic appearance of the areas of increased lung lucency. The vessels are significantly smaller in the abnormally lucent lung (*yellow arrow*) as compared with the normal opaque lung (*red arrow*).

B). During expiration, normal lung usually shows an increase in attenuation of 100 to 200 HU. When airways disease is present, air trapping causes affected regions to show little or no increase in attenuation on expiratory images. Vascular causes of mosaic perfusion generally do not show air trapping on mosaic perfusion, although this may occasionally be seen in patients with pulmonary embolism.

Stability of Mosaic Attenuation Over Time

Ground glass opacity usually changes in distribution or severity over time, unless it is due to fibrosis. Mosaic perfusion, on the other hand, may be stable when followed on multiple HRCT examinations. When HRCT shows heterogeneous lung attenuation that has been stable on serial examinations, mosaic perfusion is the most likely etiology (Fig. 5.9A, B).

Differential Diagnosis of Mosaic Perfusion

The differential diagnosis of mosaic perfusion is broad and includes many causes of airway and pulmonary vascular disease (Table 5.2). There may be other HRCT findings present, such as centrilobular nodules, tree-in-bud sign, bronchiectasis, airway wall thickening, air trapping, and pulmonary hypertension that may be helpful in diagnosis and may suggest a specific diagnosis (Fig. 5.10A, B).

5

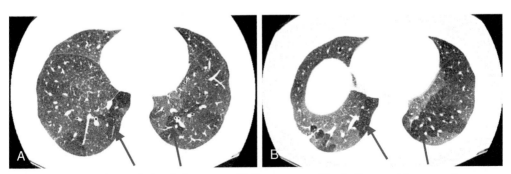

FIGURE 5.8 · **Mosaic perfusion in hypersensitivity pneumonitis. A.** Geographic areas of decreased lung attenuation (arrows) are present on the inspiratory images. **B.** On expiratory images, the normal (i.e., denser) lung shows the normal expected increase in attenuation, whereas the areas of mosaic perfusion (*arrows*) remain lucent.

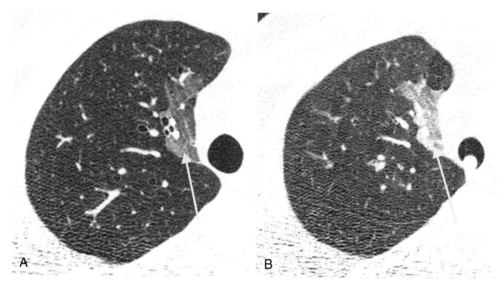

FIGURE 5.9 · Mosaic perfusion, stability over time. HRCT in this patient showed heterogenous lung density, which was thought to represent ground glass opacity. On a 6-month follow-up CT an inspiratory image **(A)** demonstrated stability of heterogenous lung attenuation with more opaque lung centrally (arrow). An expiratory image **(B)** confirmed extensive air trapping with the normal lung (arrow) showing a normal increase in attenuation. This represented constrictive bronchiolitis due to graft-versus-host disease.

TABLE 5.2	Differential diagnosis of mosaic perfusion when it is an isolated or predominant abnormality

Asthma
Hypersensitivity pneumonitis
Constrictive bronchiolitis (bronchiolitis obliterans)
Chronic pulmonary embolism
Vasculitis

When mosaic perfusion is the predominant abnormality, and little else is visible on HRCT, the differential diagnosis includes asthma, hypersensitivity pneumonitis, constrictive bronchiolitis, chronic pulmonary embolism, and vasculitis.

Differentiating Airways and Vascular Causes of Mosaic Perfusion

In most cases, a distinction can be made between mosaic perfusion resulting from airways disease and vascular disease. The presence of large airway abnormalities (bronchiectasis or bronchial wall thickening) suggests airway disease as the cause; the presence

of pulmonary artery dilatation is more typical of vascular disease.

As discussed previously, vascular disease does not generally result in air trapping on expiratory imaging (Fig. 5.11A, B). The presence of at least one lucent region that is lobular (i.e., it can be recognized as corresponding to a secondary pulmonary lobule) suggests that airways disease is the cause. Occlusion of lobular bronchioles is common in patients with airways disease. Vascular disease, in contradistinction, typically demonstrates larger, often peripheral areas of decreased attenuation without a lobular appearance (Fig. 5.12A, B).

THE HEADCHEESE SIGN

Headcheese is a sausage made from chopped parts of an animal's head, including muscle, fat, brain, ears, and snout; it is a mosaic of meats and various tissues, having different colors, shapes, and textures. The term *headcheese sign* is used to describe a mosaic appearance of lung parenchyma, consisting of geographic areas of both increased

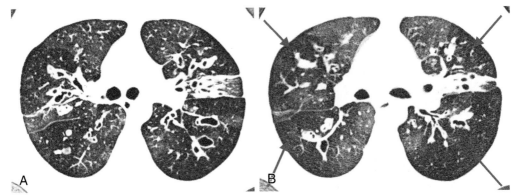

FIGURE 5.10 · **Mosaic perfusion in cystic fibrosis. A.** HRCT shows heterogeneous lung attenuation on inspiration. Airway abnormalities are obvious. **B.** Expiratory HRCT shows patchy air trapping (*arrows*). There is extensive bronchiectasis and airway wall thickening present. In this case, mosaic perfusion should be ignored in terms of differential diagnosis, and the emphasis should be placed on the large airway abnormalities.

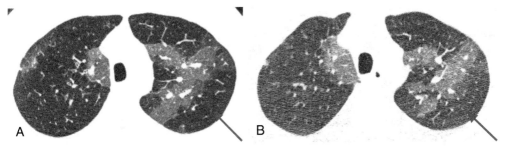

FIGURE 5.11 · **Mosaic perfusion without air trapping in chronic pulmonary embolism.** Air trapping in a patient with mosaic perfusion indicates the presence of airways disease. In patients with mosaic perfusion resulting from vascular disease, air trapping is not usually present, as in this patient with chronic pulmonary embolism. There is an increase in attenuation of the more lucent lung when comparing inspiratory (**A**, *arrow*) and expiratory (**B**, *arrow*) images.

5

attenuation (ground glass opacity and sometimes consolidation) and decreased attenuation (mosaic perfusion). It resembles headcheese but in black, white, and shades of gray (Fig. 5.13). Visible attenuation differences are accentuated on expiratory scans in which both the normal and opaque lung become denser, but areas of mosaic perfusion stay lucent (Fig. 5.14A, B).

The headcheese sign is important in that it indicates the presence of a mixed obstructive and infiltrative disease. The obstructive abnormality is manifested by mosaic perfusion, and is characteristically associated with small airways disease. The infiltrative disorder results in ground glass opacity or consolidation.

There are a limited number of diseases that have both a significant obstructive and infiltrative component, and this limits the differential diagnosis of the headcheese sign (Table 5.3). These include hypersensitivity pneumonitis, respiratory bronchiolitis and desquamative interstitial pneumonia in smokers, follicular bronchiolitis and lymphoid interstitial pneumonia (LIP), sarcoidosis, and atypical infections. Moreover, it is possible for patients with the headcheese sign to have two entirely separate diseases such as pulmonary edema and asthma.

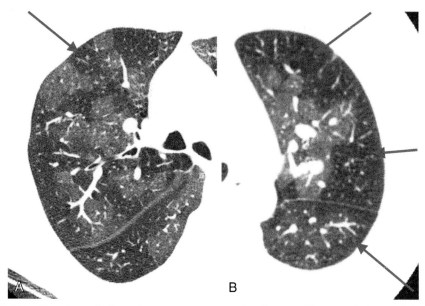

FIGURE 5.12 · **Mosaic perfusion: airways versus vascular disease.** The morphology of the lucent lung in mosaic perfusion may differ between airways and vascular disease. In airways disease **(A)**, the lucent lung often appears lobular (*arrow*) compared with the larger, peripheral, nonlobular appearance (*arrows*) in vascular disease **(B)**.

5

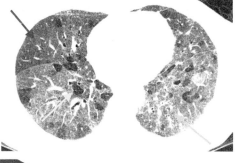

classic

FIGURE 5.13 · **The "headcheese" sign in hypersensitivity pneumonitis: Classic appearance.** Three densities of lung are present: ground glass opacity (*blue arrow*), mosaic perfusion (*yellow arrow*), and normal lung (*red arrow*). This pattern is very suggestive of hypersensitivity pneumonitis.

Furthermore, the majority of patients who show the headcheese sign have hypersensitivity pneumonitis (Fig. 5.15). The other diseases in the differential diagnosis only rarely present with this pattern, and when they do, either the ground glass or mosaic perfusion is usually limited in its severity or distribution.

CYSTIC LUNG DISEASE

A lung cyst is defined, somewhat arbitrarily, as a round, air-filled lesion, greater than 1 cm in diameter, and with a thin but recognizable wall.

On HRCT, a few lung cysts may be seen in patients who are otherwise normal, but the presence of more than a few cysts suggests a cystic lung disease. Cystic lung diseases are rare and should not be confused with other causes of lung cysts such as emphysema (i.e., bullae are cysts), honeycombing (fibrosis with cystic regions of lung destruction), and bronchiectasis (Fig. 5.16A–D).

Cystic lung disease typically presents in one of several ways. Spontaneous pneumothorax may develop with any cause of cystic lung disease if a cyst ruptures into the pleural space. When cystic lung disease is extensive, replacing a significant volume of normal lung, patients may present with dyspnea and symptoms similar to other chronic lung diseases. Pulmonary hypertension is not an uncommon sequela of extensive cystic lung disease. Cystic lung disease may also be detected as an incidental finding.

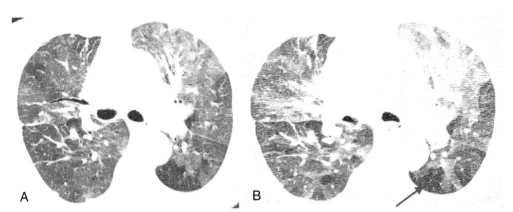

FIGURE 5.14 · **The "headcheese" sign.** Inspiratory **(A)** and expiratory **(B)** HRCT in a patient with the "headcheese" sign resulting from hypersensitivity pneumonitis. During expiration **(B)**, the areas of decreased attenuation do not change in attenuation and remain lucent (arrow). Both the normal lung and ground glass opacity increase in attenuation.

TABLE 5.3	Differential diagnosis of the "headcheese" sign

Hypersensitivity (most common)
Respiratory bronchiolitis/desquamative interstitial
   pneumonia
Follicular bronchiolitis/lymphoid interstitial
   pneumonia
Atypical infections (e.g., viral)
Sarcoid
Two separate processes (e.g., edema and asthma)

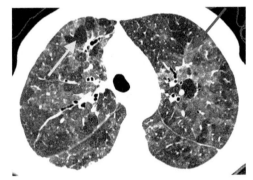

FIGURE 5.15 · **Headcheese sign in hypersensitivity pneumonitis.** The combination of ground glass opacity (*red arrow*) and mosaic perfusion/air trapping (*yellow arrow*) is highly suggestive of hypersensitivity pneumonitis. There are other causes of the "headcheese" sign, but they are much less common.

Differential Diagnosis

The differential diagnosis of cystic lung disease includes Langerhans cell histiocytosis (LCH), lymphangioleiomyomatosis (LAM), LIP, pneumatoceles from prior infection such as pneumocystis pneumonia, treated cystic metastases, benign metastasizing leiomyoma, neurofibromatosis, barotrauma in scuba divers, pulmonary papillomatosis, Birt–Hogg–Dubé disease, and amyloidosis and light-chain deposition disease (Table 5.4). These diseases are discussed in detail in other chapters. LCH and LAM produce the most extensive abnormalities, and in some cases, the lungs may be nearly entirely replaced by cysts. LCH, LAM, and LIP are most commonly encountered in clinical practice.

LCH is usually seen in cigarette smokers. On HRCT, cysts appear irregular in shape,

predominate in the upper lobes, and may be thick or thin walled in different stages of the disease. Small nodules, solid or cavitary, may be associated with the cysts or may precede the development of cysts (Figs. 5.17A and 5.18). Extensive cystic disease in LCH may be difficult to distinguish from extensive CLE (Fig. 5.17A, B). However, the cysts of LCH have visible walls, whereas CLE generally does not.

LAM is seen in women of childbearing age and is not commonly associated with

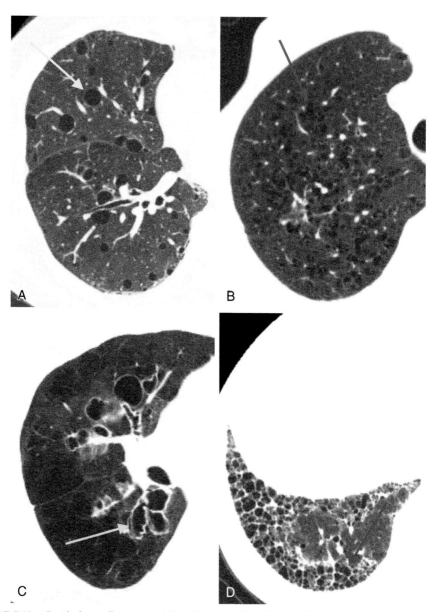

FIGURE 5.16 · Cystic lung disease and its mimics. A. Cystic lung disease in a patient with lymphoid interstitial pneumonia. Cysts are round with well-defined thin walls (*arrow*) and, as distinct from honeycombing or panlobular emphysema, do not predominate in the subpleural lung. **B.** The lucencies of centrilobular emphysema (*arrow*) lack distinct walls. Bronchiectasis **(C)** may appear cystic when dilated bronchi are seen in cross section; however, on some images the tubular or branching nature of the airways (*arrow*) should be evident. Honeycombing **(D)** is usually subpleural, stacked in layers (*arrow*), and walls are thicker than simple lung cysts.

nodules. Cysts are round in shape, thin walled, and as numerous in the lung bases as in the upper lobes. LAM is also seen in patients with tuberous sclerosis, usually women (Fig. 5.19A, B). Pleural effusions are common in LAM but rare with LCH. Angiomyolipoma of the kidney may be associated.

LIP is usually associated with a history of connective tissue disease or immunosuppression. Sjögren's disease, in particular, may present with cysts as the only manifestation of LIP (Fig. 5.20). Cysts are often associated with, or adjacent to, vessels, predominate in the lung bases and are limited to a few dozen.

TABLE 5.4	Differential diagnosis of primary cystic lung disease

Langerhans cell histiocytosis
Lymphangioleiomyomatosis
Lymphoid interstitial pneumonia
Pneumatoceles from prior infection
Treated cystic metastases
Benign metastasizing leiomyoma
Papillomatosis
Neurofibromatosis
Birt–Hogg–Dubé disease
Amyoidosis and light-chain deposition disease

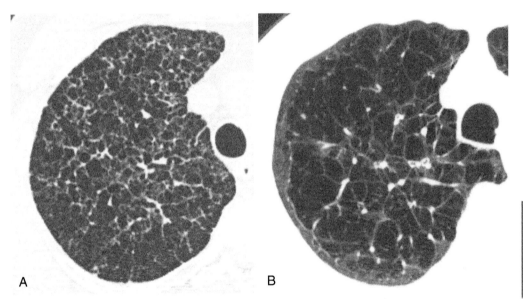

A   B

FIGURE 5.17 · **Cystic lung disease versus emphysema.** When cystic lung disease is extensive, it may be difficult to distinguish from centrilobular emphysema. The presence of clearly defined walls suggests cystic lung disease. **A.** Cysts in a patient with Langerhans cell histiocytosis demonstrate discrete walls. Centrilobular emphysema **(B)** demonstrates lucencies without well-defined walls, although some areas of emphysema show thin walls, which likely represent interlobular septa.

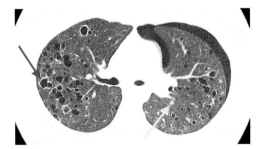

FIGURE 5.18 · **Langerhans cell histiocytosis.** Irregularly shaped cysts are present, some of which have thin walls and others have thicker walls (*red arrow*). Nodules are also seen (*yellow arrow*). This patient presented with a pneumothorax.

5

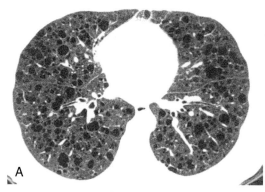
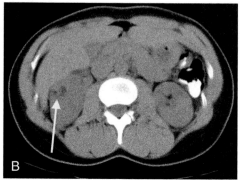

FIGURE 5.19 · **Lymphangioleiomyomatosis. A.** In a patient with tuberous sclerosis, HRCT shows diffuse, round, well-defined cysts without associated nodules. **B.** An angiomyolipoma (*arrow*) is present in the right kidney.

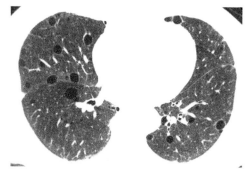

FIGURE 5.20 · **Lymphoid interstitial pneumonia.** The cysts of lymphoid interstitial pneumonia are not nearly as numerous as those in Langerhans cell histiocytosis or lymphangioleiomyomatosis. Of the connective tissue diseases, lymphoid interstitial pneumonia is most commonly seen in association with Sjögren's disease.

FURTHER READING

Arakawa H, Webb WR. Air trapping on expiratory high-resolution CT scans in the absence of inspiratory scan abnormalities: correlation with pulmonary function tests and differential diagnosis. *AJR Am J Roentgenol*. 1998;170:1349-1353.

Arakawa H, Webb WR, McCowin M, Katsou G, Lee KN, Seitz RF. Inhomogeneous lung attenuation at thin-section CT: diagnostic value of expiratory scans. *Radiology*. 1998;206:89-94.

Austin JH, Müller NL, Friedman PJ, et al. Glossary of terms for CT of the lungs: recommendations of the Nomenclature Committee of the Fleischner Society. *Radiology*. 1996;200:327-331.

Foster WL Jr, Gimenez EI, Roubidoux MA, et al. The emphysemas: radiologic-pathologic correlations. *Radiographics*. 1993;13:311-328.

Gupta N, Vassallo R, Wikenheiser-Brokamp KA, et al. Diffuse cystic lung disease. Part I. *Am J Respir Crit Care Med*. 2015;191:1354-1366.

Gupta N, Vassallo R, Wikenheiser-Brokamp KA, et al. Diffuse cystic lung disease. Part II. *Am J Respir Crit Care Med*. 2015;192:17-29.

Hansell DM, Bankier AA, MacMahon H, et al. Fleischner society: glossary of terms for thoracic imaging. *Radiology*. 2008;246:697-722.

Im JG, Kim SH, Chung MJ, Koo JM, Han MC. Lobular low attenuation of the lung parenchyma on CT: evaluation of forty-eight patients. *J Comput Assist Tomogr*. 1996;20:756-762.

Lynch DA. Imaging of small airways disease and chronic obstructive pulmonary disease. *Clin Chest Med*. 2008;29:165-179.

Müller NL, Miller RR. Diseases of the bronchioles: CT and histopathologic findings. *Radiology*. 1995;196:3-12.

Padley SPG, Adler BD, Hansell DM, Müller NL. Bronchiolitis obliterans: high-resolution CT findings and correlation with pulmonary function tests. *Clin Radiol*. 1993;47:236-240.

Park CS, Müller NL, Worthy SA, et al. Airway obstruction in asthmatic and healthy individuals: inspiratory and expiratory thin-section CT findings. *Radiology*. 1997;203:361-367.

Sherrick AD, Swensen SJ, Hartman TE. Mosaic pattern of lung attenuation on CT scans: frequency among patients with pulmonary artery hypertension of different causes. *AJR Am J Roentgenol*. 1997;169:79-82.

Thurlbeck WM, Müller NL. Emphysema: definition, imaging, and quantification. *AJR Am J Roentgenol*. 1994;163:1017-1025.

Webb WR. Thin-section CT of the secondary pulmonary lobule: anatomy and the image—the 2004 Fleischner lecture. *Radiology*. 2006;239:322-338.

Worthy SA, Müller NL, Hartman TE, Swensen SJ, Padley SP, Hansell DM. Mosaic attenuation pattern on thin-section CT scans of the lung: differentiation among infiltrative lung, airway, and vascular diseases as a cause. *Radiology*. 1997;205:465-470.

5

SPECIFIC DISEASES

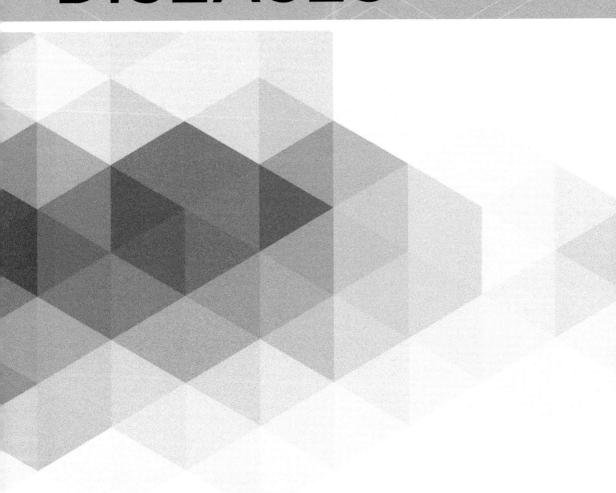

Airways Diseases

INTRODUCTION

Airways disease may have a variety of causes and associations, including inhalation of organic or inorganic materials, systemic diseases, infection, tumor, and congenital defects. Airways diseases are broadly categorized by the size of airways involved as large airways disease (affecting bronchi) or small airways disease (affecting bronchioles).

Bronchi are characterized by the presence of cartilage in their walls; they are usually larger than 3 mm and the most peripheral airways visible on CT. *Bronchioles* lack cartilage in their walls; they are usually less than 3 mm in diameter and invisible on CT.

The terms *large airways* and *small airways,* which are commonly used, are less precisely defined (i.e., they are not defined based on histology). "Small airways" are currently defined in various reviews as being less than 2 mm in diameter, although this definition is arbitrary and has changed over the years. Small airways are present within a few centimeters of the pleural surface. Generally speaking, "small airway" can be considered synonymous with "bronchiole." Although "large" and "small" airways abnormalities often occur together, many diseases show predominant involvement of one or the other.

This chapter reviews the HRCT findings of airways diseases, typical patterns of airways disease, and common airways diseases.

LARGE AIRWAYS (BRONCHIAL) DISEASES

HRCT Findings

HRCT findings indicative of large airways disease include airway dilatation, airway inflammation or infiltration with wall thickening,

and mucoid impaction of the airway lumen. Large airways diseases include *bronchiectasis* and *bronchitis*, which may occur separately or in combination.

Airway Dilatation

Irreversible dilatation of the bronchi is termed *bronchiectasis*. Bronchiectasis is usually defined by an increased bronchoarterial ratio (BAR) (described below) or specific contour abnormalities that indicate the presence of bronchial dilatation. Bronchiectasis has a variety of causes (Table 6.1), including infections, chronic inflammatory disease, bronchial obstruction, and morphologic bronchial abnormalities. Bronchiectasis is usually associated with bronchial wall destruction, fibrosis, and loss of elasticity.

There are two caveats to keep in mind in the diagnosis of bronchiectasis. *Traction bronchiectasis* (bronchial dilatation associated with lung fibrosis; see Chapter 2) is not considered an airway disease because the airway itself is not abnormal. Secondly, a transient increase in bronchial diameter may be seen in patients who have atelectasis or inflammatory lung disease; this is sometimes referred to using the oxymoronic term *reversible bronchiectasis*. The dilated airway may return to normal with resolution of the acute process.

Bronchoarterial Ratio and the "Signet Ring Sign"

The ratio of the internal bronchial diameter (i.e., the diameter of the bronchial lumen) to the diameter of the adjacent pulmonary artery branch is termed the *bronchoarterial ratio*. A normal BAR is approximately 0.7.

TABLE 6.1	Differential diagnosis of large airways disease (bronchitis and bronchiectasis)

Infection (viral, bacterial, mycobacterial, fungal)
Asthma
Aspiration
Constrictive bronchiolitis
Collagen vascular disease
Allergic bronchopulmonary aspergillosis
Cystic fibrosis
Immunodeficiency
Primary ciliary dyskinesia
Marfan syndrome
Inflammatory bowel disease
Alpha-1-antitrypsin
Yellow nail lymphedema syndrome
Young syndrome
Tracheobronchomegaly
Williams–Campbell syndrome

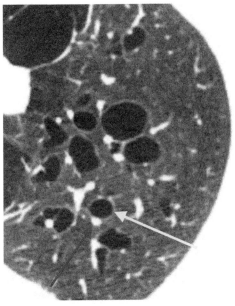

FIGURE 6.1 · **Bronchiectasis with a broncho-arterial ratio >1.5.** The diameter of the lumen of the bronchus (*yellow arrow*) is significantly greater than the adjacent artery (*red arrow*) in a patient with a disorder of bronchial cartilage. Although a bronchoarterial ratio of 1–1.5 is occasionally seen in normal patients, a ratio >1.5 is almost always abnormal.

A BAR greater than 1.0 is usually considered abnormal (Fig. 6.1), but, sometimes, this may be a normal finding in elderly patients and patients living at high altitudes (e.g.,

Denver, the mile-high city). Also, the BAR may be elevated in patients with normal bronchi and abnormally small arteries. This may be seen in processes such as alpha-1-antitrypsin deficiency or chronic pulmonary embolism.

A BAR greater than 1.5 is usually specific for bronchiectasis. In patients with a BAR between 1.0 and 1.5, the presence of airway wall thickening or impaction, or mosaic perfusion and air trapping (other findings of airway disease), makes it likely that true bronchiectasis is present. The term *signet ring sign* has been used to describe the presence of airway dilatation with an increased BAR. The ring represents a dilated bronchus, whereas the signet or stone represents the smaller adjacent pulmonary artery.

Contour Abnormalities in the Diagnosis of Bronchiectasis

Bronchiectasis is classified into three categories depending on the morphology and severity of airway dilatation. Three specific contour abnormalities may be used to diagnose the presence of bronchiectasis.

1. *Cylindrical bronchiectasis* (Fig. 6.2A, B) is characterized by relatively mild bronchial dilatation and smooth, parallel bronchial walls, without normal tapering in the lung periphery. This appearance is nonspecific and may be seen with most causes of bronchiectasis or with "reversible bronchiectasis."
2. *Varicose bronchiectasis* (Fig. 6.3) is associated with more severe, long-standing, or recurrent airway inflammation and injury. The contour of the bronchial walls appears irregular with focal areas of dilatation intermixed with regions of narrowing (similar to varicose veins). This form of bronchiectasis may be seen with many causes of bronchiectasis. It is referred to as having a "string of pearls" appearance.
3. *Cystic bronchiectasis* (Fig. 6.4) is the most severe form of airway dilatation and is seen only with long-standing bronchiectasis, often dating from childhood. Morphologically, it is characterized by

6

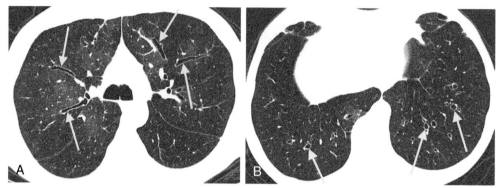

FIGURE 6.2 · Cylindrical bronchiectasis. Mild bronchial dilatation is present without evidence of strictures or saccular dilatations. When the bronchi lie within the axial plane **(A)** they appear tubular, with parallel walls (*arrows*). When they are oriented perpendicular to the axial plane **(B)** they appear circular (*arrows*), and the signet ring sign is characteristically present.

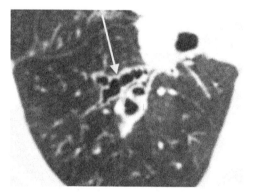

FIGURE 6.3 · Varicose bronchiectasis.
Bronchial dilatation with an irregular contour and wall thickening (*arrow*) are present. This appearance, while nonspecific, reflects a more severe and long-standing process.

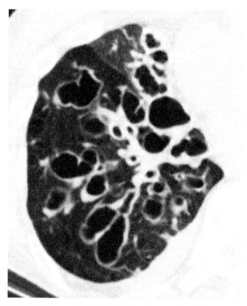

FIGURE 6.4 · Cystic bronchiectasis. The bronchi are markedly enlarged with multiple saccular dilatations and air/fluid levels. This appearance reflects severe, chronic airways inflammation and is seen with a limited number of diseases.

large saccular dilatation of airways, which may contain air/fluid levels. It may be focal or diffuse. The differential diagnosis of cystic bronchiectasis is limited because only a limited number of diseases cause such severe large airway remodeling. It is sometimes described as having a "cluster of grapes" appearance.

Airway Inflammation with Wall Thickening

Airway wall thickening is commonly seen in patients with bronchiectasis, due to chronic bronchial inflammation, infection, or fibrosis. Bronchial wall thickening without bronchial dilatation can be seen in patients with

the same diseases typically associated with bronchiectasis, in patients with acute bronchial inflammation (i.e., with viral infection), and in those with a history of smoking and chronic obstructive pulmonary disease (Fig. 6.5). *Bronchitis* (bronchial wall thickening without dilatation) should be distinguished from *bronchiectasis* (bronchial dilatation with or without wall thickening).

Often the diagnosis of bronchial wall thickening is subjective and based on experience or on a comparison of bronchi in one lung region with those in another lung region; airways disease is often patchy in distribution.

Attempts have been made to measure bronchial wall thickness. In a normal subject, the ratio of the thickness of the bronchial wall to the diameter of the bronchus is approximately 0.1 to 0.2. When this ratio is increased, bronchial wall thickening is usually present. However, keep in mind that this measurement may be normal in patients with bronchial wall thickening associated with bronchial dilatation (i.e., bronchiectasis).

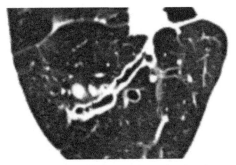

FIGURE 6.5 · Bronchial wall thickening in varicose bronchiectasis. The bronchial wall in this patient with atypical mycobacterial infection is >5 mm in maximum thickness. In some regions, the ratio of the thickened wall to the air-filled lumen is greater than 1:1.

Airway Lumen Impaction

Airway impaction results from filling of the airway lumen by mucus, infectious debris, or other substances. Depending on the orientation of the airways with respect to the image, airway impaction will appear as circular or tubular structures (Fig. 6.6A, B) that connect to more central bronchi. Luminal impaction may be present with bronchitis or bronchiectasis.

Specific Causes of Large Airways Disease and Bronchiectasis

There is a broad differential diagnosis for large airways diseases, including bronchiectasis and bronchitis (Table 6.1).

Infectious Diseases

Infection is the most common cause of large airways disease. Any type of infection may be associated with airway dilatation and inflammation. Childhood infections are a common cause of bronchiectasis.

Airway abnormalities seen in bacterial, mycobacterial, and fungal infections are usually associated with patchy lung consolidation, centrilobular nodules, or tree-in-bud (TIB) opacities. Viral infections may present with findings of large airways abnormalities as an isolated abnormality (Fig. 6.7) or in association with lung parenchymal findings. Bronchiectasis associated with remote or chronic infection is often lobar, multilobar, or patchy.

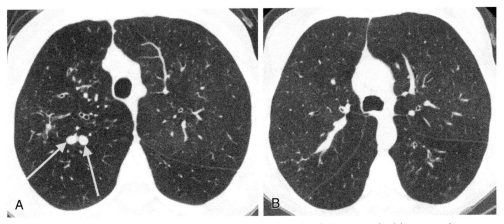

FIGURE 6.6 · Airway impaction. When an airway is completely impacted with mucus, its appearance varies depending on its orientation. **A.** Airways perpendicular to the axial plane will appear circular (*arrows*). **B.** Airways parallel to the axial plane will appear tubular (*arrows*).

In most cases, the findings of large airways disease associated with acute infection are mild and reversible. The presence of more extensive or severe abnormalities, such as varicose or cystic bronchiectasis, should suggest a remote (i.e., childhood) infection or a different etiology.

Severe or chronic airway infection may be seen with tuberculosis or nontuberculous mycobacterial infection (Fig. 6.8A, B), chronic aspiration, or acquired or congenital abnormalities that impair immunity or ciliary clearance (discussed below). Constrictive bronchiolitis (CB) may also predispose patients to chronic airway infection and mucostasis.

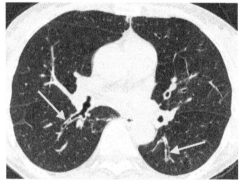

FIGURE 6.7 · **Viral infection with bronchial dilatation and wall thickening** (*arrows*). Among acute infections, viral organisms are most likely to produce isolated abnormalities of the large airways such as in this patient with dilated and thickened airways (*arrows*).

Allergic Bronchopulmonary Aspergillosis

Allergic bronchopulmonary aspergillosis (ABPA), discussed in Chapter 13, is a disorder seen predominantly in asthmatics or patients with cystic fibrosis (CF). It is a hypersensitivity reaction to *Aspergillus* that colonizes the lumen of the airways, without invasion into the lung parenchyma. The diagnosis of ABPA is predominantly clinical, but typical HRCT findings may also be diagnostic.

The most characteristic HRCT finding in patients with ABPA is unilateral or asymmetric, central (parahilar) bronchiectasis, associated with mucoid impaction (Fig. 6.9). The mid- or upper lungs are typically involved. High-attenuation (100 HU) mucous plugs (Fig. 6.10) are particularly suggestive of this diagnosis. This finding, seen in about 25% of patients with ABPA, reflects concentration of calcium salts and metallic ions by the fungus.

Although large airway abnormalities usually predominate in ABPA, small airways may also be affected. Small airway abnormalities appear as bronchiolectasis, centrilobular nodules, and TIB opacities.

Cystic Fibrosis

CF is a congenital disorder that results in impaired clearance of bronchial secretions. This predisposes patients to chronic

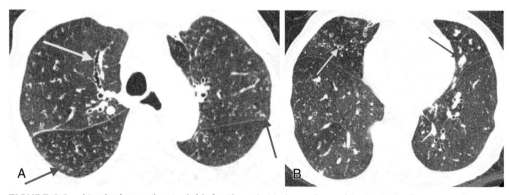

FIGURE 6.8 · **Atypical mycobacterial infection. A.** Varicose bronchiectasis (*yellow arrow*) is associated with small clusters of centrilobular nodules or tree-in-bud (*red arrows*). **B.** Bronchiectasis (*yellow arrow*) and bronchial impaction (*red arrow*) are typically most severe in the right middle lobe and lingua.

mucostasis and airway infection. Although classically presenting in a young patient population (less than 20 years of age), a greater understanding of the genetic heterogeneity and variable penetrance of this disease has led to the first diagnosis of patients later in life. Also, improvement in treatment has allowed many young patients with CF to survive into adulthood.

Typical HRCT findings include symmetric, upper lobe predominant, central bronchiectasis, bronchial wall thickening, and luminal impaction (Fig. 6.11A, B). The right upper lobe is often involved first, and most severely. The bronchiectasis varies in severity,

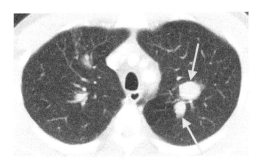

FIGURE 6.9 · **Allergic bronchopulmonary aspergillosis.** Asymmetric central bronchiectasis and mucoid impaction is seen in the upper lobes (*arrows*). No significant abnormalities were visible in the lower lobes. This distribution of varicose or cystic bronchiectasis is most typical of allergic bronchopulmonary aspergillosis and tuberculosis.

but varicose or cystic bronchiectasis is most characteristic in advanced cases. Findings of small airways disease (bronchiolectasis, centrilobular nodules, and TIB) are often present in association with the large airways abnormalities. Mosaic perfusion and air trapping are usually present. Hilar enlargement may be due to reactive lymphadenopathy or pulmonary arterial enlargement.

Immunodeficiency

Congenital or acquired immunodeficiency predisposes patients to chronic airways infection. Congenital immunodeficiencies that commonly lead to large airways disease include agammaglobulinemia, hypogammaglobulinemia, and common variable immunodeficiency. HRCT findings are similar to those seen in other causes of chronic large airways disease and include bronchiectasis (often cystic), bronchial wall thickening, and mucoid impaction. The distribution tends to be symmetric and lower lobe predominant.

The most common acquired disorder to result in large airways disease is the acquired immunodeficiency syndrome (AIDS). *AIDS-related airways disease* is most likely due to chronic airway infection by pyogenic organisms. It manifests as symmetric bilateral bronchiectasis, usually lower lobe predominant, bronchial wall thickening, and impaction. Although cystic bronchiectasis is rare, varicose bronchiectasis is common

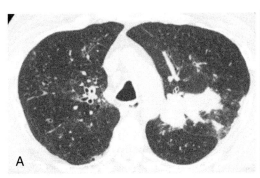

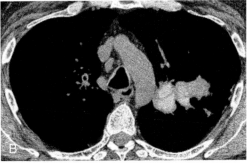

A **B**

classic

FIGURE 6.10 · **Allergic bronchopulmonary aspergillosis: Classic appearance. A.** Lung window shows a tubular branching structure in the left upper lobe representing focal bronchiectasis and mucoid impaction. **B.** Soft tissue window shows that the mucus in the lumen of this dilated bronchus is high in attenuation. This strongly suggests allergic bronchopulmonary aspergillosis.

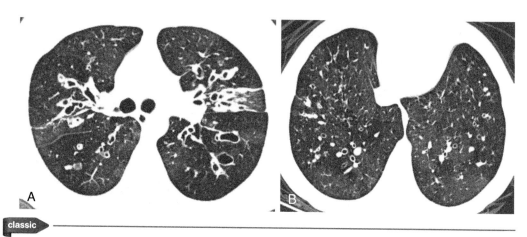

classic

FIGURE 6.11 · **Cystic fibrosis: Classic appearance.** Extensive varicose and cystic bronchiectasis, bronchial wall thickening, and mucous impaction are noted in the upper lobes **(A)**. The process is symmetric and relatively spares the lower lobes **(B)**. This pattern is most typical of cystic fibrosis.

and its presence reflects the chronicity of findings.

Primary Ciliary Dyskinesia

Primary ciliary dyskinesia or immotile cilia syndrome is a congenital disorder causing reduced or absent ciliary motion. This leads to abnormal mucociliary clearance affecting the lungs, sinuses, inner ear, and reproductive systems. Impaired airway mucociliary clearance results in chronic mucostasis, recurrent infections, and bronchiectasis.

The HRCT findings are very similar to those seen with congenital immunodeficiency. Abnormalities usually are symmetric and affect the lower lobes. Cystic or varicose bronchiectasis is typical and associated with airway wall thickening and mucous impaction (Fig. 6.12). Findings of small airways disease may also be present but do not predominate. Situs inversus is seen in 50% of patients, in which case the disease is termed *Kartagener syndrome* (Fig. 6.13A, B).

Williams–Campbell Syndrome

Williams–Campbell syndrome is a rare congenital disorder characterized by the absence of cartilage in the fourth through sixth order bronchi. It typically presents in children, but a rare initial presentation in adults has been described. Lack of supporting cartilage causes weakness and dilatation

of affected bronchi. Over time, this eventually leads to chronic mucostasis and infection.

Cystic bronchiectasis with a mid- to lower lung predominance is characteristic. Focal mid-lung bronchiectasis may be present or there may be more extensive dilatation beginning in the central lung and extending peripherally (Fig. 6.14). As is typical of other disorders of cartilage, there may be severe cystic bronchiectasis with relatively little airway inflammation. The airways show significant increase in size during inspiration and collapse on expiration. This is in contrast to immunodeficiency syndromes and primary ciliary disorders.

Tracheobronchomegaly

Tracheobronchomegaly or *Mounier–Kuhn syndrome* is a rare condition in which there is atrophy of portions of the tracheal and bronchial walls. Typical HRCT findings include thinning of the walls of the trachea and bronchi. The airways are dilated and show dynamic collapse during expiration. Scalloping of the walls of the affected airways may be seen because of restriction of the lumen by cartilage rings (Fig. 6.15A, B). As with Williams–Campbell syndrome, there may be a relative lack of inflammatory abnormalities, even in cases of severe dilatation.

6

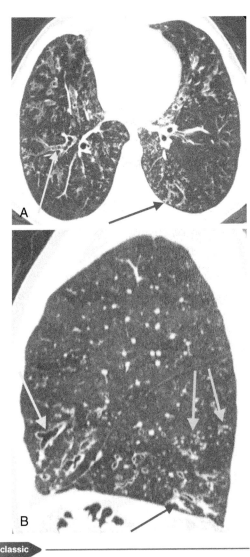

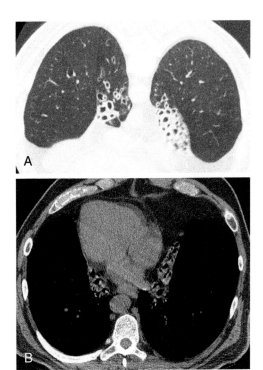

FIGURE 6.13 · **Kartagener syndrome.** Prone HRCT (**A**) shows extensive bilateral lower lobe cystic bronchiectasis and collapse. Supine HRCT image (**B**) shows situs inversus and dextrocardia.

classic

FIGURE 6.12 · **Primary ciliary dyskinesia: Classic appearance. A.** Bilateral and symmetrical airway abnormalities are typical, with bronchiectasis (*yellow* arrow), bronchial wall thickening, and tree-in-bud opacities (*red arrow*). **B.** Sagittal reformatted HRCT shows lower lobe predominant bronchiectasis (*yellow arrow*), airway impaction (*red arrow*), centrilobular nodules, and tree-in-bud (*blue arrows*). A bilateral, lower lobe distribution is typical of primary ciliary dyskinesia, immunodeficiency, and other causes of chronic infection.

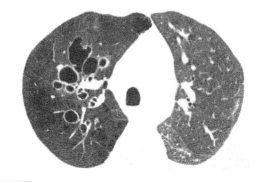

classic

FIGURE 6.14 · **Williams–Campbell syndrome: Classic appearance.** HRCT in a patient with Williams–Campbell syndrome, status-post left lung transplant. The native right lung shows extensive cystic bronchiectasis and diffuse lung lucency. Note the lack of inflammation and airway wall thickening.

Other Causes of Large Airways Disease

There are many other causes of diffuse or extensive bilateral large airways disease including connective tissue disease, recurrent and chronic aspiration, CB, Marfan syndrome, alpha-1-antitrypsin deficiency, yellow nail lymphedema syndrome, and Young syndrome. Most of these disorders present with

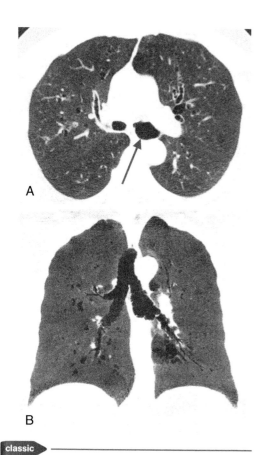

A

B

classic

FIGURE 6.15 · Tracheobronchomegaly: Classic appearance. Marked dilatation of the left main bronchus (*red arrow*) is noted in association with bronchiectasis predominantly within the central lung regions **(A)**. There is a relative paucity of airways inflammation and wall thickening. Coronal reformatted minimum intensity projection image **(B)** shows scalloping of the tracheal wall and thin-walled bronchiectasis in the central lung regions.

nonspecific findings and the diagnosis is often based on the clinical presentation.

Recurrent or chronic aspiration often shows consolidation and/or fibrosis involving the dependent lung regions. Marfan syndrome may show bullous emphysema out of proportion to the patient's age. Alpha-1-antitrypsin deficiency shows diffuse lung lucency with a lower lobe predominance.

HRCT Diagnosis of Large Airways Diseases and Bronchiectasis

Bronchial wall thickening without bronchial dilatation (i.e., bronchitis) may be seen with

infection or noninfectious inflammatory diseases, such as chronic bronchitis related to smoking, asthma, inflammatory bowel disease, or many of the diseases associated with bronchiectasis. Mucus may be visible within the abnormal airways.

Cylindrical bronchiectasis is a nonspecific finding, and in patients who show this finding, the diagnosis is usually based on a combination of the clinical presentation, sputum analysis, and/or pathologic findings. In some patients, this appearance may resolve.

Varicose or cystic bronchiectasis suggests a long-standing or chronic process. Two diseases that not uncommonly produce varicose bronchiectasis include mycobacterial infection and recurrent/chronic aspiration. Of note, any cause of cystic bronchiectasis may present at an earlier stage, at which point varicose bronchiectasis is the predominant abnormality. The differential diagnosis of cystic bronchiectasis is more limited including ABPA (Figs. 6.9 and 6.10), CF (Fig. 6.11), primary ciliary dyskinesia (Figs. 6.12 and 6.13), immunodeficiency, childhood infection, and abnormalities of the cartilage including Williams-Campbell syndrome and tracheobronchomegaly.

The distribution of abnormalities can be helpful in diagnosis. Diseases that lead to mid- or upper lung bronchiectasis include CF, ABPA, and tuberculosis (Fig. 6.16). Lower lobe bronchiectasis may be due to chronic infection, aspiration, immunodeficiency, and primary ciliary dyskinesia (Fig. 6.12). Bronchiectasis that is most severe in the middle lobe and lingula suggests atypical mycobacterial infection. Unilateral bronchiectasis is often due to infection (Fig. 6.16) or bronchial obstruction. Bilateral bronchiectasis suggests a systemic or congenital abnormality, or immunodeficiency.

High-density mucus within areas of bronchiectasis is suggestive of ABPA (Fig. 6.10A, B). Situs inversus suggests primary ciliary dyskinesia. The absence of airway wall thickening or mucoid impaction in the presence of severe bronchiectasis suggests a cartilage abnormality (Figs. 6.14 and 6.15) or CB with associated large airway abnormalities.

6

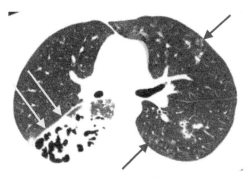

FIGURE 6.16 · **Tuberculosis.** Focal cystic bronchiectasis is seen in the superior segment of the right lower lobe (*yellow arrows*). Small clusters of centrilobular nodules (*red arrows*) are seen elsewhere, reflecting endobronchial spread of tuberculosis.

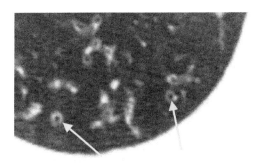

FIGURE 6.17 · **Bronchiolectasis.** Dilatation of small peripheral airways (*arrows*) is seen in a patient with cystic fibrosis. Airways are seen in the peripheral 1–2 cm of the lung, which is not normal, and their lumens are significantly larger than the adjacent arteries.

SMALL AIRWAYS (BRONCHIOLAR) DISEASES

HRCT Findings

Analogous to findings seen in large airways disease, HRCT findings indicative of small airways disease include bronchiolectasis, bronchiolar inflammation with wall thickening, and bronchiolar impaction with TIB (see Chapter 3). Other findings of small airways disease include centrilobular nodules and mosaic perfusion with air trapping (see Chapter 5). Also, keep in mind that patients with small airways disease commonly show large airway abnormalities as well.

Bronchiolectasis and Tree-in-Bud

Bronchiolectasis is defined as dilatation of small airways (Fig. 6.17). There are no specific criteria for bronchiolectasis on HRCT, but normal airways should not be visible in the peripheral 1 to 2 cm of the lung. When they are seen in this location, bronchiolectasis with wall thickening is likely present.

Dilated bronchioles may be air filled or filled with secretions. Bronchiolectasis with luminal impaction results in the appearance of TIB. TIB is an important finding in making the diagnosis of small airways disease.

Centrilobular Nodules

Infectious or inflammatory diseases involving the centrilobular bronchiole may spread to the surrounding lung regions, resulting in

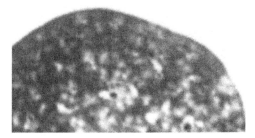

FIGURE 6.18 · **Centrilobular nodules of soft tissue attenuation.** Centrilobular nodules of soft tissue attenuation are most typical of endobronchial spread of infection or tumor, or aspiration. The nodules spare the subpleural lung. This patient has a bacterial bronchopneumonia.

centrilobular nodules visible on HRCT (Fig. 6.18). Centrilobular nodules may be of soft tissue attenuation or of ground glass opacity (GGO) (see Chapter 3).

Mosaic Perfusion and Air Trapping

Mosaic perfusion is caused by decreased blood flow to localized lung regions. In the case of airways disease, hypoxia resulting from airway narrowing or obstruction results in reflex vasoconstriction and reduced perfusion. HRCT shows focal regions of decreased attenuation; vessels within these regions appear relatively small. When due to small airways disease, mosaic perfusion is often associated with air trapping. The HRCT features of mosaic

6

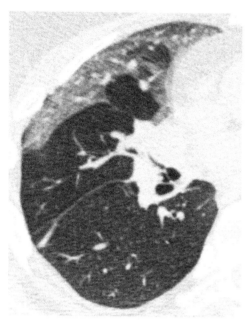

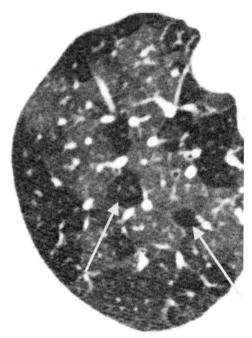

FIGURE 6.19 · **Air trapping due to central airways stenosis.** Expiratory HRCT in a lung transplant recipient with a stricture of the bronchus intermedius shows focal air trapping involving the right middle and lower lobes. A portion of the anterior right upper lobe shows a normal increase in attenuation on expiration. Air trapping that involves a segment, lobe, or lung suggests large airways disease.

FIGURE 6.20 · **Mosaic perfusion due to small airways disease.** Inspiratory HRCT shows very well-defined lobular regions of decreased lung attenuation (*arrows*) in a patient with constrictive bronchiolitis. A lobular distribution of mosaic perfusion or air trapping suggests small airways disease.

perfusion and air trapping are discussed in greater detail in Chapter 5.

Mosaic perfusion may be seen with both small and large airways disease but is more commonly seen with the former. Mosaic perfusion and air trapping in the setting of large airways disease are segmental or lobar in distribution (Fig. 6.19) or may involve an entire lung. Small airways disease typically demonstrates lobular regions of increased lung lucency (Fig. 6.20), although when abnormalities are extensive, larger regions of the lung may be involved (Fig. 6.21A, B).

HRCT Classification of Small Airways Disease

Pathologically small airways disease (i.e., bronchiolitis) is classified as *cellular bronchiolitis*, characterized by the presence of inflammation, and *constrictive bronchiolitis*, characterized by fibrotic obliteration of

bronchioles. The HRCT classification of small airways disease (i.e., bronchiolitis) is based on the recognition of specific findings, which correlate, to some extent, with these two pathologic categories.

Four major patterns of small airways disease are shown in Table 6.2. Recognition of one of these patterns allows for formulation of a focused differential diagnosis that may be further refined using clinical information.

Bronchiolitis with Centrilobular Nodules of Ground Glass Opacity

Pathologically, centrilobular nodules of GGO generally represent inflammation (or sometimes fibrosis) surrounding centrilobular bronchioles. This pattern generally indicates a cellular bronchiolitis. Impaction of bronchioles is typically absent. The nodules tend to be fairly homogeneous in size and may be diffuse or patchy in distribution (Fig. 6.22).

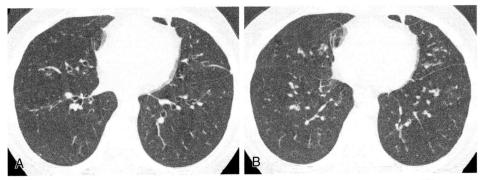

FIGURE 6.21 · Constrictive bronchiolitis. Rarely small airways disease may have a diffuse and uniform distribution. This is most typical of constrictive bronchiolitis. In such cases, inspiratory HRCT **(A)** shows diffusely increased lung lucency and attenuated vessels. Expiratory image **(B)** shows diffuse air trapping that may be difficult to distinguish from a poor expiratory effort.

TABLE 6.2	**HRCT patterns of small airways disease**

HRCT finding	Pathophysiology	Common diseases
Centrilobular nodules of ground glass opacity	Peribronchiolar inflammation or fibrosis	Hypersensitivity pneumonitis, respiratory bronchiolitis, follicular bronchiolitis, atypical infections, pneumoconioses
Centrilobular nodules of soft tissue attenuation	Bronchiolar impaction with spread into adjacent alveoli	Endobronchial infection, tumor, aspiration
Tree-in-bud opacities	Infectious mucoid impaction of bronchioles	Endobronchial infection, aspiration
Mosaic perfusion or air trapping	Bronchiolar narrowing or occlusion	Asthma, hypersensitivity pneumonitis, constrictive bronchiolitis

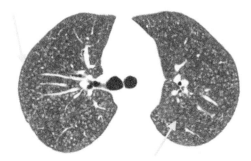

FIGURE 6.22 · Centrilobular nodules of ground glass attenuation. Symmetric, similar-sized nodules of ground glass opacity are present in a patient with subacute hypersensitivity pneumonitis. Note sparing of the subpleural regions (*arrows*) and even spacing of the nodules; this is typical of a centrilobular distribution of nodules.

The differential diagnosis of bronchiolitis with centrilobular GGO nodules (Table 6.3) includes hypersensitivity pneumonitis (HP), respiratory bronchiolitis (RB), follicular bronchiolitis (FB), pneumoconioses, and atypical infections. Langerhans cell histiocytosis (LCH), other infections, and endobronchial spread of tumor rarely present with centrilobular ground glass nodules as the predominant abnormality; soft-tissue attenuation nodules are more common.

Some patients with this pattern have a clinical history that suggests a specific diagnosis. HP, the most common cause of this pattern, has an identifiable exposure in 50% of patients. When an exposure is present, this HRCT pattern is considered diagnostic of HP. In smokers, RB is most likely. FB is seen in patients with connective tissue disease or immunocompromise. Patients with pneumoconiosis have a long-term exposure history. Patients with acute symptoms are most likely to have either an atypical infection or HP.

6

TABLE 6.3	Differential diagnosis of centrilobular nodules of ground glass opacity

Hypersensitivity pneumonitis
Respiratory bronchiolitis
Follicular bronchiolitis
Pneumoconioses
Atypical infections
Langerhans cell histiocytosis (usually soft tissue nodules)
Bacterial, mycobacterial infections (usually soft tissue nodules)
Endobronchial spread of tumor (usually soft tissue nodules)

TABLE 6.4	Differential diagnosis of centrilobular nodules of soft tissue attenuation

Endobronchial spread of infection (bacterial, mycobacterial, fungal)
Endobronchial spread of tumor (invasive mucinous adenocarcinoma)
Aspiration

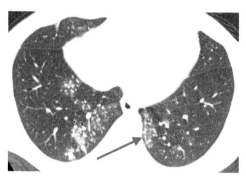

FIGURE 6.24 · **Bronchopneumonia with centrilobular nodules of soft tissue attenuation.** Nodules are patchy, asymmetric, and heterogeneous in size. Note that the nodules are separated from the pleural surface (*red arrow*). This appearance is typical of endobronchial spread with bronchiolar impaction such as in this patient with bacterial bronchopneumonia.

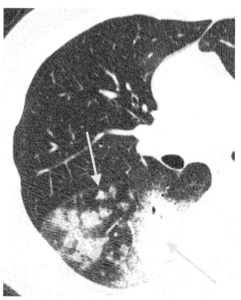

FIGURE 6.23 · **Centrilobular nodules of soft tissue attenuation in invasive mucinous adenocarcinoma.** The centrilobular distribution of nodules on this HRCT is indicated by relative sparing of the subpleural lung (*yellow arrow*). As the process extends outward from the centrilobular region, it may reach the pleural surface (*red arrow*). When adjacent lobules coalesce, confluent areas of consolidation may be present (*blue arrow*).

Bronchiolitis with Centrilobular Nodules of Soft Tissue Attenuation

Centrilobular nodules of soft tissue attenuation are generally a reflection of cellular bronchiolitis, with bronchiolar impaction and consolidation of peribronchiolar alveoli (Fig. 6.23). With progression, consolidation may involve entire pulmonary lobules, or multiple lobules. In this case, abnormalities may be segmental or subsegmental.

Centrilobular nodules of soft tissue attenuation tend to be patchy and heterogeneous in size. The differential diagnosis (Table 6.4) includes diseases that spread via the small airways (Fig. 6.24), including infections (bacterial, mycobacterial, fungal, and viral) and tumor (invasive mucinous adenocarcinoma [IMA]). Aspiration without pneumonia is also included in this category. Infection and aspiration typically present with acute symptoms, whereas tumor typically presents with chronic symptoms.

Bronchiolitis with TIB Opacities

On HRCT, TIB manifests as tubular, branching opacities with associated nodules (Fig. 6.25). Pathologically, this represents a cellular

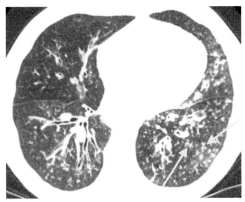

FIGURE 6.25 · **Tree-in-bud sign.** Several good examples of the tree-in-bud are visible, with branching, tubular opacities (*yellow arrows*) representing dilated and impacted bronchioles. This finding is highly specific for infection as in this case of bacterial bronchopneumonia. Patchy, bilateral centrilobular nodules of soft tissue attenuation are also present.

TABLE 6.5	Differential diagnosis of the tree-in-bud sign

Bacterial infection
Mycobacterial infection
Fungal infection
Viral infection
Cystic fibrosis
Allergic bronchopulmonary aspergillosis
Primary ciliary dyskinesia
Immunodeficiency
Diffuse panbronchiolitis
Follicular bronchiolitis
Invasive mucinous adenocarcinoma
Aspiration

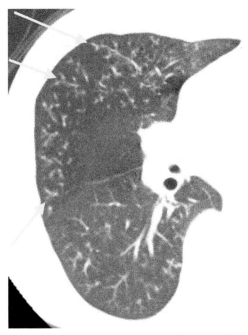

FIGURE 6.26 · **Diffuse panbronchiolitis with the tree-in-bud.** Centrilobular nodules and tree-in-bud opacities (*arrows*) are classic findings of diffuse panbronchiolitis. This disease is most common in Asian patients.

and ABPA (Fig. 6.27A, B). The etiology of diffuse panbronchiolitis is unclear, but it is likely that chronic infection plays a significant role. Noninfectious causes of airways disease rarely produce TIB; causes include FB, sarcoidosis, and IMA.

Bronchiolitis with Mosaic Perfusion or Air Trapping

Mosaic perfusion associated with airways disease reflects bronchiolar narrowing or occlusion and reflex vasoconstriction. It is a nonspecific finding and may be seen with any cause of small or large airways disease. In most cases, other findings (e.g., large airway abnormalities, centrilobular nodules, TIB) predominate. For instance, mosaic perfusion may be seen in patients with atypical mycobacterial infections, but in this disease, bronchiectasis, nodules, and TIB are usually the most significant findings (Fig. 6.28).

bronchiolitis. TIB is almost always (>90%) due to infection (Table 6.5) or aspiration, although it is not specific with regard to the type of infection present. TIB is most commonly seen with bacterial and mycobacterial infections; however, it may also be seen with fungal and viral infections.

Chronic causes of airways infection may demonstrate TIB; these include CF, ciliary disorders, and immunodeficiency. In such cases, large airways findings are also usually present (Fig. 6.12). Additional causes of TIB include diffuse panbronchiolitis (Fig. 6.26)

6

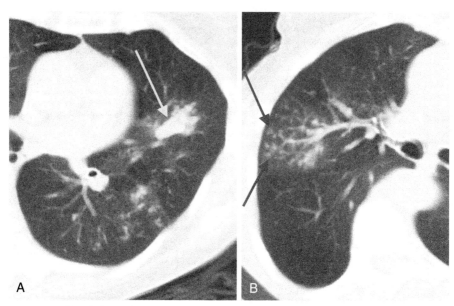

FIGURE 6.27 · **Allergic bronchopulmonary aspergillosis (ABPA). A.** ABPA is most commonly seen in asthmatics and in most cases large airways findings of bronchiectasis and bronchial impaction (*arrow*) predominate. **B.** Small airways abnormalities such as tree-in-bud opacities (*arrows*) may also be present.

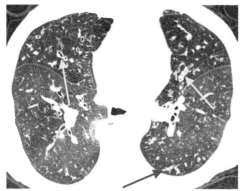

FIGURE 6.28 · **Mosaic perfusion associated with other findings of airways disease.** HRCT shows focal areas of decreased lung attenuation representing mosaic perfusion in a patient with atypical mycobacterial infection. However, other findings of airways disease are the predominant abnormality, including bronchiectasis (*yellow arrows*), bronchial wall thickening, and tree-in-bud opacities (*red arrow*). In this case, the mosaic perfusion should be ignored and diagnosis is driven by the other findings.

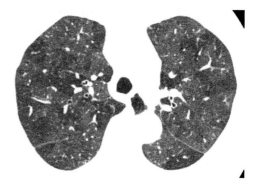

FIGURE 6.29 · **Mosaic perfusion as the predominant finding.** HRCT displayed with a narrow window accentuates the finding of bilateral mosaic perfusion in isolation. Note the patchy distribution suggesting small airways disease. This patient has constrictive bronchiolitis.

is quite limited and includes asthma, hypersensitivity pneumonia, and CB as common causes.

Specific Small Airways Diseases
Infections

Infections commonly involve the small airways and (infections are discussed in greater

When mosaic perfusion or air trapping is the only or predominant finding (Fig. 6.29), the differential diagnosis (Table 6.6)

TABLE 6.6	Differential diagnosis of isolated mosaic perfusion

Asthma
Hypersensitivity pneumonitis
Constrictive bronchiolitis
Vascular diseases (chronic pulmonary thrombo-
embolism, vasculitis)

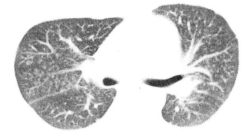

FIGURE 6.31 · **Viral infection with centrilobular nodules of ground glass opacity.** Although some overlap exists, atypical infections are more likely to produce centrilobular nodules of ground glass attenuation in comparison with bacterial, mycobacterial, and fungal infections. The density of these nodules reflects peribronchiolar inflammation without bronchiolar impaction.

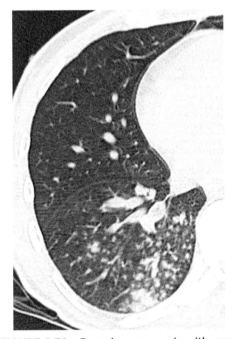

FIGURE 6.30 · **Bronchopneumonia with centrilobular nodules of soft tissue attenuation.** Focal centrilobular nodules of soft tissue attenuation are seen in the right lower lobe. Note the sparing of the subpleural regions and the heterogeneous size of the nodules. In the acute setting, these findings are suggestive of either infection or aspiration.

detail in Chapter 14). The HRCT manifestations of infection depend on the mechanism of spread.

Endobronchial spread of infection is characteristic of bacterial bronchopneumonia and mycobacterial and fungal infections. With endobronchial spread, a cellular bronchiolitis is the initial abnormality present, often appearing on HRCT as bronchiolar impaction with TIB; centrilobular nodules of soft tissue attenuation may also be seen (Fig. 6.30) as the infection spreads from the

bronchiole to alveoli adjacent to the center of the pulmonary lobule. Nodules of infection may enlarge until they involve the entire pulmonary lobule or multiple lobules. When consolidation in adjacent lobules coalesces, confluent areas of consolidation will develop. These findings are often associated with bronchiolar wall thickening and dilatation. The findings are typically unilateral or bilateral and asymmetric.

Peribronchiolar inflammation without bronchiolar impaction and TIB is characteristic of atypical infections. It is manifested by centrilobular nodules of GGO (Fig. 6.31). As the abnormality progresses, patchy areas of GGO and eventually consolidation will develop, representing more generalized areas of infection and diffuse alveolar damage. Bronchial/bronchiolar wall thickening and dilatation with mosaic perfusion/air trapping may be associated findings. The findings are typically bilateral and symmetric, although occasionally may be asymmetric or even unilateral.

Hypersensitivity Pneumonitis

HP is discussed in greater detail in Chapter 13. It represents a reaction to inhaled organic antigens. Airway abnormalities are most evident in the subacute stage of HP. Centrilobular nodules of GGO are characteristically visible on HRCT and represent peribronchiolar

6

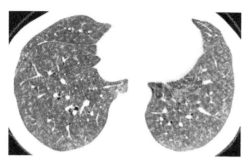

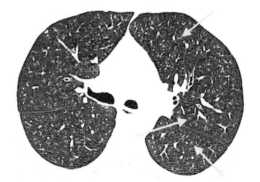

FIGURE 6.32 · **Hypersensitivity pneumonitis (HP) with centrilobular nodule of ground glass opacity (GGO).** When centrilobular nodules of GGO are present, HP is the most likely diagnosis. When there is a clear exposure, such as in this patient with an exposure to birds, the HRCT is considered diagnostic of HP.

FIGURE 6.33 · **Respiratory bronchiolitis with centrilobular nodules of ground glass opacity (GGO).** Centrilobular nodules of GGO (*arrows*) seen in smokers suggest respiratory bronchiolitis. Note the sparing of the subpleural regions.

inflammation and cellular infiltration. The centrilobular nodules are often diffuse or symmetric in distribution (Fig. 6.32), similar to the distribution of nodules in RB, FB, and atypical infections.

HP commonly presents with mosaic perfusion and/or air trapping due to bronchiolitis and bronchiolar narrowing. This finding may be seen in isolation or may be associated with nodules. When seen in isolation, the differential diagnosis includes CB and asthma. Air trapping and mosaic perfusion are also commonly present in association with fibrosis in patients with chronic HP. In fact, this combination is highly suggestive of HP.

Respiratory Bronchiolitis and Desquamative Interstitial Pneumonia

RB is a disease of cigarette smokers in which cellular infiltration and/or inflammation occurs around bronchioles as a reaction to smoke inhalation. This is discussed in greater detail in Chapter 11. The classic HRCT finding of RB is centrilobular nodules of GGO (Fig. 6.33), a finding that is shared with HP. RB may also show mosaic perfusion and/or air trapping; however, the severity of these findings is usually less than with HP.

Desquamative interstitial pneumonia (DIP), also a smoking-related disease, is closely

related to RB. RB and DIP, in fact, are thought to represent different points on a spectrum of the same pathologic process. Thus, HRCT features of both may coexist. When there is overlap, HRCT may demonstrate peripheral or generalized GGO with or without associated cysts or emphysema.

Follicular Bronchiolitis

FB is seen in patients with connective tissue disease or immunocompromise and is characterized by cellular bronchiolitis with lymphoid follicles. This is discussed in greater detail in Chapter 17. Similar to RB, the characteristic finding of FB is centrilobular nodules of GGO (Fig. 6.34). Also similar to RB, FB may have associated mosaic perfusion and/or air trapping; however, it is rarely as severe as in patients with HP. Lymphoid interstitial pneumonia is a more generalized lymphoproliferative disorder seen in the same groups of patients as FB. FB and lymphoid interstitial pneumonia are thought to represent different distributions or severity of the same disease; thus, radiographic overlap may be present as is the case for RB and DIP.

Invasive Pulmonary Mucinous Adenocarcinoma

The multifocal or diffuse type of IMA commonly involves small airways by endobronchial

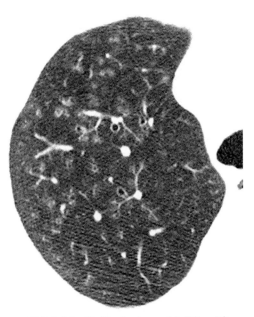

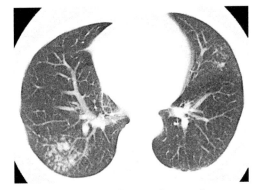

FIGURE 6.35 · Invasive mucinous adenocarcinoma with centrilobular nodules. Patchy bilateral centrilobular nodules are present. Note sparing of the subpleural lung and even spacing of the nodules. Many of the nodules are of soft tissue attenuation.

FIGURE 6.34 · Follicular bronchiolitis with centrilobular nodule of ground glass opacity (GGO). HRCT through the right upper lobe shows centrilobular nodules of GGO in a patient with follicular bronchiolitis associated with connective tissue disease.

spread. Spread of the tumor involves small airways and alveoli. IMA produces quantities of both mucin and fluid, which, in turn, result in bronchiolar impaction and alveolar consolidation. These appear on HRCT as centrilobular nodules of soft tissue attenuation or GGO. The tumor, which primarily spreads along alveolar walls, eventually can involve entire pulmonary lobules, producing confluent areas of consolidation (Fig. 6.35). This mechanism of spread shares features with infection; thus, significant radiographic overlap between these two entities is often present. IMA will be discussed in greater detail in Chapter 17.

Asthma

Asthma is characterized by recurrent or chronic airway hyperreactivity. The primary features of this disease include small airway inflammation and obstruction. The initial diagnosis is usually made in young patients (less than 40 years) with typical symptoms, physical-examination findings, and an obstructive defect on pulmonary function tests that is at least partially reversible. Patients with asthma are not commonly imaged because the diagnosis in most cases is straightforward, and symptoms in the majority of patients are well controlled on currently available therapies. The HRCT findings of asthma are typically mild and include bronchial wall thickening, mild bronchiectasis, and mosaic perfusion or air trapping (Fig. 6.36A, B). As mosaic perfusion and air trapping are often the predominant findings, the differential includes HP and CB.

Constrictive Bronchiolitis

CB is also known as obliterative bronchiolitis or bronchiolitis obliterans. Pathologically, CB is characterized by fibrosis of the bronchiolar wall and peribronchiolar tissues with bronchiolar obstruction.

There are multiple causes of CB, the most common of which is prior severe viral infection. Other etiologies include connective tissue disease, drug toxicity, toxic inhalations such as chlorine gas and smoke, graft-versus-host disease, chronic rejection in lung transplant recipients, and neuroendocrine hyperplasia (Table 6.7). The end result of these insults is irreversible obstruction of the small airways by fibrosis.

Fibrosis of the small airways cannot be directly visualized on HRCT. The secondary effects of airway obstruction are the primary

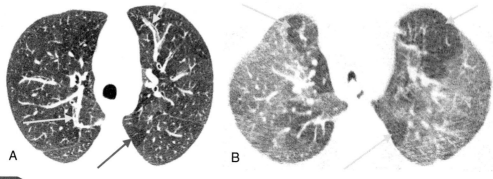

classic

FIGURE 6.36 · **Asthma: Classic appearance.** Inspiratory HRCT **(A)** shows mosaic perfusion (*red arrow*) and mild bronchial wall thickening (*yellow arrows*) as the predominant findings in this patient with asthma. Note air trapping (*blue arrows*) on the dynamic expiratory image **(B)** in the same distribution as the mosaic perfusion on inspiration.

TABLE 6.7	Cause of constrictive bronchiolitis

Postviral infection
Connective tissue disease
Drug toxicity
Toxic inhalations
Graft-versus-host disease
Chronic rejection in lung transplant recipients
Neuroendocrine hyperplasia

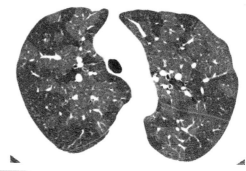

classic

FIGURE 6.37 · **Constrictive bronchiolitis: Classic appearance.** Constrictive bronchiolitis due to neuroendocrine hyperplasia. Inspiratory HRCT shows heterogeneous lung density with sharply demarcated regions of decreased lung attenuation compatible with mosaic perfusion. Note the lobular nature of these regions, highly suggestive of small airways disease.

HRCT findings of CB. These findings include mosaic perfusion and/or air trapping, which may be lobular or diffuse (Figs. 6.37 and 6.38). Bronchial wall thickening and bronchiectasis may be seen in severe, long-standing disease (Fig. 6.38C).

Although the large majority of cases are bilateral, unilateral CB with decreased lung volume and reduction in the size of pulmonary artery branches has been referred to as *Swyer–James syndrome.*

HP and asthma usually show a limited distribution of mosaic perfusion and air trapping; thus, when findings of mosaic perfusion or air trapping are extensive, CB is the favored diagnosis. Extensive lung involvement by CB may show a diffuse decrease in lung attenuation. Without any normal lung present, this finding may be difficult to recognize. Mosaic perfusion is best appreciated when it is contrasted against adjacent normal lung, but when normal lung is absent the finding may go unnoticed. Furthermore, diffuse air trapping on expiratory images may be difficult to differentiate from a poor expiratory effort (Fig. 6.39A, B). Correlation with pulmonary function tests may be helpful to confirm the presence of extensive small airways disease in questionable cases.

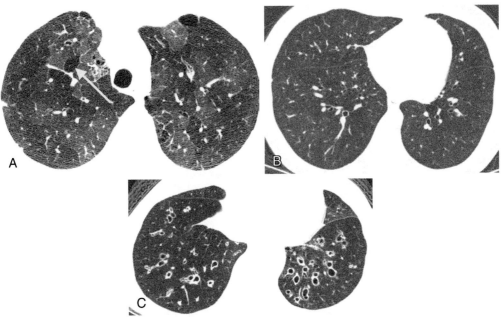

FIGURE 6.38 · Constrictive bronchiolitis: spectrum of lung abnormalities. A. Patchy lobular mosaic perfusion (*arrow*) is visible, representing constrictive bronchiolitis associated with connective tissue disease. Only minimal bronchiectasis is present **(B).** Diffuse lung involvement is seen in a lung transplant recipient with constrictive bronchiolitis associated with chronic rejection. Diffuse lung lucency is present. This may be difficult to distinguish from normal. **C.** Bronchiolitis obliterans due to rheumatoid arthritis. Diffuse lung lucency is associated with bronchiectasis and bronchial wall thickening.

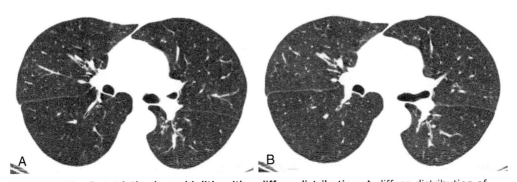

FIGURE 6.39 · Constrictive bronchiolitis with a diffuse distribution. A diffuse distribution of constrictive bronchiolitis appears as extensive lung lucency on inspiratory HRCT **(A).** Diagnosis of diffuse involvement may be challenging as there is no normal lung with which to compare the affected regions. Correlation with expiratory images **(B)**, showing no change in lung attenuation, and pulmonary function tests is helpful to confirm diffuse constrictive bronchiolitis.

FURTHER READING

Arakawa H, Webb WR. Air trapping on expiratory high-resolution CT scans in the absence of inspiratory scan abnormalities: correlation with pulmonary function tests and differential diagnosis. *AJR Am J Roentgenol.* 1998;170:1349-1353.

Cartier Y, Kavanagh PV, Johkoh T, et al. Bronchiectasis: accuracy of high-resolution CT in the differentiation of specific diseases. *AJR Am J Roentgenol.* 1999;173:47-52.

Im JG, Kim SH, Chung MJ, Koo JM, Han MC. Lobular low attenuation of the lung parenchyma on CT: evaluation of forty-eight patients. *J Comput Assist Tomogr.* 1996;20:756-762.

Kang EY, Miller RR, Müller NL. Bronchiectasis: comparison of preoperative thin-section CT and pathologic findings in resected specimens. *Radiology.* 1995;195:649-654.

Kang EY, Woo OH, Shin BK, et al. Bronchiolitis: classification, computed tomographic and histopathologic features, and radiologic approach. *J Comput Assist Tomogr.* 2009;33:32-41.

Lynch DA. Imaging of small airways disease. *Clin Chest Med.* 1993;14:623-634.

Lynch DA. Imaging of small airways disease and chronic obstructive pulmonary disease. *Clin Chest Med.* 2008;29:165-179.

McGuinness G, Naidich DP, Leitman BS, McCauley DI. Bronchiectasis: CT evaluation. *AJR Am J Roentgenol.* 1993;160:253-259.

Milliron B, Henry TS, Veeraraghavan S, Little BP. Bronchiectasis: mechanisms and imaging clues of associated common and uncommon diseases. *Radiographics.* 2015;35:1011-1030.

Müller NL, Miller RR. Diseases of the bronchioles: CT and histopathologic findings. *Radiology.* 1995;196:3-12.

O'Donnell AE. Bronchiectasis. *Chest.* 2008;134:815-823.

Padley SPG, Adler BD, Hansell DM, Müller NL. Bronchiolitis obliterans: high-resolution CT findings and correlation with pulmonary function tests. *Clin Radiol.* 1993;47:236-240.

Park CS, Müller NL, Worthy SA, et al. Airway obstruction in asthmatic and healthy individuals: inspiratory and expiratory thin-section CT findings. *Radiology.* 1997;203:361-367.

Shah RM, Sexauer W, Ostrum BJ, et al. High-resolution CT in the acute exacerbation of cystic fibrosis: evaluation of acute findings, reversibility of those findings, and clinical correlation. *AJR Am J Roentgenol.* 1997;169:375-380.

Ward S, Heyneman L, Lee MJ, et al. Accuracy of CT in the diagnosis of allergic bronchopulmonary aspergillosis in asthmatic patients. *AJR Am J Roentgenol.* 1999;173:937-942.

Winningham PJ, Martínez-Jiménez S, Rosado-de-Christenson ML, et al. Bronchiolitis: a practical approach for the general radiologist. *Radiographics.* 2017;37:777-794.

6

Pulmonary Vascular Diseases and Pulmonary Hemorrhage

Pulmonary vascular diseases may affect pulmonary arteries (PAs), veins, and/or capillaries. Large vessel abnormalities are primarily evaluated using modalities such as contrast-enhanced computed tomography (CT), magnetic resonance imaging (MRI), echocardiography, and conventional angiography. However, in selected cases, high-resolution computed tomography (HRCT) may provide insights not provided by other imaging studies. In particular, HRCT allows an accurate assessment of lung abnormalities, which may result in or are associated with pulmonary vascular disease and are helpful in the diagnosis of some pulmonary vasculitis syndromes and pulmonary hemorrhage.

PULMONARY HYPERTENSION

Pulmonary hypertension (PH) is defined as the presence of an elevated mean pulmonary arterial pressure ≥ 25 mm Hg. The most accurate method of determining this is right-sided heart catheterization. The 2013 Nice (France) classification divides PH into five categories (Table 7.1) based on similar pathophysiology. The term pulmonary arterial hypertension (PAH) is used in this classification to refer to PH resulting from diseases of the PAs.

HRCT Findings

PH may be associated with a variety of diseases that affect the lung parenchyma, PAs, pulmonary veins, and heart. While PA pressures cannot be directly estimated using HRCT, several CT findings may suggest the presence and relative severity of PH (Table 7.2).

Enlargement of the Main PA

Main PA diameter correlates with the presence or absence of PAH. This correlation is significantly more accurate in patients without parenchymal lung disease than in those with associated lung disease.

PA diameter should be measured perpendicular to the long axis of the vessel. Although the reported threshold of main PA diameter, above which PH can be said to be present, varies among studies, a diameter of 3.3 cm or more is relatively specific. As a method of quick assessment, the PA diameter should appear smaller than that of the adjacent aorta on the same slice (Fig. 7.1).

Increased Right Ventricular Size

Right ventricular (RV) size may be difficult to assess on HRCT images obtained without contrast injection; however, in many cases the location of the interventricular septum may be estimated even on noncontrast images (Fig. 7.2). The transverse diameter of the RV should be less than the left ventricle. PH is a common cause of RV enlargement.

Increased Size of the Right Atrium, Superior Vena Cava, and Inferior Vena Cava

In the setting of PH, the right atrium (Fig. 7.2), superior vena cava, and inferior vena cava are often enlarged owing to tricuspid regurgitation. The size of these structures can often be determined, even on noncontrast images. There are no specific size thresholds used to determine their dilatation, and enlargement is diagnosed based on reader experience. Keep in mind that these signs of PH are nonspecific.

TABLE 7.1	2013 Nice classification of pulmonary hypertension (PH)

Category	Description	Causes
1	Pulmonary arterial hypertension (PAH)	Idiopathic PAH; heritable PAH; drug and toxin induced; associated with connective tissue disease, HIV infection, portal hypertension, congenital heart disease, or schistosomiasis
1′	Pulmonary veno-occlusive disease and/or pulmonary capillary hemangiomatosis	
2	PH due to left-sided heart disease	Systolic or diastolic dysfunction; valvular heart disease
3	PH due to lung diseases and/or hypoxia	Chronic obstructive pulmonary disorders; interstitial lung disease; mixed restrictive and obstructive disease; sleep-disordered breathing (e.g., obstructive sleep apnea); alveolar hypoventilation syndromes; high altitude; developmental
4	Chronic thromboembolic PH	
5	PH with unclear or multifactorial mechanisms	Hematologic disorders; systemic diseases (e.g., sarcoidosis, Langehans cell histiocytosis, lymphangioleiomyomatosis); metabolic disorders; obstruction (e.g., neoplasm, fibrosing mediastinitis)

Modified from Simonneau G, Gatzoulis MA, Adatia I, et al. Updated clinical classification of pulmonary hypertension. *J Am Coll Cardiol.* 2013;62(suppl 25):D34-D41.

TABLE 7.2	HRCT findings that may be associated with pulmonary hypertension

Enlargement of the main pulmonary artery
Increased right ventricular size
Increased right atrial size
Increased size of superior/inferior vena cava
Mosaic perfusion
Centrilobular nodules

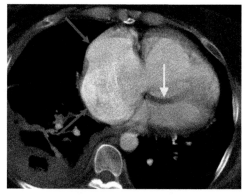

FIGURE 7.2 · **Right ventricular and right atrial enlargement.** The diameters of the right ventricle and right atrium (*red arrows*) are enlarged in a patient with pulmonary hypertension due to chronic pulmonary thromboembolism. Bowing of the interventricular septum toward the left ventricle (*yellow arrow*) is also seen.

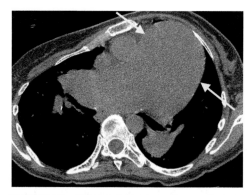

FIGURE 7.1 · **Main pulmonary artery enlargement.** There is marked dilatation of the main pulmonary artery (*arrows*) in a patient with idiopathic pulmonary arterial hypertension.

Mosaic Perfusion

Heterogeneous lung attenuation due to regional differences in blood flow is termed "mosaic perfusion"; reduced blood flow in specific lung regions results in decreased lung attenuation on CT. *Mosaic perfusion* is characterized by decreased vascular size in areas of reduced lung density. It is most common in association with small airway disease but may also be seen with vascular diseases and in the setting of PH.

The term "mosaic attenuation" is less specific, referring only to regional or geographic differences in lung density without

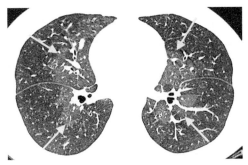

FIGURE 7.3 · **Mosaic perfusion.** Heterogeneous lung attenuation is present with peripheral lung appearing decreased in attenuation and central lung regions (*arrows*) appearing to be of increased attenuation. In this case, the lower attenuation lung is abnormal, resulting from decreased perfusion due to vasculitis.

a consideration of vascular size or etiology. *Mosaic attenuation* may be due to lung diseases associated with patchy ground glass opacity, airway disease, or vascular disease with mosaic perfusion (see Chapters 5 and 6). In patients with vascular disease associated with PH, mosaic perfusion is most common with chronic pulmonary thromboembolic embolism (CPTE).

The morphology of the mosaic perfusion may help to distinguish CPTE from airways obstruction. CPTE usually results in large, segmental, lobar, or peripheral regions of decreased lung attenuation (Fig. 7.3). Small airways disease typically shows smaller, patchy, and, in particular, lobular areas of decreased attenuation.

Centrilobular Nodules

The distal PAs are centrilobular in location, and diseases that affect the pulmonary arterial system may be associated with centrilobular nodules. Centrilobular nodules resulting from a vascular etiology are often of ground glass opacity (Fig. 7.4). These may be seen in association with PAH of any cause, but they are most common with idiopathic pulmonary arterial hypertension (IPAH), capillary hemangiomatosis, pulmonary veno-occlusive disease (PVOD), and various other causes of vasculitis. They often reflect the presence of pulmonary edema or hemorrhage, or cholesterol

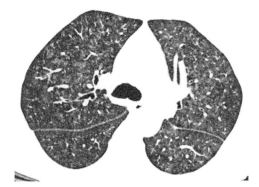

FIGURE 7.4 · **Centrilobular nodules of ground glass opacity in pulmonary hypertension.** Ill-defined centrilobular ground glass opacity nodules are often seen in primary and secondary causes of pulmonary hypertension. They may represent focal areas of edema, hemorrhage, or cholesterol granuloma formation.

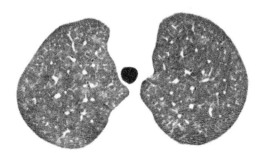

FIGURE 7.5 · **Centrilobular nodules of ground glass opacity.** The nodules in this patient represented pulmonary hemorrhage due to systemic lupus erythematosus. Nodules of this type commonly have causes other than pulmonary hypertension. These include edema and hemorrhage unrelated to pulmonary vascular disease, hypersensitivity pneumonitis, and respiratory bronchiolitis.

granulomas, which are an indication of previous hemorrhage.

Centrilobular nodules are not specific for vascular disease and are more commonly associated with pulmonary edema, pulmonary hemorrhage (Fig. 7.5), airway diseases such as hypersensitivity pneumonitis, and infections.

Diseases Associated with PH

The differential diagnosis of PH is broad (Table 7.1). HRCT may be obtained in the diagnostic evaluation of a patient with PH of unknown cause. In this setting, its major

7

TABLE 7.3	Causes of pulmonary hypertension that may be associated with findings suggestive of a specific diagnosis
Disease	**HRCT finding**
Parenchymal lung disease	Fibrosis, emphysema, or cystic lung disease
Chronic pulmonary thromboembolism	Pulmonary artery filling defects or occlusion; mosaic perfusion
Idiopathic pulmonary arterial hypertension	Dilated main pulmonary artery; centrilobular nodules of ground glass opacity
Pulmonary veno-occlusive disease	Smooth interlobular septal thickening; dilated main pulmonary artery; normal-sized pulmonary veins
Pulmonary capillary hemangiomatosis	Centrilobular nodules of ground glass opacity; progression of findings after treatment with vasodilators
Intravenous injection of oral medications	Diffuse, small, homogeneous, branching centrilobular nodules
Sickle cell disease	Dense bones, rugger jersey spine
Liver disease	Small, nodular liver
Left-sided heart disease	Left atrial or ventricular dilatation; smooth interlobular septal thickening (pulmonary edema)

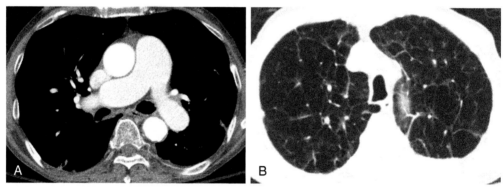

FIGURE 7.6 · Pulmonary hypertension due to emphysema. A. The main pulmonary artery is enlarged in this patient with pulmonary hypertension. **B.** On lung windows, extensive centrilobular emphysema is visible.

role is in the detection of diffuse lung disease (category 3), primarily emphysema and lung fibrosis, which may be associated with PH. HRCT may also be used to evaluate for interlobular septal thickening or centrilobular ground glass nodules associated with PVOD or capillary hemangiomatosis (category 1'). Contrast-enhanced CT may also be obtained to evaluate for chronic pulmonary thromboembolism (category 4).

There are many causes of PH that are not well evaluated using HRCT. These include systolic or diastolic left ventricular dysfunction, valvular heart disease, cardiovascular shunts, hypoventilation disorders, and sleep disorders. The discussion of specific diseases associated with PH will be restricted to those

that commonly show lung abnormalities on HRCT (Table 7.3).

Parenchymal Lung Disease

PH may result from parenchymal lung disease because of hypoxia (with vasoconstriction) or obliteration of the pulmonary capillary bed. The most common lung parenchymal processes to result in PH are emphysema (Fig. 7.6A, B) and diffuse lung fibrosis (Fig. 7.7A, B). Cystic lung disease is a rare cause of PH.

Lung fibrosis causing PH is most commonly due to idiopathic pulmonary fibrosis, connective tissue disease, or sarcoidosis. Chronic airways disease, such as cystic fibrosis, and cystic lung disease, such as

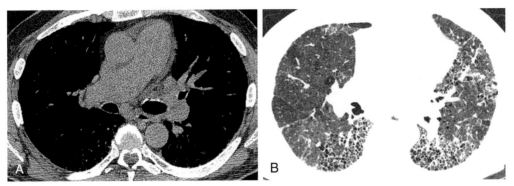

FIGURE 7.7 · **Pulmonary hypertension associated with lung fibrosis.** Mild main pulmonary artery enlargement **(A)** is associated with fibrosis **(B)** in this patient with idiopathic pulmonary fibrosis.

lymphangioleiomyomatosis or Langerhans cell histiocytosis, may also be associated with PH. As lung disease associated with PH is typically extensive, it should be evident on HRCT. The lack of significant abnormality on HRCT makes a lung etiology of PH unlikely. In general, the severity of lung disease correlates with the degree of PH.

Sarcoidosis and connective tissue disease–related interstitial lung disease (Fig. 7.8A–C) may show PH out of proportion to the extent of lung disease. In these cases, vasculitis, thrombosis, stenosis, or occlusion of small PAs likely contribute. Of note, in the presence of lung disease, there is a poor correlation between main PA diameter and the severity of PH. This is in contrast to IPAH and other diseases without significant lung manifestations in which pulmonary arterial diameter shows better correlation with the presence and severity of PH.

Chronic Pulmonary Thromboembolism

The diagnosis of CPTE may be challenging. Patients present with nonspecific symptoms, and initial objective examinations, such as pulmonary function tests, are nonspecific. Contrast-enhanced CT pulmonary angiography, although effective in the setting of acute pulmonary thromboembolism, has limited sensitivity in the diagnosis of CPTE.

Despite this fact, contrast-enhanced CT is often obtained in the evaluation of suspected CPTE. Findings that may be seen include eccentric filling defects in PAs with or without calcification, artery wall thickening, and PA webs. Enlargement of the main PA,

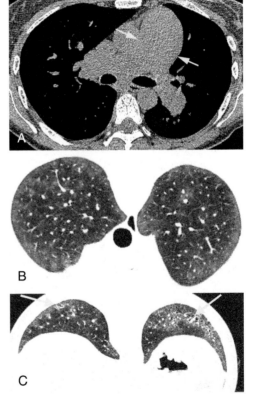

FIGURE 7.8 · **Pulmonary hypertension in connective tissue disease.** This patient with scleroderma and pulmonary hypertension shows enlargement of the main pulmonary artery (*arrow*) **(A)**. A prone scan through the upper lobes **(B)** shows lobular areas of ground glass opacity, perhaps pulmonary edema or hemorrhage related to pulmonary hypertension. In the lower lobes **(C)**, mild fibrosis is present (*arrows*); it is too mild to explain the pulmonary hypertension. This patient likely has vasculitis contributing to pulmonary hypertension.

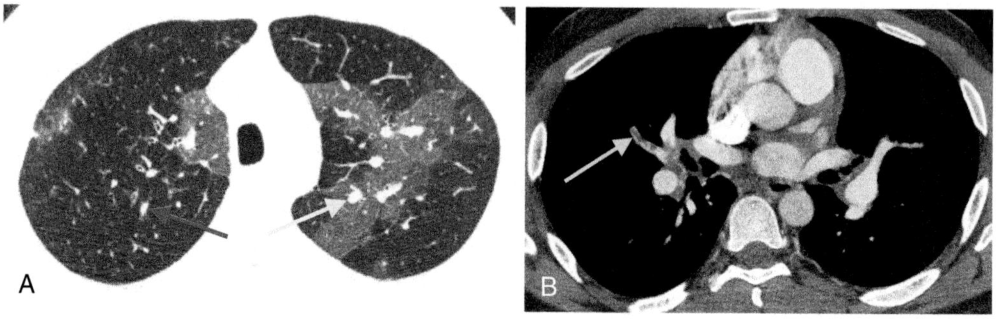

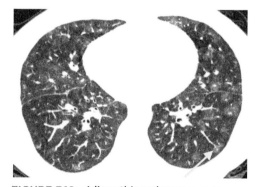

classic

FIGURE 7.9 · Chronic pulmonary thromboembolism: Classic appearance. A. Mosaic perfusion is present with lucent regions of lung reflecting decreased perfusion. Note that the vessels are significantly larger in areas of normal lung (*yellow arrow*) than in lucent lung regions (*red arrow*). **B.** CT with contrast shows irregular filling defects in pulmonary artery branches (*blue arrow*).

RV, and right atrium are common findings. Narrowing of the distal pulmonary arterial branches and bronchial artery enlargement may also be seen.

The principal lung parenchymal finding of CPTE is mosaic perfusion due to vascular stenoses and/or occlusions. Mosaic perfusion tends to be more severe in CPTE than in other causes of PAH. The distribution of mosaic perfusion is peripheral and usually affects larger geographic areas of lung as compared with airways disease (Fig. 7.9A, B). Lobular areas of decreased lung attenuation are not typical.

Idiopathic Pulmonary Arterial Hypertension

IPAH is a disease that typically affects young females with a peak onset of 30 to 40 years of age. It is a diagnosis of exclusion but occurs in an age-group in which other causes of PAH are uncommon. Plexogenic arteriopathy, a disordered proliferation of capillary-like vessels, is the typical histologic abnormality in these patients, although it may also be seen with other causes of PAH.

Enlargement of the main PA is a common finding in IPAH and is seen in more than 90% of patients with this disease. Centrilobular nodules of ground glass opacity may be present (Fig. 7.10). These may represent focal hemorrhage or edema, cholesterol granulomas, or perhaps plexogenic lesions. When present in this clinical setting, centrilobular nodules should be assumed to be related to the PAH

FIGURE 7.10 · Idiopathic pulmonary arterial hypertension. Centrilobular nodules of ground glass opacity (*arrow*) are seen in a patient with pulmonary arterial hypertension. These nodules may be seen with both primary and secondary causes of pulmonary hypertension and often reflect edema or hemorrhage.

and not due to an alternative disease such as hypersensitivity pneumonitis.

Other findings that may be seen in IPAH include mosaic perfusion, interlobular septal thickening, and air trapping. These are typically mild in severity and not useful in diagnosis. Significant mosaic perfusion, in particular, is atypical for IPAH and suggests an alternative disease, particularly pulmonary thromboembolic disease.

Pulmonary Veno-Occlusive Disease

PVOD is a rare cause of PAH characterized by idiopathic obliteration of the pulmonary venules, which leads to pulmonary edema,

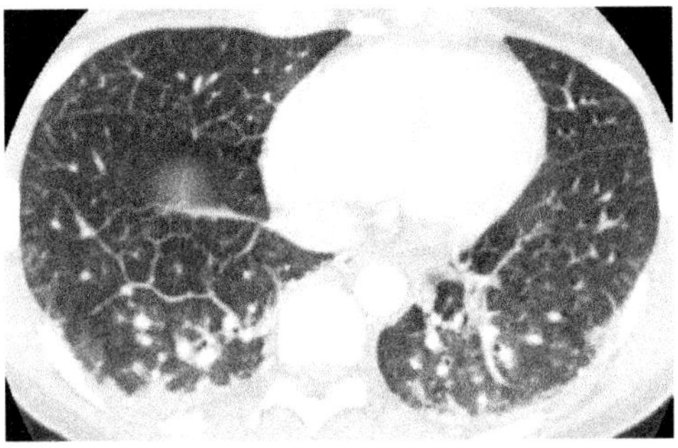

FIGURE 7.11 · **Pulmonary veno-occlusive disease.** Smooth interlobular septal thickening is present in a patient with pulmonary veno-occlusive disease (PVOD). This finding represents pulmonary edema and in a patient with pulmonary hypertension without left-sided heart disease suggests PVOD.

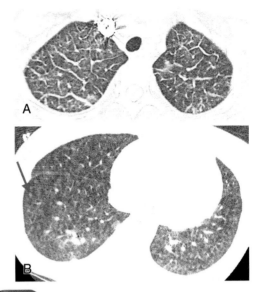

A

B

classic

FIGURE 7.12 · **Pulmonary veno-occlusive disease: Classic appearance. A.** Smooth interlobular septal thickening is present in a patient with pulmonary veno-occlusive disease (PVOD). **B.** After treatment, the septal thickening resolved and centrilobular nodules of ground glass opacity were evident (*arrow*). This represents an overlap of PVOD and capillary hemangiomatosis.

hemorrhage, and/or venous infarcts proximal to the level of obstruction. This disease is seen in patients of various ages but most commonly presents in children and young adults. It portends a poor prognosis with an average survival of 2 years after presentation. Clinically PVOD closely mimics IPAH, and in some cases, HRCT may be the only examination to suggest the correct diagnosis. This distinction is clinically important, as some patients with PVOD worsen clinically with vasodilatory therapy.

The most characteristic finding of PVOD is smooth interlobular septal thickening (Fig. 7.11), resembling pulmonary edema from heart failure. This finding is suggestive of PVOD in patients with known PAH and no evidence of left-sided heart disease. Ground glass opacity may also be present in a diffuse, patchy, or lobular distribution. Centrilobular nodules of ground glass opacity can also be seen and may reflect the overlap between this disease and capillary hemangiomatosis (Fig. 7.12A, B). Supportive findings include enlargement of the main PA and normal-sized or small pulmonary veins.

Pulmonary Capillary Hemangiomatosis

Pulmonary capillary hemangiomatosis (PCH) is a rare cause of PAH characterized by an idiopathic proliferation of capillaries within the alveolar walls. It has a similar demographic to PVOD. In fact, PCH and PVOD

are likely a spectrum of the same disease, as there is significant overlap of these entities both clinically and pathologically. As with PVOD, PCH is often confused clinically with IPAH. As with PVOD, symptoms may worsen after the initiation of vasodilatory therapy.

The most characteristic HRCT finding of PCH is centrilobular nodules of ground glass opacity (Fig. 7.13A, B). These resemble the nodules seen in IPAH, and it is unclear if HRCT is able to make a distinction between these two entities. Other findings include ground glass opacity, pleural effusions, and lymphadenopathy. The presence of smooth interlobular septal thickening may also be seen and likely represents an overlap with PVOD.

Intravenous Injection of Oral Medications

Oral medications contain binders, such as talc or cellulose, that are not absorbed through the gastrointestinal tract. When these medications

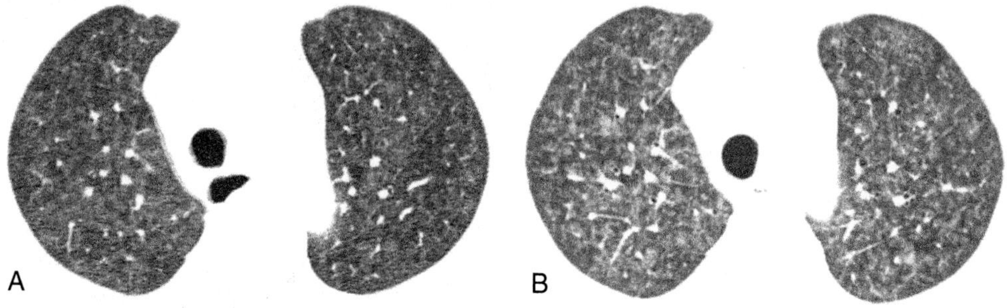

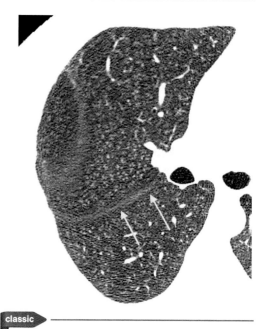

classic

FIGURE 7.13 · **Capillary hemangiomatosis: Classic appearance. A.** Centrilobular nodules of ground glass opacity are seen in a patient with pulmonary arterial hypertension. **B.** After the initiation of vasodilator therapy, the patient clinically worsened and the nodules became larger and denser.

are injected intravenously, the binders may embolize to the lungs and deposit in small pulmonary arterial branches. Over time, these may induce an inflammatory lung response that causes vascular and lung fibrosis. While this entity is commonly called *talcosis*, talc is but one of many materials contained in oral medications that may cause this disease. Alternative names for this entity include injection granulomatosis and excipient lung disease.

Centrilobular nodules or branching structures are the earliest HRCT manifestations of the intravenous injection of oral medications. These may resemble tree-in-bud opacities (Fig. 7.14). In contrast to infectious causes of tree-in-bud, the nodules or branching opacities are diffuse in distribution, small, and not associated with significant consolidation. Diffuse or symmetric ground glass opacity may also be present, but this finding is nonspecific. Over time, fibrosis may develop in areas affected by nodules. This fibrosis may progress even after the cessation of injection. When fibrosis occurs, irregular reticulation, traction bronchiectasis, and progressive massive fibrosis are seen.

Panlobular emphysema is another manifestation of the intravenous injection of oral medications. This is most closely associated with the intravenous injection of oral methylphenidate (Ritalin). HRCT shows a diffuse increase in lung lucency and attenuated vessels with a basilar predominance.

classic

FIGURE 7.14 · **Talcosis: Classic appearance.** Diffuse, small centrilobular nodules are noted. Note sparing of the subpleural lung (*yellow arrows*) reflecting their centrilobular distribution. Some of the centrilobular opacities have a branching appearance (*red arrow*). These are due to injected material embolized in small pulmonary arterial branches and an associated inflammatory reaction and fibrosis.

Miscellaneous Diseases

There are many other causes of PH including familial PAH, left-sided heart disease, hypoxemia without parenchymal lung disease, vasculitis, liver disease, human immunodeficiency

TABLE 7.4	Classification of pulmonary vasculitides and their most common HRCT findings

Size of vessels involved	Associated diseases	HRCT findings
Large	Takayasu arteritis	Pulmonary artery wall thickening, thrombosis, stenosis, or obstruction Infarcts Mosaic perfusion
	Giant cell arteritis	Same as Takayasu arteritis
	Behçet's disease	Pulmonary artery aneurysms Hemorrhage
Medium	Polyarteritis nodosa	Hemorrhage
	Kawasaki disease	Pulmonary involvement rare
Small	Granulomatosis with polyangiitis (Wegener's granulomatosis)	Nodules often with cavitation Hemorrhage Patchy consolidation
	Eosinophilic granulomatosis with polyangiitis (Churg–Strauss granulomatosis)	Peripheral/lobular consolidation or ground glass opacity Nodules often without cavitation Bronchial wall thickening Interlobular septal thickening
	Microscopic polyangiitis	Hemorrhage

virus, congenital systemic to pulmonary shunts, drugs, sickle cell anemia, and other rare congenital disorders. In most cases, lung findings are either absent or nonspecific, and making a correct diagnosis depends on the clinical history. There may be extrapulmonary findings that suggest a specific diagnosis, such as dense bones in patients with sickle cell disease. Findings suggestive of the appropriate diagnosis may be outside the chest, such as a cirrhotic liver. Left-sided heart disease may be accompanied by chamber dilatation or evidence of pulmonary edema such as smooth interlobular septal thickening.

VASCULITIS

The term vasculitis refers to a group of systemic disorders that cause inflammation of vessel walls and may eventually lead to vessel dilatation, stenosis, or hemorrhage. Some vasculitis syndromes have pulmonary manifestations.

Vasculitis is classified by the size of vessels involved: large, medium, or small (Table 7.4). Large vessel vasculitis syndromes include giant cell arteritis, Takayasu arteritis, and Behçet's disease. Medium vessel vasculitis includes polyarteritis nodosa and Kawasaki disease. Small vessel vasculitis includes granulomatosis with polyangiitis (GPA; also termed

Wegener's granulomatosis), eosinophilic granulomatosis with polyangiitis (EGPA; also termed Churg–Strauss granulomatosis), and microscopic polyangiitis.

HRCT Findings

In patients with pulmonary vasculitis, HRCT may show abnormalities of PAs or lung parenchyma. In general, large vessel vasculitis shows predominant involvement of the PAs and their branches, while small vessel vasculitis shows predominant pulmonary parenchymal involvement. Medium vessel vasculitis only rarely affects the PAs or lungs.

Pulmonary arterial involvement may be manifested by stenosis, dilatation, thrombosis, or aneurysm. PA dilatation and aneurysm may eventually lead to rupture and hemorrhage. When stenosis predominates, mosaic perfusion may be present, reflecting regional decreases in blood flow.

Parenchymal manifestations of vasculitis include pulmonary hemorrhage, infarcts, and/or inflammation. Pulmonary hemorrhage results in ground glass opacity or consolidation that is often diffuse but may, in selected cases, be focal, patchy, or centrilobular. Infarcts and inflammation may appear on HRCT as

7

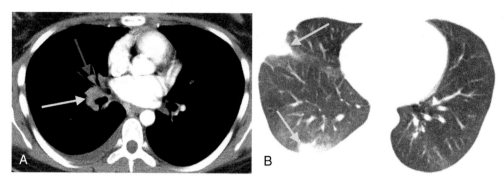

FIGURE 7.15 • **Takayasu arteritis. A.** Postcontrast CT shows occlusion of the right lower lobe (*yellow arrow*) and right middle lobe (*red arrow*) pulmonary arteries. **B.** Lung windows show infarcts (*blue arrows*) in the affected lobes.

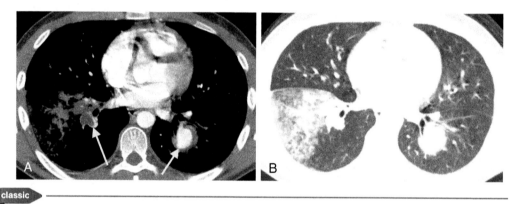

classic

FIGURE 7.16 • **Behçet's disease: Classic appearance. A.** Postcontrast CT shows pulmonary artery aneurysms (*arrows*) with both peripheral and central thrombus. **B.** Lung window ground glass opacity around the aneurysm in the right lower lobe from acute hemorrhage.

nodules with or without cavitation. These nodules vary in size from less than 1 to 10 cm or more. Consolidation may also be present.

The vasculitis syndromes that most commonly present with pulmonary manifestations are discussed below.

Specific Vasculitis Syndromes
Giant Cell and Takayasu Arteritis

These are both large vessel vasculitides that predominantly affect the large systemic thoracic arteries, including branches of the aorta and carotid arteries. Takayasu arteritis typically affects women under the age of 40 years, whereas giant cell arteritis affects patients over the age of 40 years. Involvement of PAs may result in wall thickening, thrombosis, stenosis, or obstruction (Fig. 7.15A, B). Associated mosaic perfusion or infarcts may also be present. Pulmonary arterial

aneurysms are less common and likely due to poststenotic dilatation.

Behçet's Disease

Behçet's disease is a rare disorder characterized by deposition of immune complexes in vessel walls. It presents clinically with oral aphthous ulcers, genital ulcers, uveitis, and skin lesions. It typically occurs in young adults of Turkish or Japanese descent.

Behçet's disease shows a predilection for pulmonary arterial involvement and is characterized by PA aneurysms that may rupture and produce hemorrhage (Fig. 7.16A, B). PA thrombosis and thrombosis of thoracic veins (i.e., superior vena cava and brachiocephalic veins) also occur. Pulmonary hemorrhage may occur because of small vessel abnormalities.

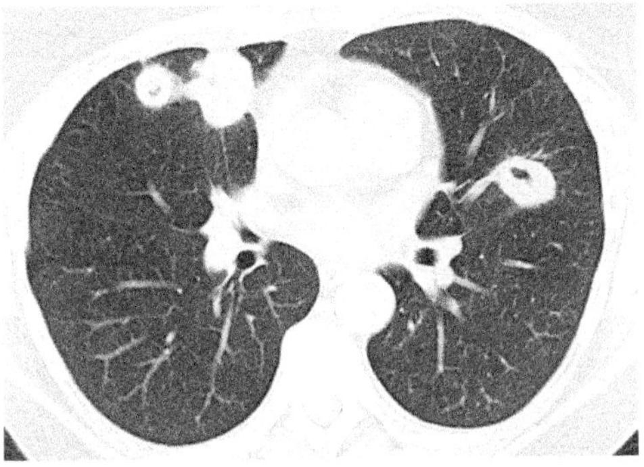

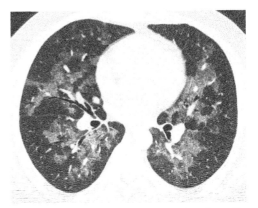

classic ▶

FIGURE 7.17 · **Granulomatosis with polyangiitis: Classic appearance.** Several nodules are seen, ranging from 1 to 3 cm in size. Early cavitation is present in two of the nodules. This is the most common manifestation of Wegener's granulomatosis.

FIGURE 7.18 · **Granulomatosis with polyangiitis.** Symmetric bilateral ground glass opacity is seen as a manifestation of pulmonary hemorrhage in a patient presenting with hemoptysis.

Hughes–Stovin syndrome is likely a forme fruste of Behçet's disease, in which PA aneurysms and systemic venous thrombosis predominate, but the other clinical manifestations of Behçet's disease are absent. Pulmonary hemorrhage may also occur because of small vessel abnormalities.

Granulomatosis with Polyangiitis (Wegener's Granulomatosis)

GPA, formerly termed Wegener's granulomatosis, is the most common vasculitis to show pulmonary parenchymal manifestations. The most frequently affected organs include the upper respiratory tract, lungs, and kidneys. Serum cystoplasmic antineutrophilic cytoplasmic antibody (C-ANCA) titers are elevated in up to 90% of patients.

The most common HRCT manifestation of GPA is pulmonary nodules, representing a combination of infarcts and inflammation. These are variable in size from less than 1 cm to large masses. The number of nodules and masses vary widely; however, innumerable nodules, as are often seen with hematogenous spread of infection or metastases, are rare in GPA. They have a variable distribution but are usually bilateral. Cavitation is common, particularly with larger nodules (Fig. 7.17).

Ground glass opacity may also be seen in patients with GPA, representing pulmonary hemorrhage (Fig. 7.18). The ground

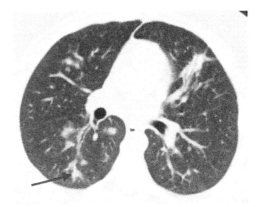

FIGURE 7.19 · **Granulomatosis with polyangiitis.** Patchy, bilateral, peribronchovascular consolidation (arrows) is present. Pathologically these abnormalities corresponded to areas of organizing pneumonia. This is a rare manifestation of Wegener's granulomatosis.

glass opacity may be focal, patchy, or diffuse. Consolidation is a less frequent finding and may be a manifestation of inflammation, hemorrhage, or organizing pneumonia (OP). OP is not uncommonly seen pathologically in association with GPA. When consolidation is due to OP, it is often peribronchovascular and subpleural (Fig. 7.19).

Eosinophilic Granulomatosis with Polyangiitis (Churg–Strauss Syndrome)

EGPA, previously known as Churg–Strauss syndrome, is a necrotizing vasculitis of small to medium size vessels with eosinophilic and granulomatous inflammation. In 50 to 75% of patients, it is associated with ANCA, usually P-ANCA (perinuclear pattern).

EGPA is characterized by asthma, hypereosinophilia, and necrotizing vasculitis. EGPA often shows findings of simple pulmonary eosinophilia or chronic eosinophilic pneumonia (i.e., peripheral areas of consolidation or ground glass opacity that are often lobular in distribution), pulmonary nodules or masses (20%), bronchial wall thickening or bronchiectasis (35%), and pulmonary edema (5%) associated with cardiac involvement. Although cavitation of nodules or masses may occur, it is much less common than with GPA. EGPA is also discussed in Chapter 13.

Microscopic Polyangiitis

Microscopic polyangiitis is a systemic small vessel vasculitis that occurs in middle-aged men. It commonly affects the kidneys, but lung involvement may be seen in up to 30% of patients. Its most common lung manifestation is that of pulmonary hemorrhage. Ground glass opacity and/or consolidation may be present in a variable distribution, similar to Wegener's granulomatosis.

PULMONARY HEMORRHAGE

Pulmonary hemorrhage may be diffuse or focal. Focal pulmonary hemorrhage is usually due to localized lung abnormalities, and an identifiable cause may be visualized. Diffuse pulmonary hemorrhage is often due to systemic processes, including a number of the vasculitis syndromes described above, and making a specific diagnosis based on HRCT findings may be challenging. As the HRCT findings overlap significantly with those of other diseases, correlation with the patient's clinical symptoms is important. Patients with pulmonary hemorrhage may present with hemoptysis, but this is not always the case.

Focal Pulmonary Hemorrhage

Findings of focal hemorrhage include consolidation, ground glass opacity, and centrilobular nodules. Sometimes, associated HRCT abnormalities may lead to the correct diagnosis (Fig. 7.20). Examples of diagnosable causes of focal hemorrhage include bronchiectasis,

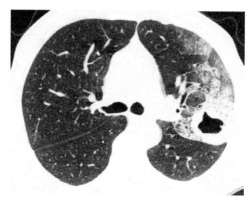

FIGURE 7.20 · Focal pulmonary hemorrhage. HRCT may be used to identify a source of bleeding in patients with hemoptysis. Focal ground glass opacity and consolidation are present in the left upper lobe surrounding a cavitary bronchogenic carcinoma.

TABLE 7.5	Causes of diffuse alveolar hemorrhage

With capillaritis
  Vasculitis
  Goodpasture syndrome
  Henoch–Schönlein purpura
  Collagen vascular disease
  Cryoglobulinemia
  Antiphospholipid syndrome
  IgA nephropathy
Without capillaritis
  Idiopathic pulmonary hemosiderosis
  Diffuse alveolar damage
  Elevated pulmonary venous pressure
  Anticoagulation
  Coagulation disorders and thromocytopenia
  Inhalation injury, toxic exposures
  Drug-associated disease (e.g., chemotherapy)
  Illicit drug use (particularly cocaine smoking)

malignancy, trauma, pneumonia, cavitary lung disease, mycetoma, and thromboembolic disease. HRCT may also be useful in localizing the approximate site of hemorrhage before angiography or bronchoscopy. Volumetric HRCT is optimal in this setting.

Diffuse Alveolar Hemorrhage (DAH)

Diffuse alveolar hemorrhage (DAH) is rare and most commonly secondary to systemic disorders or conditions (Table 7.5). In many cases, diffuse hemorrhage may be the only lung manifestation of disease, and findings that suggest a specific diagnosis are absent.

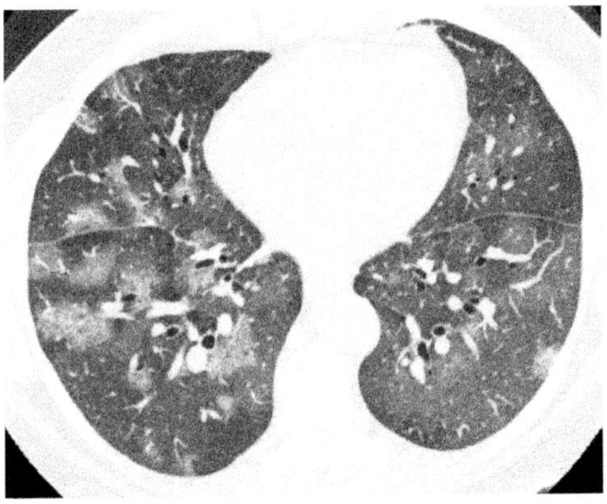

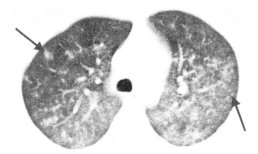

classic

FIGURE 7.21 · **Diffuse pulmonary hemorrhage: Classic appearance.** Patchy bilateral ground glass opacity is seen as a manifestation of diffuse pulmonary hemorrhage in a patient with systemic lupus erythematosus.

FIGURE 7.22 · **Pulmonary hemorrhage with centrilobular nodules.** Nodules of ground glass opacity (*arrows*) may be a manifestation of pulmonary hemorrhage and are often associated with more generalized ground glass opacity. The centrilobular distribution may reflect bleeding around the centrilobular artery or blood spreading via the airways.

In some patients, DAH results from capillaritis, with inflammation of pulmonary capillaries and alveolar interstitium, disruption of the epithelial–endothelial basement membrane, and leakage of red blood cells into the alveolar spaces. Capillaritis may be associated with vasculitis, involving small vessels (e.g., Behçet's disease, GPA, microscopic polyangiitis) or may result from circulating immune complexes (e.g., Goodpasture syndrome, Henoch–Schönlein purpura, collagen vascular disease, mixed cryoglobulinemia, antiphospholipid syndrome, IgA nephropathy).

Causes of DAH without capillaritis include idiopathic pulmonary hemosiderosis (IPH), diffuse alveolar damage (DAD), elevated pulmonary venous pressure, anticoagulation and coagulation disorders, inhalation injury, and illicit drug use.

HRCT findings in any of these entities include diffuse or symmetric ground glass opacity progressing to consolidation (Fig. 7.21). Ground glass may be lobular in distribution. Centrilobular nodules of ground glass opacity may be present in isolation or may be associated with more diffuse hemorrhage (Fig. 7.22). Smooth interlobular septal thickening may be seen in association with ground glass opacity (i.e., the crazy paving pattern) (Fig. 7.23). Isolated septal thickening is uncommon.

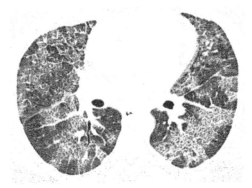

FIGURE 7.23 · **Pulmonary hemorrhage with crazy paving.** A combination of ground glass opacity and smooth interlobular septal thickening is seen in a patient with pulmonary hemorrhage from vasculitis. Other causes of the crazy paving pattern in the acute setting include edema, atypical infection, and diffuse alveolar damage.

HRCT findings show significant overlap with other causes of diffuse ground glass opacity such as pulmonary edema, DAD, and atypical infections.

Goodpasture Syndrome

Goodpasture syndrome is an autoimmune disorder characterized by antibodies against the glomerular basement membrane. It primarily affects the kidneys and lungs. The combination of renal and pulmonary disease in Goodpasture syndrome is most common in young males, 20 to 30 years of age. Isolated renal disease may be seen in elderly females, 60 to 70 years of age.

7

Pulmonary capillaritis results in pulmonary hemorrhage. The HRCT findings are identical to other causes of pulmonary hemorrhage. Ground glass opacity and consolidation are most often diffuse but may be asymmetric or focal.

Idiopathic Pulmonary Hemosiderosis

IPH is a rare disease of unknown origin characterized by recurrent episodes of diffuse pulmonary hemorrhage without associated glomerulonephritis or a serologic abnormality.

IPH most commonly occurs in children or young adults. IPH may sometimes be associated with conditions such as milk allergy, immunoglobulin A gammopathy, and exposure to toxic mold.

IPH is a diagnosis of exclusion in which there is no evidence of other causes of pulmonary hemorrhage, such as GPA. HRCT findings are the same as Goodpasture syndrome and other causes of diffuse pulmonary hemorrhage. Recurrent episodes of hemorrhage may eventually lead to emphysema, cysts, or fibrosis (Fig. 7.24).

MISCELLANEOUS VASCULAR DISEASES

Hepatopulmonary Syndrome

Liver dysfunction may result in pulmonary vascular dilatation, causing hypoxemia. This is termed hepatopulmonary syndrome (HPS).

It is hypothesized that nitric oxide or other vasoactive substances, which are not metabolized by the liver, have a vasodilatory effect on the lungs that causes these abnormalities. Patients with liver disease may present with a clinical syndrome that includes hypoxemia, platypnea (dyspnea with sitting up), and orthodeoxia (desaturation with sitting up). Dilated vessels at the lung bases are better perfused with sitting, and shunting increases in this position.

In patients with HPS, HRCT typically shows dilated vessels, 1 to 2 mm in diameter, in the lung periphery, particularly in the lower lobes (Fig. 7.25). The dilated vessels in patients with HPS may extend to the pleural surface. The severity of vascular dilatation correlates with the severity of hypoxemia, but not all patients with HPS will show this finding. In 15% of cases of HPS, frank arteriovenous fistulas are present. Angiography is likely more sensitive than HRCT in the detection of these abnormalities.

Metastatic Calcification

Metastatic calcification occurs in disorders that lead to abnormal calcium or phosphorus metabolism. It is most frequently seen in patients with renal failure. Other disorders with which it is associated include hyperparathyroidism, osseous malignancies, and hypervitaminosis D. In these conditions, calcium is deposited within the lung interstitium adjacent to pulmonary vessels. Most patients are asymptomatic, even with extensive disease; however, this disorder may occasionally lead to symptoms and even death.

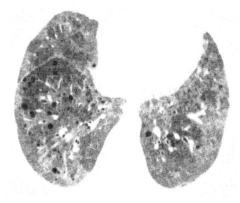

FIGURE 7.24 · Idiopathic pulmonary hemosiderosis. Recurrent episodes of alveolar hemorrhage have resulted diffuse ground glass opacity associated with lung cysts.

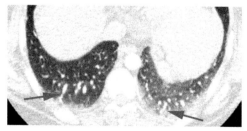

FIGURE 7.25 · Hepatopulmonary syndrome. Enhanced HRCT at the lung bases in a 33-year-old woman with liver disease, platypnea, and orthodeoxia. Dilated vessels (*arrows*) in the posterior lung are typical of hepatopulmonary syndrome.

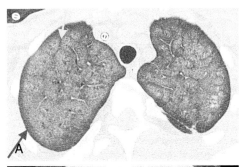

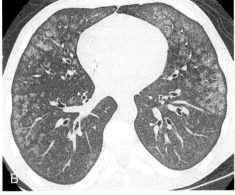

FIGURE 7.26 · Metastatic calcification. A.
Symmetric bilateral ground glass opacity
is present. Note sparing of the subpleural
region (*red arrow*) reflecting a centrilobular
distribution. Linear areas of sparing represent
the interlobular septa at the periphery of the
lobules (*yellow arrow*). **B.** Findings in the mid-
lung are much less severe but show the lobular nature of the ground glass opacity.

Typical HRCT findings include centrilobular nodules of ground glass opacity. The
nodules are symmetric bilaterally and variable
in size but may eventually involve the entire
pulmonary lobule (Fig. 7.26A, B). The process
is usually upper lobe predominant. Frank calcification may or may not be seen.

FURTHER READING

Akyar S, Ozbek SS. Computed tomography findings in
idiopathic pulmonary hemosiderosis. *Respiration.*
1993;60:63-64.

Bergin CJ, Rios G, King MA, Belezzuoli E, Luna J, Auger
WR. Accuracy of high-resolution CT in identifying
chronic pulmonary thromboembolic disease. *AJR Am
J Roentgenol.* 1996;166:1371-1377.

Brown KK. Pulmonary vasculitis. *Proc Am Thorac Soc.*
2006;3:48-57.

Castañer E, Alguersuari E, Gallardo X, et al. When to
suspect pulmonary vasculitis: radiologic and clinical
clues. *Radiographics.* 2010;30:33-53.

Cheah FK, Sheppard MN, Hansell DM. Computed
tomography of diffuse pulmonary haemorrhage with
pathological correlation. *Clin Radiol.* 1993;48:89-93.

Collard HR, Schwarz MI. Diffuse alveolar hemorrhage.
Clin Chest Med. 2004;25:583-592.

Connolly B, Manson D, Eberhard A, et al. CT appearance of pulmonary vasculitis in children. *AJR Am J
Roentgenol.* 1996;167:901-904.

Cordier JF, Valeyre D, Guillevin L, et al. Pulmonary
Wegener's granulomatosis. A clinical and imaging
study of 77 cases. *Chest.* 1990;97:906-912.

Engelke C, Schaefer-Prokop C, Schirg E, Freihorst J,
Grubnic S, Prokop M. High-resolution CT and CT
angiography of peripheral pulmonary vascular disorders. *Radiographics.* 2002;22:739-764.

Galiè N, Hoeper MM, Humbert M, et al. Guidelines for
the diagnosis and treatment of pulmonary hypertension: the Task Force for the Diagnosis and Treatment
of Pulmonary Hypertension of the European Society
of Cardiology (ESC) and the European Respiratory
Society (ERS), endorsed by the International Society
of Heart and Lung Transplantation (ISHLT). *Eur Heart
J.* 2009;30:2493-2537.

Hansell DM. Small-vessel diseases of the lung:
CT-pathologic correlates. *Radiology.* 2002;225:639-653.

Hiller N, Lieberman S, Chajek-Shaul T, Bar-Ziv J, Shaham
D. Thoracic manifestations of Behcet disease at CT.
Radiographics. 2004;24:801-808.

Hoffman GS, Kerr GS, Leavitt RY, et al. Wegener granulomatosis: an analysis of 158 patients. *Ann Intern Med.*
1992;116:488-498.

Ioachimescu OC, Sieber S, Kotch A. Idiopathic pulmonary haemosiderosis revisited. *Eur Respir J.*
2004;24:162-170.

Johkoh T, Ikezoe J, Nagareda T, et al. Metastatic pulmonary calcification: early detection by high resolution
CT. *J Comput Assist Tomogr.* 1993;17:471-473.

Lee KN, Lee HJ, Shin WW, Webb WR. Hypoxemia and
liver cirrhosis (hepatopulmonary syndrome) in eight
patients: comparison of the central and peripheral
pulmonary vasculature. *Radiology.* 1999;211:549-553.

Lee KS, Kim TS, Fujimoto K, et al. Thoracic manifestation of Wegener's granulomatosis: CT findings in 30
patients. *Eur Radiol.* 2003;13:43-51.

Marten K, Schnyder P, Schirg E, Prokop M, Rummeny
EJ, Engelke C. Pattern-based differential diagnosis in
pulmonary vasculitis using volumetric CT. *AJR Am J
Roentgenol.* 2005;184:720-733.

Mayberry JP, Primack SL, Müller NL. Thoracic manifestations of systemic autoimmune diseases: radiographic
and high-resolution CT findings. *Radiographics.*
2000;20:1623-1635.

Ng CS, Wells AU, Padley SP. A CT sign of chronic pulmonary arterial hypertension: the ratio of main pulmonary artery to aortic diameter. *J Thorac Imaging.*
1999;14:270-278.

Ozer C, Duce MN, Ulubas B, et al. Inspiratory and expiratory HRCT findings in Behcet's disease and correlation with pulmonary function tests. *Eur J Radiol.*
2005;56:43-47.

Primack SL, Müller NL, Mayo JR, Remy-Jardin M, Remy
J. Pulmonary parenchymal abnormalities of vascular
origin: high-resolution CT findings. *Radiographics.*
1994;14:739-746.

7

Primack SL, Miller RR, Müller NL. Diffuse pulmonary hemorrhage: clinical, pathologic, and imaging features. *AJR Am J Roentgenol.* 1995;164:295-300.

Reuter M, Schnabel A, Wesner F, et al. Pulmonary Wegener's granulomatosis: correlation between high-resolution CT findings and clinical scoring of disease activity. *Chest.* 1998;114:500-506.

Schwickert HC, Schweden F, Schild HH, et al. Pulmonary arteries and lung parenchyma in chronic pulmonary embolism: preoperative and postoperative CT findings. *Radiology.* 1994;191:351-357.

Seo JB, Im JG, Chung JW, et al. Pulmonary vasculitis: the spectrum of radiological findings. *Br J Radiol.* 2000;73:1224-1231.

Simonneau G, Gatzoulis MA, Adatia I, et al. Updated clinical classification of pulmonary hypertension. *J Am Coll Cardiol.* 2013;62(suppl 25):D34-D41.

Tunaci A, Berkmen YM, Gokmen E. Thoracic involvement in Behcet's disease: pathologic, clinical, and imaging features. *AJR Am J Roentgenol.* 1995;164:51-56.

Weir IH, Müller NL, Chiles C, et al. Wegener's granulomatosis: findings from computed tomography of the chest in 10 patients. *Can Assoc Radiol J.* 1992;43:31-34.

Pulmonary Edema, Acute Lung Injury, Diffuse Alveolar Damage, and the Acute Respiratory Distress Syndrome

PULMONARY EDEMA

Pulmonary edema may result from changes in pulmonary venous pressure, increased permeability of capillary endothelium, or a combination of both. The high-resolution computed tomography (HRCT) features of these two processes show significant overlap and are often difficult to distinguish. The most important role of HRCT is in making a distinction between edema and other causes of pulmonary symptoms, such as pneumonia.

Hydrostatic Pulmonary Edema

An alteration of the hydrostatic or oncotic pressure within pulmonary capillaries may result in pulmonary edema. Increased hydrostatic pressure is significantly more common and usually results from pulmonary venous hypertension due to left heart disease. Left heart failure and valvular heart disease are the most frequent causes. Decreased oncotic pressure due to low albumin may also result in edema accumulation, but this is less common.

The HRCT findings of hydrostatic pulmonary edema associated with pulmonary venous hypertension are shown in Table 8.1. Hydrostatic pulmonary edema may be interstitial or alveolar. Both are typically diffuse or symmetrical and may be associated with vascular congestion and pulmonary veins enlargement, particularly in the upper lobes.

Interstitial Pulmonary Edema

Edema fluid may accumulate within the interlobular septa, subpleural interstitium, and peribronchovascular interstitium.

On HRCT, interlobular septal edema appears as smooth interlobular septal thickening (IST; Fig. 8.1). Keep in mind that a few interlobular septa may be seen in normal patients; they appear very thin. However, when multiple, easily seen, interlobular septa are visible, the septa are abnormally thickened.

A reticular abnormality visible on HRCT can be diagnosed as IST if the lines outline what can be recognized as pulmonary lobules because of their typical size and polygonal shape. Centrilobular arteries may be seen as small dots at the center of these polygonal structures and may appear prominent because of surrounding edema. Interlobular septal thickening as a result of edema is often best seen in the upper lobes because septa are best developed in this location. Subpleural edema (Fig. 8.2), equivalent to interlobular septal thickening, may be seen as thickening of fissures.

Edema fluid may also accumulate in the peribronchovascular interstitium. On HRCT, thickening of the interstitium surrounding the central bronchi gives the appearance of bronchial wall thickening and a corresponding increase in the diameter of pulmonary arteries (Fig. 8.3).

TABLE 8.1	HRCT findings of pulmonary venous hypertension
Stage of pulmonary venous hypertension	**HRCT finding**
Vascular congestion	Enlarged pulmonary veins Upper lobe vessels particularly involved
Interstitial edema	Smooth interlobular septal thickening Subpleural edema (thickening of fissures) Peribronchovascular interstitial thickening Typically diffuse or symmetric
Alveolar edema	Ground glass opacity and consolidation Typically diffuse or symmetric

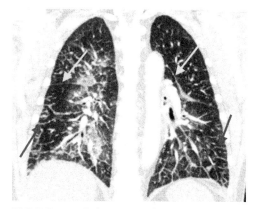

FIGURE 8.2 · Pulmonary edema with interlobular septal and fissural thickening. Coronal reformatted CT shows thickening of the fissures (*yellow arrows*). This represents fluid in the subpleural interstitium. Smooth interlobular septal thickening is also noted (*red arrows*) in this patient with interstitial pulmonary edema.

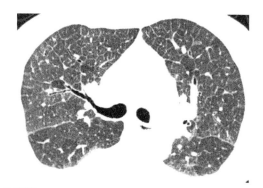

classic

FIGURE 8.1 · Interstitial pulmonary edema with interlobular septal thickening: Classic appearance. Multiple, smooth, thin, interconnecting linear opacities are noted, outlining polygonal structures, which can be identified as pulmonary lobules because of their characteristic size and shape and the presence of a centrilobular artery. These are the interlobular septa that marginate the pulmonary lobule. Pulmonary edema is the most common cause of this finding. Thickening of the major fissures is also seen.

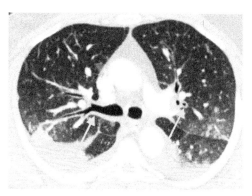

FIGURE 8.3 · Pulmonary edema with peribronchovascular interstitial thickening. Fluid is seen in the interstitium adjacent to or surrounding the bronchi and arteries (*arrows*). This is easily confused with bronchial wall thickening. Note the lack of narrowing of the lumen of the bronchi. Ground glass opacity and pleural effusion are also present.

Their distribution of interstitial edema is variable, but abnormalities tend to be bilateral and symmetric. While edema is often most severe in the dependent lung regions, this is not a constant feature.

Alveolar Edema

Severe pulmonary edema results in alveolar flooding. Ground glass opacity and consolidation are the most common findings (Fig. 8.4). Centrilobular nodules of ground glass attenuation may also be seen with mild or early alveolar edema (Fig. 8.5).

Findings of interstitial and alveolar edema frequently coexist. Smooth interlobular septal and/or peribronchovascular interstitial thickening may be associated with areas of ground glass opacity or consolidation (Figs. 8.6 and 8.7). The "crazy paving" sign, representing a combination of ground

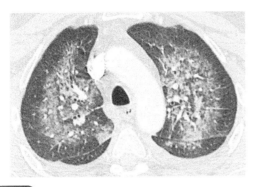

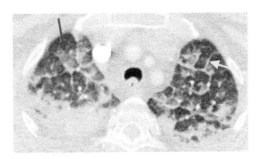

classic

FIGURE 8.6 · Interstitial and alveolar pulmonary edema: Classic appearance. Smooth interlobular septal thickening (*yellow arrow*) is seen as a manifestation of interstitial pulmonary edema. Additionally, there is patchy bilateral ground glass opacity (*red arrow*) and consolidation (*blue arrow*) compatible with alveolar edema. Abnormalities of both interstitial and alveolar edema often coexist.

classic

FIGURE 8.4 · Pulmonary edema with symmetric ground glass opacity: Classic appearance. Symmetric parahilar ground glass opacity is seen as a manifestation of pulmonary edema.

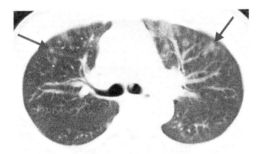

FIGURE 8.5 · Pulmonary edema with centrilobular nodules. Ill-defined centrilobular nodules of ground glass opacity (*arrows*) are seen in the anterior lungs bilaterally. This is not an uncommon manifestation of edema and is often seen in association with other findings of alveolar edema.

glass opacity and interlobular septal thickening visible in the same lung regions, is not uncommon in patients with pulmonary edema (Fig. 8.7).

Distribution of Hydrostatic Edema

In patients with hydrostatic edema, the distribution of abnormalities is typically diffuse or symmetric. More severe abnormalities may be seen in the dependent lung because of the normal hydrostatic pressure gradient, but this is not always present. Lymphatic drainage in the upper lobes may, in some cases, be less efficient than that in the lower lobes leading to an upper lung distribution of edema.

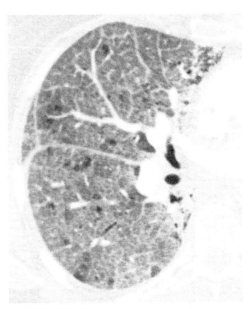

FIGURE 8.7 · Pulmonary edema with crazy paving. A combination of ground glass opacity and smooth interlobular septal thickening is seen in the right lung. This finding is nonspecific, but pulmonary edema is one of the most common causes of this pattern in the acute setting.

A patchy or lobular distribution of abnormalities may sometimes be present (Figs. 8.6 and 8.8), and in some patients, edema may

8

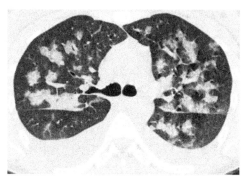

FIGURE 8.8 · Pulmonary edema with lobular opacities. Lobular areas of ground glass opacity are present. The process is symmetric and associated with pleural effusions. Occasionally, causes of alveolar disease such as pulmonary edema may be very geographic such as in this case.

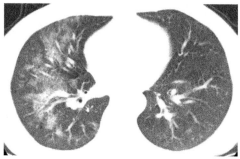

FIGURE 8.9 · Asymmetric pulmonary edema. While edema is typically a symmetric process, unilateral or asymmetric edema is not uncommon. This patient was placed in a right-side-down decubitus position for a surgical procedure, explaining the unilateral right-sided edema. Patchy ground glass opacity and crazy paving are visible.

be asymmetric (Fig. 8.9). Causes of asymmetric or focal pulmonary edema include the following:

1. **Patient position.** Pulmonary edema may occur in dependent lung regions because of gravitational effects. Patient positioning may have an influence on the location of pulmonary edema. For example, right-sided pulmonary edema may be seen in patients who lay on their right side while sleeping.
2. **Asymmetric emphysema/bullous disease.** Emphysema, particularly when associated with bulla, may be asymmetric. Edema will show relative sparing of areas of emphysema and will appear more severe on the contralateral side.
3. **Mitral regurgitation.** Focal right upper lobe pulmonary edema may occur in the setting of mitral regurgitation, particularly when associated with acute papillary muscle rupture after a myocardial infarction. The regurgitant jet is directed into the right superior pulmonary vein.
4. **Pulmonary embolism or vascular obstruction.** In patients with pulmonary embolism or other causes of pulmonary artery obstruction, edema predominates in well-perfused lung regions and may appear patchy.
5. **Neurogenic pulmonary edema.** An unusual distribution of pulmonary edema may be seen in patients with intracranial abnormalities associated with trauma,

hemorrhage, or seizure. The exact mechanism by which this occurs is poorly understood, but it often occurs in patients without heart disease. Approximately 50% of patients show focal bilateral upper lobe abnormalities while the remainder of cases are indistinguishable from other causes of pulmonary edema. Opacities may show rapid shifting from one location to another, a feature uncommon in pulmonary edema from other causes.

Differential Diagnosis of Hydrostatic Edema

In the acute setting, pulmonary edema is the most common cause of isolated smooth IST and peribronchovascular interstitial thickening. Lymphangitic spread of tumor is another cause of this appearance, but such patients usually have a known malignancy or have chronic and progressive symptoms. Lymphangitic spread of tumor often results in unilateral or asymmetric abnormalities, while hydrostatic edema is usually symmetrical.

IST that is not an isolated or predominant feature is nonspecific and should be ignored in formulating a differential diagnosis. Some septal thickening is present in a variety of lung diseases.

Peribronchovascular interstitial thickening is easily confused with bronchial wall thickening from bronchial inflammation.

8

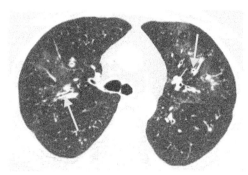

TABLE 8.2	HRCT findings of diffuse alveolar damage (DAD)
Early	Diffuse or symmetric ground glass opacity and consolidation May show peripheral distribution Lack of interlobular septal thickening
Late	Fibrosis (irregular reticulation, traction bronchiectasis, honeycombing) Anterior/subpleural distribution

FIGURE 8.10 · Bronchial wall thickening in a patient with airways disease. Thickening of the bronchial wall may resemble fluid in the peribronchovascular interstitium. When narrowing of the airway lumen is present (*arrows*), bronchial wall thickening is the likely etiology.

When mucous impaction or luminal narrowing is present, bronchial inflammation is the most likely cause (Fig. 8.10).

Ground glass opacity and consolidation are nonspecific findings in the acute setting and may be seen with infection, aspiration, acute lung injury (diffuse alveolar damage [DAD]), and hemorrhage. The diagnosis is driven by the clinical presentation rather than the HRCT findings. When ground glass opacity is associated with significant smooth interlobular septal thickening, however, pulmonary edema is the most likely etiology.

Increased Permeability Edema Without Diffuse Alveolar Damage

Increased permeability edema results from injury to capillary endothelium with increased capillary permeability. It is usually associated with DAD. Increased permeability edema unassociated with DAD is uncommon and usually is seen in association with drugs, transfusion reactions, toxic shock syndrome, air embolism, and hantavirus pulmonary syndrome. HRCT findings closely mimic those of hydrostatic pulmonary edema with smooth interlobular septal thickening and ground glass opacity.

Increased Permeability Edema with DAD (Acute Lung Injury)

Increased permeability edema is often, but not always, associated with DAD on histopathology. DAD is characterized by an acute injury to alveoli and capillary end (by a variety of mechanisms), followed by organization and eventual healing or fibrosis. *Acute lung injury* is a term used to refer to a clinical syndrome of respiratory insufficiency associated with DAD on pathology.

Histologically, DAD has several stages, and its appearance varies with the time interval between lung injury and biopsy.

The *exudative stage* of DAD is associated with pulmonary edema and pulmonary hemorrhage; it develops within hours of lung injury. It is followed by alveolar and capillary necrosis with progressive edema, hemorrhage, and formation of alveolar hyaline membranes.

The *proliferative (reparative or organizing) stage* of DAD is associated with regrowth of alveolar lining cells, organization of alveolar exudates, and fibroblast proliferation within the interstitium and air spaces. It is seen within days of lung injury.

These abnormalities may largely resolve, or there may be progression to the *chronic or fibrotic stage*, typically 2 weeks or more after lung injury. This stage is associated with progressive lung fibrosis and collagen deposition.

The HRCT findings of DAD (Table 8.2) resemble those of hydrostatic pulmonary edema, although some differences exist. Diffuse or symmetric consolidation and ground glass opacity are most characteristic (Fig. 8.11). In early stages of DAD, these abnormalities may have a peripheral distribution, but they eventually become diffuse and confluent. Abnormalities often demonstrate a gradient of opacity from anterior to posterior, with the anterior lung showing near-normal findings and the posterior lung showing dense consolidation (Fig. 8.11). Interlobular septal thickening is characteristically absent.

Not infrequently DAD coexists with organizing pneumonia (OP). When significant OP

exists, patchy, focal areas of consolidation may be seen in association with the other findings of DAD. Nonpulmonary (systemic) causes of DAD, such as sepsis, tend to show opacities that are bilateral and symmetric on HRCT. Pulmonary causes of DAD, such as pneumonia, typically show asymmetric or focal abnormalities.

While the HRCT findings of DAD are nonspecific at presentation, their evolution over time may be characteristic. Within 1 to 3 weeks, irregular reticulation and traction bronchiectasis often appear within areas of ground glass opacity and consolidation (Fig. 8.12). Focal areas of consolidation corresponding, in some cases, to OP, may resolve in patients treated with corticosteroids.

In patients who survive, findings that suggest fibrosis, developing 1 to 3 weeks after presentation, are often reversible and show improvement over the following weeks to months. However, residual fibrosis is not uncommon; it tends to be mild and predominates in the anterior subpleural lung (Fig. 8.13). This evolution of findings over time may be used to distinguish fibrotic DAD from alternative causes of diffuse lung opacities such as infection and pulmonary edema.

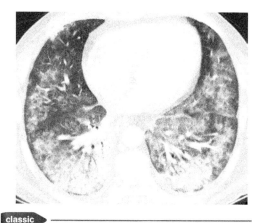

classic

FIGURE 8.11 · **Diffuse alveolar damage resulting in ARDS: Classic appearance.** Diffuse consolidation and ground glass opacity in a patient with sepsis are nonspecific but typical of DAD and acute respiratory distress syndrome (ARDS). Note more severe involvement in the lung periphery and in dependent lung regions.

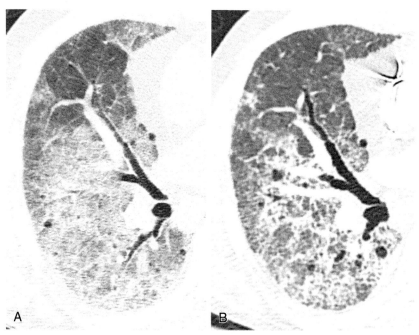

A   B

FIGURE 8.12 · **Diffuse alveolar damage (DAD): Baseline CT (A) demonstrates extensive ground glass opacity.** Three weeks later **(B)**, there has been interval development of irregular reticulation and traction bronchiectasis. This is a typical evolution of DAD over time.

8

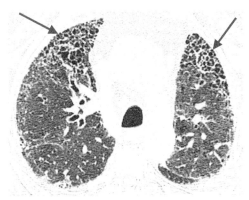

FIGURE 8.13 · Post-ARDS fibrosis. Patients who survive an episode of acute respiratory distress syndrome may develop fibrosis as a sequela. This fibrosis typically has an anterior distribution. Typical findings include irregular reticulation, traction bronchiectasis, and/or honeycombing (*arrows*).

Acute Respiratory Distress Syndrome (ARDS)

Acute respiratory distress syndrome (ARDS) is a clinical syndrome that may be associated with DAD. Current clinical criteria for the diagnosis of ARDS (i.e. the Berlin classification) are primarily clinical and include 3 grades. These are as follows:

1. Acute onset of symptoms (within 1 week of known insult or new symptoms)
2. Bilateral opacities on chest radiographs (not explained by effusions, collapse, or nodules)
3. Exclusion of cardiac failure or fluid overload as an etiology (echocardiography is often required)
4. Reduced ratio of partial pressure of oxygen in arterial blood to fraction of inspired oxygen (Pao_2/Fio_2)
   a. Mild ARDS: Pao_2/Fio_2 ≤300 mm Hg but >200 mm Hg
   b. Moderate ARDS: Pao_2/Fio_2 ≤200 mm Hg but >100 mm Hg
   c. Severe ARDS: Pao_2/Fio_2 ≤100 mm Hg

This definition of ARDS is intended to capture patients with severe DAD; however, only about half the patients with ARDS will have DAD on pathology. The most common causes of ARDS without DAD include infection, emphysema, cardiogenic pulmonary edema, hemorrhage, and interstitial lung disease. Conversely, not all patients with DAD will meet clinical criteria for ARDS. When describing typical HRCT findings, it is more accurate to say they are consistent with DAD or acute lung injury rather than ARDS.

The causes of ARDS are largely the same as those of DAD. They can be divided into systemic processes and processes that directly involve the lungs. Systemic processes resulting in DAD and ARDS include sepsis, shock, disseminated intravascular coagulation, drugs, pancreatitis, and severe burns. Processes that involve the lungs and result in ARDS include pneumonia, aspiration, trauma, and toxic inhalations. Acute worsening in patients with known interstitial lung disease is another cause of DAD. This is most frequently seen in patients with idiopathic pulmonary fibrosis and is called an acute exacerbation. DAD without a known inciting cause is termed *acute interstitial pneumonia (AIP)* or Hamman–Rich syndrome. This is discussed in more detail in Chapter 9.

On HRCT, the differential diagnosis of DAD includes other causes of extensive consolidation such as hydrostatic pulmonary edema, infection, and hemorrhage. There is significant overlap of the findings in these diseases and, not infrequently, more than one process is present. Early DAD may have a peripheral distribution as opposed to pulmonary edema, which is typically diffuse or central. Significant smooth interlobular septal thickening suggests pulmonary edema rather than DAD. Centrilobular nodules of soft tissue attenuation, airways inflammation, and tree-in-bud opacities suggest infection.

FURTHER READING

ARDS Definition Task Force; Ranieri VM, Rubenfeld GD, Thompson BT, et al. Acute respiratory distress syndrome: the Berlin definition. *JAMA.* 2012;307: 2526-2533.

Desai SR, Wells AU, Rubens MB, Evans TW, Hansell DM. Acute respiratory distress syndrome: CT abnormalities at long-term follow-up. *Radiology.* 1999;210:29-35.

Fan E, Brodie D, Slutsky AS. Acute respiratory distress syndrome: advances in diagnosis and treatment. *JAMA.* 2018;319:698-710.

8

Gluecker T, Capasso P, Schnyder P, et al. Clinical and radiologic features of pulmonary edema. *Radiographics.* 1999;19:1507-1531.

Goodman LR. Congestive heart failure and adult respiratory distress syndrome. New insights using computed tomography. *Radiol Clin North Am.* 1996;34:33-46.

Goodman LR, Fumagalli R, Tagliabue P, et al. Adult respiratory distress syndrome due to pulmonary and extrapulmonary causes: CT, clinical, and functional correlations. *Radiology.* 1999;213:545-552.

Ketai LH, Godwin JD. A new view of pulmonary edema and acute respiratory distress syndrome. *J Thorac Imaging.* 1998;13:147-171.

Storto ML, Kee ST, Golden JA, Webb WR. Hydrostatic pulmonary edema: high-resolution CT findings. *AJR Am J Roentgenol.* 1995;165:817-820.

The Interstitial Pneumonias

INTRODUCTION

The interstitial pneumonias (IPs), or idiopathic interstitial pneumonias (IIPs), are a heterogeneous group of diffuse lung diseases characterized by varying degrees of lung inflammation and fibrosis. They are best thought of as reactions to lung injury, presenting with specific histologic patterns. They are loosely unified by several characteristics including clinical presentation, radiographic manifestations, and pathologic appearance and may be idiopathic or associated with specific diseases. In this chapter, we intend to provide a general understanding of the IPs and the clinical disorders with which they may be associated.

CLASSIFICATION

The IPs were originally classified by Liebow in the 1960s. As an understanding of their patterns has been refined, they have been redefined and reclassified several times. Although some of the terms in the original classification have remained the same, others have been changed or deleted.

It is important to recognize that the IPs are defined as histologic patterns and not diseases. Each IP pattern may be the result of an idiopathic clinical syndrome (thus representing an IIP) or may be associated with a specific disease and not be idiopathic. The current classification is shown in Table 9.1.

The IPs and IIPs are referred to using both their full name and acronyms. Acronyms are usually used to refer to these entities, even in reports.

The IPs include usual interstitial pneumonia (UIP), nonspecific interstitial pneumonia (NSIP), organizing pneumonia (OP), desquamative interstitial pneumonia (DIP), lymphoid interstitial pneumonia (LIP), diffuse alveolar damage (DAD) and acute interstitial pneumonia (AIP), and pleuroparenchymal fibroelastosis (PPFE). DIP, along with respiratory bronchiolitis interstitial lung disease (RB-ILD), is usually related to smoking and is also discussed in Chapter 11. LIP is best thought of as a lymphoproliferative disorder that will be discussed in detail in Chapter 17.

HRCT IN THE IPs

In the interpretation of high-resolution computed tomography (HRCT) in a patient with a suspected IP, it is important to understand the relationship between the imaging pattern and the pathology and clinical syndrome present. In classic cases, the HRCT pattern may be used to predict the pathologic pattern.

Take, for example, UIP. When classic findings of UIP are present on HRCT (i.e., we say a "UIP pattern" is present), there is a high degree of certainty that a surgical lung biopsy will also show UIP.

However, several different diseases may be associated with a UIP pattern on HRCT and pathology. If the abnormality is idiopathic, UIP is considered to represent idiopathic pulmonary fibrosis (IPF). On the other hand, UIP may be associated with connective tissue diseases, drug toxicity, and asbestosis. UIP associated with each of these may

TABLE 9.1	Classification of interstitial pneumonia

Histologic pattern	Idiopathic clinical syndrome	Associated diseases or conditions
Usual interstitial pneumonia	Idiopathic pulmonary fibrosis	Connective tissue disease, drug toxicity, asbestosis
Nonspecific interstitial pneumonia (NSIP)	Idiopathic NSIP	Connective tissue disease, drug toxicity, hypersensitivity pneumonitis
Organizing pneumonia	Cryptogenic organizing pneumonia	Drugs, infections, toxic inhalations
Desquamative interstitial pneumonia (DIP)/respiratory bronchiolitis interstitial lung disease	Idiopathic DIP	Cigarette smoking, toxic fumes
Diffuse alveolar damage	Acute interstitial pneumonia	Known causes of acute respiratory distress syndrome
Lymphoid interstitial pneumonia (LIP)	Idiopathic LIP	Connective tissue disease, immunodeficiency
Pleuroparenchymal fibroelastosis (PPFE)	Idiopathic PPFE	Chronic infection, drugs, connective tissue disease, bone marrow transplant, chronic rejection in lung transplant

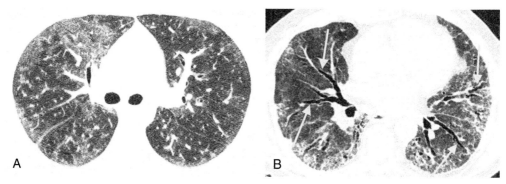

A B

FIGURE 9.1 · **Inflammation versus fibrosis on HRCT.** The interstitial pneumonias present with varying degrees of inflammation and fibrosis. Two patients with nonspecific interstitial pneumonia from connective tissue disease are depicted. **A.** HRCT shows ground glass opacity without definite signs of fibrosis, representing potentially reversible inflammatory abnormalities. **B.** HRCT shows fibrosis as manifested by traction bronchiectasis (*arrows*) and irregular reticulation. These findings reflect irreversible lung scarring that would be unresponsive to treatment.

be indistinguishable on HRCT and pathologically. Clinical correlation is important in distinguishing the various causes of a UIP pattern. Similar relationships exist for each of the different IPs.

The IPs are a common cause of diffuse lung disease and should be considered as a possible etiology whenever a patient has chronic symptoms or HRCT findings of fibrosis or lung infiltration. HRCT findings vary depending on the degree of inflammation or fibrosis that is present. Cases that are predominantly inflammatory result in ground glass opacity (GGO) and/or consolidation. Cases that are predominantly fibrotic are associated with irregular reticulation, traction bronchiectasis, and/or honeycombing.

Although there may be significant components of both inflammation and fibrosis in selected cases, most of the IPs present at the extremes of this spectrum (Fig. 9.1A, B). UIP is a pattern characterized predominantly by fibrosis. NSIP may be fibrotic, cellular, or a combination of both. The remaining IPs are predominantly inflammatory, although they may show progression to fibrosis in some cases.

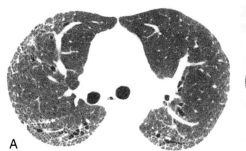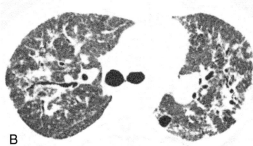

A   B

FIGURE 9.2 · **Distribution of HRCT abnormalities in diagnosis. A.** In this patient with fibrotic nonspecific interstitial pneumonia (NSIP) related to scleroderma, HRCT shows a peripheral and subpleural predominance of abnormalities. **B.** HRCT in a patient with sarcoidosis shows central and peribronchial abnormalities, with relative sparing of the subpleural lung. In the setting of chronic symptoms, a subpleural and basilar predominance of abnormalities suggests usual interstitial pneumonia, NSIP, or desquamative interstitial pneumonia. A diffuse or central axial distribution is atypical for an interstitial pneumonia and suggests alternative diseases such as hypersensitivity pneumonitis or sarcoidosis.

Distribution can be helpful in distinguishing the different IPs and in differentiating them from other causes of diffuse lung disease (Fig. 9.2A, B). UIP, NSIP, and DIP often demonstrate a peripheral predominance of abnormalities, with involvement of the lung bases, including the costophrenic angles. The other IPs typically demonstrate equal involvement of both the peripheral and central lung. Other causes of diffuse lung disease, such as hypersensitivity pneumonitis (HP) or sarcoidosis, are often diffuse or central in axial distribution and show sparing of the inferior costophrenic angles.

USUAL INTERSTITIAL PNEUMONIA

UIP (Table 9.2) is common and accounts for approximately 50% of cases of IP. Pathologically, UIP has a typical appearance (Fig. 9.3) that is characterized by the following:

1. Areas of established fibrosis that are patchy and nonuniform (reflecting spatial and temporal heterogeneity of lung involvement)
2. Microscopic honeycombing (air-filled cysts, lined by bronchial epithelium and surrounded by fibrosis)
3. Fibroblastic foci (the active phase of fibrosis deposition)

4. Normal lung (also reflecting spatial and temporal heterogeneity)
5. Subpleural lung predominance without relation to bronchioles

The most common disease associated with UIP is IPF, but there are several specific diseases that may also result in this pattern, including connective tissue diseases, drug toxicity, and asbestosis.

TABLE 9.2	Features of usual interstitial pneumonia
Frequency	Most common interstitial pneumonia; 50% of cases
HRCT findings	Subpleural, basilar predominant Honeycombing Other signs of fibrosis (traction bronchiectasis, irregular reticulation) Absence of mosaic perfusion, air trapping, diffuse nodules, ground glass opacity outside of areas of fibrosis
Idiopathic syndrome	Idiopathic pulmonary fibrosis
Associated diseases	Connective tissue disease Drug toxicity (rare) Asbestosis (rare) Hypersensitivity pneumonitis (usually has HRCT findings atypical for usual interstitial pneumonia [UIP]) Sarcoidosis (usually has HRCT findings atypical for UIP)

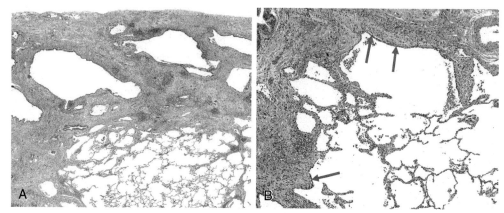

FIGURE 9.3 · **A and B. Pathology of usual interstitial pneumonia.** On low power **(A)**, the spatial and temporal heterogeneity of usual interstitial pneumonia is apparent with subpleural microscopic honeycombing (air-filled cysts) and less-fibrotic central lung tissue. On higher power view **(B)**, fibroblast foci are noted (*arrows*) at the interface between the fibrotic and less-involved lung tissue.

HRCT Findings

In patients with UIP, HRCT typically shows reticulation with a subpleural and basilar predominance. The reticular opacities are often irregular in appearance. Traction bronchiectasis is often associated with reticular opacities. Honeycombing is present in about 70% of cases and is important in making a definite diagnosis of UIP (Fig. 9.4A–D). Honeycombing results in the presence of clustered, cystic airspaces, with well-defined walls, usually 3 to 10 mm in diameter, and predominating in the subpleural lung. As with the overall extent of abnormalities, honeycombing, when present, is most severe and extensive at the lung bases (Fig. 9.5A–E). In patients with early or mild UIP, reticulation with or without traction bronchiectasis may be visible on HRCT, without honeycombing.

Isolated areas of GGO (i.e., unassociated with reticulation) are rare in UIP. GGO is usually seen only in lung regions that also show findings of fibrosis (i.e., reticulation, traction bronchiectasis, or honeycombing) and, in UIP, typically reflects the presence of microscopic fibrosis.

Although the upper lobes are usually abnormal in patients with UIP, findings of fibrosis predominate in the lung bases, and the posterior costophrenic angles are typically involved. The findings of fibrosis are often patchy in distribution but involve the posterior and subpleural lung to the greatest degree.

To standardize the HRCT interpretation of suspected UIP and IPF, two major HRCT classification schemes have been developed. These use combinations of findings and the distribution of those findings within the lung to determine the overall confidence in the diagnosis of UIP (high, intermediate, or low). The American Thoracic Society along with European, Japanese, and Latin American respiratory societies guidelines were published in 2011 (ATS criteria). The Fleischner Society (FS) published modified criteria in 2018 (FS criteria), which will be subject to review. These are both summarized in Table 9.3.

Criteria for High Confidence in the Diagnosis of UIP

An HRCT diagnosis of a UIP pattern can be made with a high degree of confidence based on four criteria:

1. Reticular opacities
2. Honeycombing
3. Subpleural and basilar distribution of abnormalities
4. Lack of features that are atypical for UIP

This combination of findings is described as "definite UIP" according to the ATS criteria

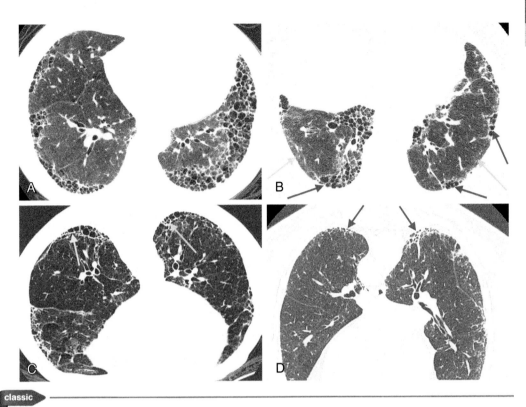

classic

FIGURE 9.4 • **Usual interstitial pneumonia (UIP): Classic appearances. A.** Extensive subpleural and basilar predominant honeycombing is noted in a patient with a UIP pattern associated with idiopathic pulmonary fibrosis. **B.** Subpleural honeycombing (*red arrows*) is present in a patchy distribution. This is interspersed with areas of relatively normal lung (*blue arrows*). **C.** Prone HRCT shows honeycombing (*arrows*) in a patient with UIP. Honeycombing may be in a single (*yellow arrow*) or multiple (*blue arrow*) layers. **D.** Early UIP shows mild subpleural reticulation and honeycombing. A confident diagnosis of honeycombing (*arrows*) can be made in this case despite the mild abnormalities.

and a "typical UIP CT pattern" according to FS criteria. When present, this HRCT pattern predicts a pathologic diagnosis of UIP with >90% certainty. Surgical lung biopsy is usually considered unnecessary for a confident diagnosis in this setting, and diagnosis is based primarily on HRCT findings.

When HRCT findings are considered diagnostic of a UIP pattern, the differential diagnosis includes IPF (Fig. 9.6A), connective tissue disease (Fig. 9.6B), asbestosis (Fig. 9.6C), and drug toxicity (Fig. 9.6D). These are often indistinguishable on HRCT and may be difficult to differentiate pathologically.

Moreover, keep in mind that not all cases of UIP meet these criteria. Although these criteria are specific, they are not sensitive (i.e., about 50 to 70%). Furthermore,

these criteria do not specify the degree of honeycombing that needs to be present to make a confident diagnosis of UIP. Mild honeycombing is all that is needed. Moreover, while traction bronchiectasis is an important finding in the diagnosis of fibrosis, it does not need to be present to make a confident diagnosis of UIP.

Criteria for Intermediate Confidence in the Diagnosis of UIP

Honeycombing is an important finding in the radiographic diagnosis of UIP, and when absent, the confidence of a UIP diagnosis decreases (Fig. 9.7). According to the ATS criteria, a "possible UIP" pattern is considered present when all of the criteria of "definite UIP" are met with the exception of honeycombing;

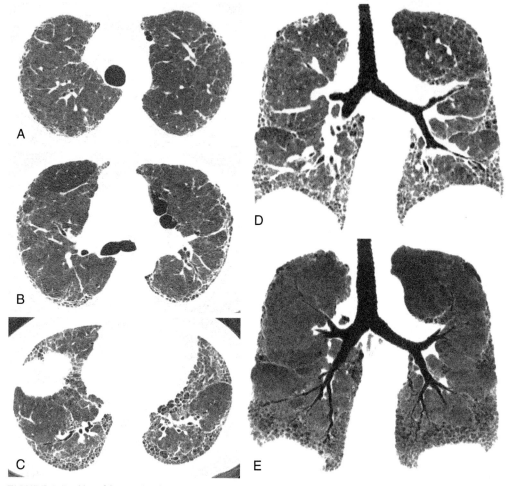

FIGURE 9.5 · **Usual interstitial pneumonia, distribution.** HRCT images through the aortic arch **(A)**, tracheal carina **(B)**, and lung bases **(C)** show a peripheral and basilar predominance of honeycombing. Coronal reformat **(D)** and coronal minimum intensity projection **(E)** images confirm the basilar distribution of disease.

TABLE 9.3	ATS/ERS/JRS/ALAT and Fleischner criteria for HRCT diagnosis of usual interstitial pneumonia based on confidence in the diagnosis of UIP

Confidence in UIP	ATS category	Fleischner category	Features[a]
High	Definite UIP	Typical UIP CT pattern	• Reticulation • Honeycombing • Subpleural/basilar distribution • Absence of atypical features
Intermediate	Possible UIP	Probable UIP CT pattern	• Reticulation • No honeycombing • Subpleural/basilar distribution • Absence of atypical features
	N/A	CT pattern indeterminate for UIP	• Findings of fibrosis • Variable or diffuse distribution • Inconspicuous features suggestive of non-UIP pattern
Low	Inconsistent with UIP	CT features most consistent with non-IPF diagnosis	• Peribronchovascular distribution • Mid- and upper lung distribution • Presence of atypical features (mosaic perfusion, air trapping, ground glass opacity, consolidation, nodules, cysts)

[a]All features must be present to be categorized as high or intermediate confidence in UIP. Only one feature needs to be present to be categorized as low confidence in UIP.

UIP, usual interstitial pneumonia; ATS, American Thoracic Society; ERS, European Respiratory Society; JRS, Japan Respiratory Society; ALAT, Latin American Thoracic Association.

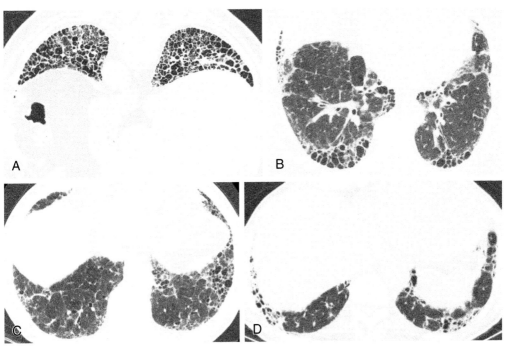

FIGURE 9.6 · **High confidence of usual interstitial pneumonia (UIP), differential diagnosis.** Four examples of UIP on HRCT are shown. Subpleural, basilar predominant fibrosis with honeycombing is seen in patients with UIP secondary to idiopathic pulmonary fibrosis **(A)**, connective tissue disease **(B)**, asbestosis **(C)**, and drug toxicity **(D)**. When presenting with a UIP pattern, these diseases are often indistinguishable on HRCT.

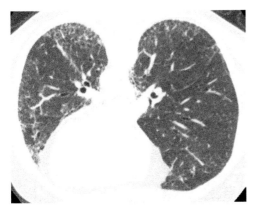

FIGURE 9.7 · **Intermediate confidence in the diagnosis of usual interstitial pneumonia.** Peripheral and subpleural reticulation are present, but honeycombing is absent.

the FS refers to this as a "probable UIP pattern." Criteria are as follows:

1. Reticular opacities
2. Absence of honeycombing
3. Subpleural and basilar distribution of abnormalities
4. Lack of features that are atypical for UIP

IPF accounts for approximately 60 to 90% of patients with this pattern. The remaining 10 to 40% are mostly compromised of hypersensitivity pneumonitis and, to a lesser extent, connective tissue disease. The use of biopsy in patients with "possible UIP" (ATS) and "probable UIP" (FS) is controversial. In practices with a relatively low incidence of HP, biopsy might not be necessary, as most of the patients will have IPF. Other radiographic or clinical features may also be used in determining the likelihood of IPF in patients with "possible/probable UIP" on HRCT. Factors that are associated with a higher risk of IPF include older age (>60 years of age), male gender, and greater degrees of traction bronchiectasis on HRCT.

The FS criteria include an additional category called a "CT pattern indeterminate for UIP" that also corresponds to an intermediate likelihood of IPF (Fig. 9.8). This pattern demonstrates the following features:

1. Findings of fibrosis: reticulation, traction bronchiectasis, and/or honeycombing
2. Variable or diffuse distribution

3. Inconspicuous features considered atypical for UIP

The key feature for a FS "CT pattern indeterminate for UIP" is the presence of one or more features that are generally NOT associated with UIP but with these features not present in amounts that would be considered significant. These features are the same ones listed under the heading of "Criteria for a low confidence in the diagnosis of UIP" (see Table 9.3).

Low Confidence in the Diagnosis of UIP

Certain HRCT features are considered atypical for UIP and suggest an alternative diagnosis. In the ATS classification this is termed "inconsistent with UIP," and in the FS classification, it is termed "CT features most consistent with a non-UIP diagnosis." These features include one or more of the following:

1. Upper or mid-lung predominance (Fig. 9.9)
2. Peribronchovascular predominance (Fig. 9.10)
3. Presence of HRCT features atypical for UIP (and more typical of another disease, including the following:
   a. Mosaic perfusion on inspiratory CT
   b. Air trapping on expiratory CT (Fig. 9.11)
   c. GGO (out of proportion to reticulation)
   d. Diffuse micronodules
   e. Consolidation
   f. Cysts (away from areas of fibrosis)

Each of these findings is typical of an IP other than UIP or a different lung disease. Any one of these is sufficient for determining if the HRCT is inconsistent with a UIP pattern (see Figs. 9.12–9.15). Of note, the atypical features must be present in "significant amounts." For instance, air trapping must be seen bilaterally and in at least three lobes to be considered a significant finding, otherwise it is ignored in terms of the pattern and diagnosis. A finding of subpleural sparing is considered "peribronchovascular" in distribution and is thus considered unlikely to be UIP. Approximately 75% of patients with in this category will have an alternative (non-IPF) diagnosis; however,

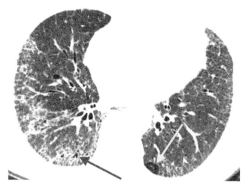

FIGURE 9.8 · Nonspecific pattern of fibrosis. HRCT shows peripheral fibrosis with irregular reticulation and mild traction bronchiectasis (*red arrow*). Minimal mosaic perfusion is present (*yellow arrow*), but no honeycombing is seen. This pattern is not diagnostic of any particular disease, and biopsy is required for definitive diagnosis.

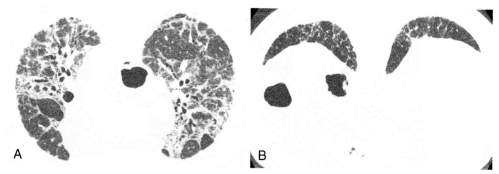

FIGURE 9.9 · Low confidence in UIP. In this patient with hypersensitivity pneumonitis, a prone HRCT demonstrates a distribution of fibrosis that is not subpleural predominant **(A)**, with sparing of the costophrenic angles **(B)**. Because of the central and upper lobe distribution in this case, it would be read as inconsistent with usual interstitial pneumonia.

25% will still have IPF. In other words, an atypical distribution or finding on HRCT does not exclude the diagnosis of IPF.

Idiopathic Pulmonary Fibrosis

IPF is a common cause of diffuse fibrotic lung disease and is the most common cause of a UIP pattern (Fig. 9.12).

A patient with idiopathic UIP has IPF. If a patient with a UIP pattern on HRCT has a disease or exposure that is known to be associated with this pattern (e.g., collagen disease and asbestos exposure), by ATS definition, the diagnosis cannot be IPF. It is important to

note that there are other fibrotic lung diseases in which clinical history does not suggest a specific diagnosis. Examples include sarcoidosis or hypersensitivity pneumonitis in which an exposure cannot be identified. In these cases, the HRCT findings are usually suggestive of a non-UIP diagnosis.

IPF primarily affects patients older than 50 years. It is progressive and patients have a poor prognosis, with a 50% 3-year survival. The disease is usually unresponsive to traditional immunosuppressive treatments, such as corticosteroids; however, two antifibrotic agents, pirfenidone and nintedanib, have been approved for the treatment of IPF and have been shown to slow the progression of fibrosis over time. At this time, these agents are not used for any other diffuse fibrotic lung diseases, although this is the subject of study.

The diagnosis of IPF, in many cases, is based solely on a combination of clinical information and typical HRCT findings (i.e., a high confidence for UIP on HRCT). Lung biopsy is not usually performed unless the HRCT findings are nondiagnostic or atypical for UIP or the patient's clinical history suggests an alternative diagnosis.

In the absence of any clinical or radiographic findings to suggest an alternative diagnosis, a patient with a UIP pattern on HRCT will be given a presumptive diagnosis of IPF (Fig. 9.13). As an HRCT may be considered diagnostic of IPF without a biopsy, it

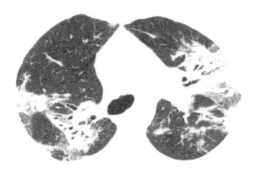

FIGURE 9.10 · **Low confidence in UIP.** HRCT in a patient with sarcoidosis shows large consolidative areas of fibrosis and architectural distortion with a peribronchovascular distribution. Because of the central and upper lobe distribution in this case, this CT would be read as inconsistent with usual interstitial pneumonia.

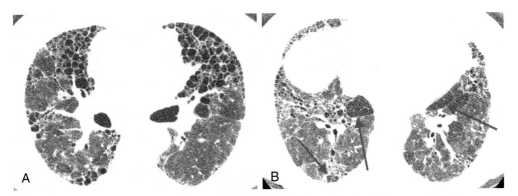

FIGURE 9.11 · **A and B. Low confidence in UIP. A.** HRCT in a patient with hypersensitivity pneumonitis demonstrates extensive honeycombing with a mid-lung predominance. **B.** Expiratory image through the lung base shows patchy bilateral air trapping (*arrows*). Despite the presence of honeycombing, the HRCT does not suggest usual interstitial pneumonia (UIP). Because of the mid-lung distribution and air trapping in this case, it would be read as inconsistent with UIP.

9

is important to be conservative in diagnosing a definite UIP pattern.

Keep in mind that not all cases of IPF show typical HRCT findings. Despite that, however, HRCT remains extremely important in making this diagnosis. Even if lung biopsy is interpreted as "UIP," a clinical diagnosis of UIP cannot be made with certainty if HRCT is interpreted as inconsistent with this diagnosis. It has been recommended that in such a case, a careful consideration of all data by a multidisciplinary group of lung disease experts is necessary.

Atypical HRCT manifestations of IPF include (1) fibrosis that is not subpleural and basilar predominant (Fig. 9.14A, B), (2) predominant GGO (Fig. 9.15), and (3) focal areas of mosaic perfusion or air trapping (Fig. 9.16A, B).

Patients with IPF may show either slow or rapid progression of their disease, with a progressive increase in findings of fibrosis. Patients with IPF also may present with an acute worsening of their symptoms. This is termed *acute exacerbation of IPF*. HRCT in such patients usually shows GGO involving areas previously affected by fibrosis or previously unaffected regions of lung (Fig. 9.17A–C). The GGO typically represents DAD on histopathology.

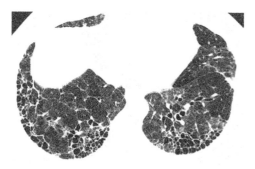

FIGURE 9.12 · **Idiopathic pulmonary fibrosis.** A typical usual interstitial pneumonia pattern is present, manifested by patchy subpleural honeycombing. Idiopathic pulmonary fibrosis is the most common cause of this pattern.

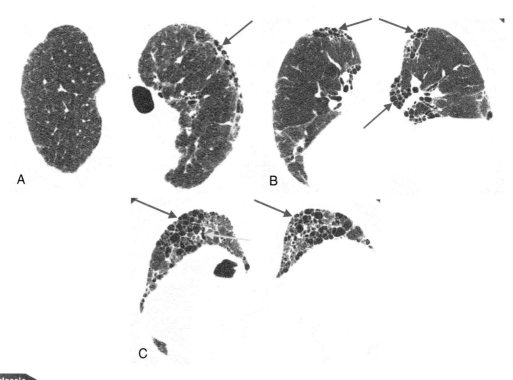

classic

FIGURE 9.13 · **Idiopathic pulmonary fibrosis (IPF): Classic appearance.** HRCT images through the upper **(A)**, mid- **(B)**, and lower **(C)** lungs show a subpleural and basilar predominance of honeycombing (*red arrows*) and traction bronchiectasis (*blue arrow*) compatible with usual interstitial pneumonia. In the absence of known diseases or exposures, this patient will be given a diagnosis of IPF.

Differential Diagnosis

The lung abnormalities of IPF are typically indistinguishable on HRCT from other causes of a UIP pattern, including connective tissue disease, drug toxicity, and asbestosis. The distinction between IPF and these diseases is primarily clinical. Patients with connective tissue disease usually have additional clinical manifestations of a systemic disorder. The possibility of drug toxicity will be discovered by an investigation of a patient's medication list. Patients with asbestosis have long-term exposure in high-risk occupations.

Asbestosis shows associated pleural disease on HRCT in more than 80% of cases. Small centrilobular nodules in the peripheral lung, reflecting peribronchiolar fibrosis, have been described with asbestosis, but this is an uncommon finding and is typically seen in early disease.

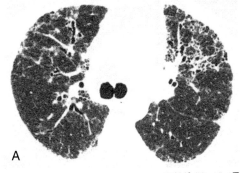

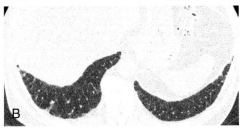

FIGURE 9.14 · **Idiopathic pulmonary fibrosis (IPF), atypical distribution.** This patient with IPF and biopsy-proven usual interstitial pneumonia (UIP) shows atypical findings, with fibrosis that is not subpleural predominant and has significant involvement of the central lung regions **(A)**. Moreover, there is relative sparing of the costophrenic angles **(B)**. Atypical manifestations of IPF are not uncommon. On the basis of HRCT, this case would be read as "inconsistent" with UIP.

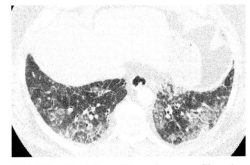

FIGURE 9.15 · **Idiopathic pulmonary fibrosis; presence of ground glass opacity (GGO).** Rarely idiopathic pulmonary fibrosis may present with GGO as a predominant abnormality without definitive signs of fibrosis. In these cases, the GGO represents fibrosis below the resolution of HRCT, and biopsy is required for definitive diagnosis.

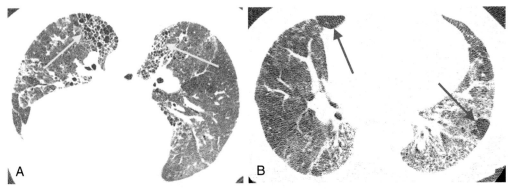

FIGURE 9.16 · **Idiopathic pulmonary fibrosis (IPF), mild air trapping. A.** Prone HRCT through the mid-lung shows peripheral fibrosis with honeycombing (*yellow arrows*) characteristic of IPF. **B.** Mild air trapping (*red arrows*) is not uncommon in patients with IPF and should not suggest an alternative diagnosis if it is limited in severity and extent.

9

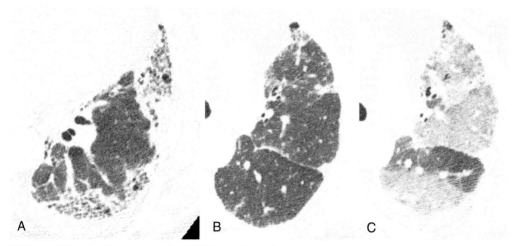

FIGURE 9.17 · **Acute exacerbation of idiopathic pulmonary fibrosis (IPF). A.** HRCT through the left lung base shows peripheral reticulation in a patient with biopsy-proven IPF. **B.** HRCT through the mid-lung shows minimal abnormality. **C.** HRCT at the same level 3 months later shows development of diffuse ground glass opacity in a patient with an acute exacerbation of IPF.

Pathology, in some cases, may be limited by sampling error. In other words, the biopsy sample may be obtained from a portion of the lung that is not representative of the overall disease. For instance, HP and sarcoidosis may show a UIP pattern pathologically if areas of severe fibrosis are sampled. HRCT's advantage is that it images the entire lung parenchyma and usually shows distinguishing features in these cases.

HP typically does not predominate in the subpleural regions but involves the entire cross section of the lung and is most severe in the mid- or upper lungs (Fig. 9.9A, B). Additionally, HRCT in a patient with HP may show centrilobular nodules or multiple areas of mosaic perfusion and/or air trapping (Fig. 9.11A, B). Sarcoidosis is often upper lobe predominant and central or peribronchovascular in distribution (Fig. 9.10). Perilymphatic nodules may be present in association with fibrosis.

NSIP may resemble UIP in some patients, as it often shows fibrosis in a subpleural and basilar distribution. However, fibrotic NSIP often shows a peribronchovascular predominance of reticulation or relative sparing of the subpleural lung; these findings are considered inconsistent with a UIP pattern. Furthermore, honeycombing is not a common finding in

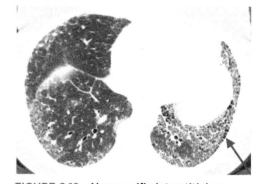

FIGURE 9.18 · **Nonspecific interstitial pneumonia (NSIP), presence of honeycombing.** Fibrotic NSIP may show honeycombing (*arrow*), but it is usually limited in severity such as in this patient with scleroderma. This is in contrast to usual interstitial pneumonia in which honeycombing is often a significant component of the abnormality present.

patients with NSIP, and when present, it tends to be mild and limited in extent (Fig. 9.18).

Familial Pulmonary Fibrosis

Some patients with pulmonary fibrosis have one or more close relatives who also have pulmonary fibrosis. This familial clustering of fibrotic lung disease is thought to be due to a genetic predisposition to various types of lung injury. A specific genetic cause has been identified in a subset of patients with disorders, such as surfactant protein C or telomerase mutations, but the majority of cases are idiopathic.

Familial pulmonary fibrosis is most closely associated with a diagnosis of IPF and is thought to account as many as 20% of cases of this disease. Familial factors may also be seen with HP, connective tissue disease, or any other cause of lung fibrosis. Familial pulmonary fibrosis is not a diagnosis per se. A patient's final diagnosis is that of the underlying disease, such as IPF. Pathologically, patients with familial fibrosis often have a pattern of UIP; however, unclassifiable pathologic findings are also common.

The HRCT findings of familial pulmonary fibrosis are those of the underlying disease; however, atypical manifestations are

more common than in nonfamilial disease (Fig. 9.19). In familial IPF, GGO and atypical distributions of fibrosis are more common than in nonfamilial IPF. There may be variable HRCT patterns within the same family.

NONSPECIFIC INTERSTITIAL PNEUMONIA

The term NSIP was originally used to describe a pathologic pattern that did not meet criteria for any of the other IPs. Over time, it has been recognized that cases classified as NSIP actually represent a specific entity with a characteristic pathologic appearance and clear associations with certain diseases. Connective tissue disease is the most common systemic abnormality to be associated with NSIP, but NSIP may also be seen as a manifestation of drug toxicity or HP or as an idiopathic disorder. Note that both connective tissue disease and drug toxicity may present with either a UIP or NSIP pattern.

On pathology, NSIP demonstrates uniform thickening of the alveolar walls owing to inflammation and/or fibrosis (Fig. 9.20). Typically, lung architecture is preserved, as opposed to UIP, in which the lung architecture is highly distorted. Lung regions affected in NSIP show a uniform histologic appearance, i.e., the disease is spatially and temporally homogeneous.

NSIP (Table 9.4) is less common than UIP and tends to present in younger patients (peak 40 to 50 years of age) with symptoms

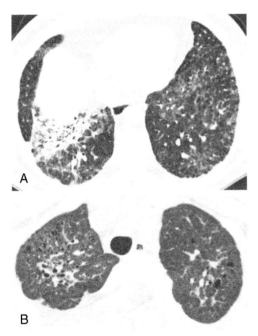

A

B

FIGURE 9.19 · **Familial pulmonary fibrosis.** Two patients in the same family with familial pulmonary fibrosis are shown (**A** and **B**). On biopsy, the histologic pattern was that of usual interstitial pneumonia. **A.** One patient shows patchy basilar predominant ground glass opacity and mild traction bronchiectasis in the lung base. **B.** The other patient shows upper lobe and centrally predominant reticulation, traction bronchiectasis, and cysts. HRCT findings are often atypical in patients with familial pulmonary fibrosis.

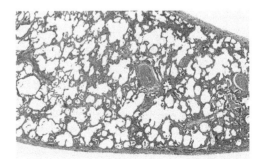

FIGURE 9.20 · **Pathology of nonspecific interstitial pneumonia.** Diffuse alveolar septal wall thickening due to fibrosis is present with little distortion of the underlying lung architecture.

TABLE 9.4 | Features of nonspecific interstitial pneumonia

Frequency	Second most common IP; 25% of IP cases
HRCT findings	Subpleural, basilar predominant
	Ground glass opacity, irregular reticulation, traction bronchiectasis
	No or minimal honeycombing
	Subpleural sparing in 20–50%
Idiopathic syndrome	Idiopathic NSIP
Associated diseases	Connective tissue disease
	Drug toxicity
	Hypersensitivity pneumonitis

IP, interstitial pneumonia; NSIP, nonspecific interstitial pneumonia.

that are less severe. There are two subtypes of NSIP, cellular and fibrotic, representing different stages of disease. The fibrotic subtype is more common in clinical practice.

In general, the prognosis of patients with NSIP is better than that of UIP (75% 5-year survival), although this survival difference is not as significant in patients with the fibrotic subtype of NSIP.

HRCT Findings
The HRCT findings in patients with NSIP depend on whether the cellular or fibrotic subtype is present. Cellular NSIP presents with GGO as the predominant abnormality, although fine reticulation is often associated, and traction bronchiectasis may also be present (Fig. 9.21A–D).

Fibrotic NSIP presents with traction bronchiectasis and irregular reticulation as the predominant findings (Fig. 9.22A–D). GGO may also be present in fibrotic NSIP, and this may reflect superimposed cellular NSIP. Honeycombing is uncommon with fibrotic NSIP, seen in only a few percent of cases, and, when present, is typically limited in severity and extent.

Acute exacerbation of NSIP, similar to acute exacerbation in IPF, may occur with DAD on histology and GGO and consolidation on HRCT.

The distribution of NSIP is similar to that of UIP, being peripheral and basilar predominant (Fig. 9.23). However, a peripheral, concentric distribution of abnormalities with relative sparing of the immediate subpleural lung (i.e., *subpleural sparing*) is a finding that

is highly predictive of NSIP; this finding is present in 20 to 50% of cases (Figs. 9.21A–C, 9.22A–C, 9.24A, B). NSIP may also show a peribronchovascular predominance.

Patients with connective tissue disease and suspected NSIP do not typically undergo lung biopsy for diagnosis, as the lung disease is assumed to be related to their systemic disorder. In the absence of a history of connective tissue disease, biopsy is usually performed when NSIP is suspected based on HRCT findings.

Differential Diagnosis
Differentiating fibrotic NSIP from UIP on HRCT may be difficult in some cases. When subpleural sparing is present and honeycombing is absent or minimal, NSIP is very likely. When there is fibrosis with minimal or no honeycombing and no subpleural sparing is present, both UIP and NSIP are possible (Fig. 9.25A, B). The greater the severity of fibrosis without honeycombing, the more likely NSIP is as a diagnosis. The presence of significant honeycombing suggests UIP. Moreover, NSIP tends to appear concentric in distribution; UIP is often patchy.

DESQUAMATIVE INTERSTITIAL PNEUMONIA

DIP (Table 9.5) is a pattern of lung injury associated with cigarette smoking and will be discussed in greater detail in Chapter 11. Rarely, DIP is seen as a reaction in connective tissue disease, drug toxicity, toxic inhalations, and surfactant protein C mutations

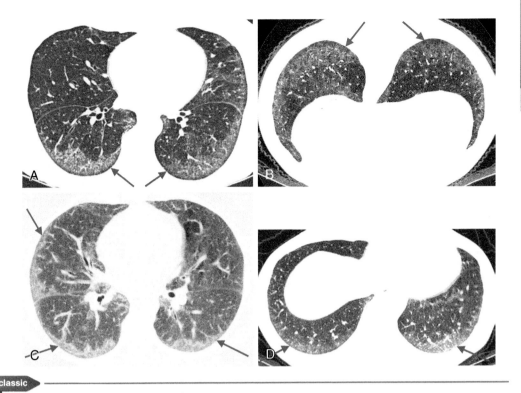

FIGURE 9.21 · **Cellular nonspecific interstitial pneumonia (NSIP): Classic appearances.** Four examples of cellular NSIP are shown. In each of these cases, ground glass opacity (*arrows*) is the most significant abnormality. Findings of fibrosis, such as traction bronchiectasis, are absent or mild in severity. Relative sparing of the immediate subpleural lung **(A–C)** is very suggestive of this diagnosis, but is absent in many cases of NSIP **(D)**.

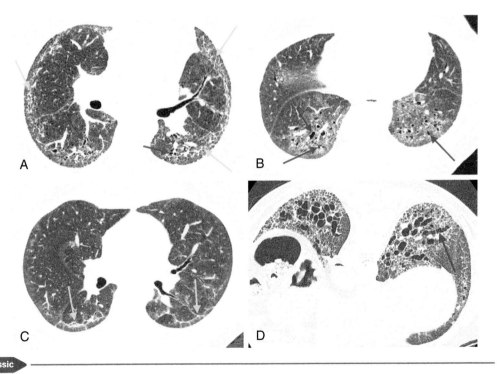

FIGURE 9.22 · **Fibrotic nonspecific interstitial pneumonia: Classic appearances.** Four examples of fibrotic nonspecific interstitial pneumonia are shown. In each of these cases, irregular reticulation (*blue arrows*) and traction bronchiectasis (*red arrows*) are the predominant findings. Sparing of the immediate subpleural lung **(A–C)** is suggestive of this diagnosis, but may be absent **(D)**. Honeycombing is absent or inconspicuous.

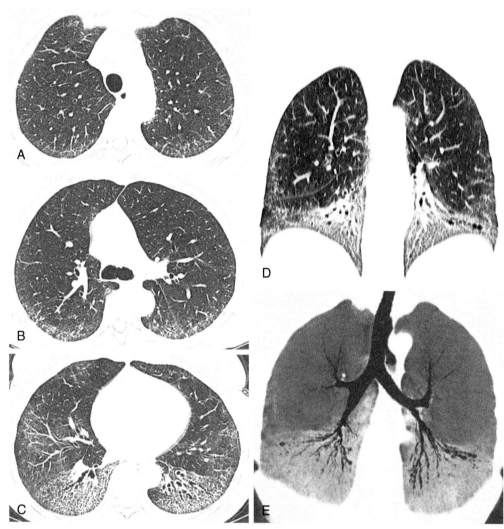

FIGURE 9.23 · **Nonspecific interstitial pneumonia, distribution.** HRCT images through the upper **(A)**, mid- **(B)**, and lower **(C)** lungs show a subpleural and basilar distribution of irregular reticulation and traction bronchiectasis. Coronal reformatted image **(D)** and coronal minimum intensity projection **(E)** confirm the basilar distribution of findings.

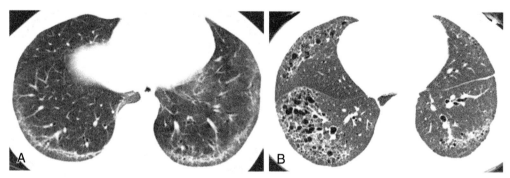

FIGURE 9.24 · **Nonspecific interstitial pneumonia (NSIP), subpleural sparing.** A peripheral distribution of findings with relative sparing of the immediate subpleural interstitium is highly suggestive of NSIP. **A.** A rim of peripheral irregular reticulation is present with relative sparing of the immediate subpleural interstitium in a patient with NSIP related to rheumatoid arthritis. **B.** More severe traction bronchiectasis and irregular reticulation is present in a patient with scleroderma. The findings are peripheral; however, the subpleural lung is relatively spared. The immediate subpleural lung is less abnormal than lung the 1 cm away from the pleura.

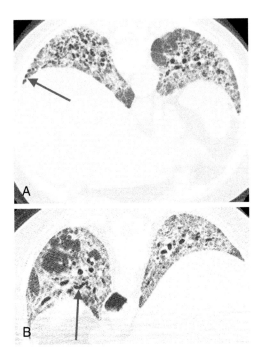

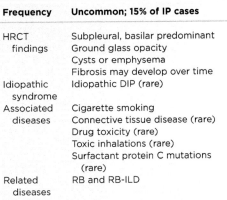

TABLE 9.5	Features of desquamative interstitial pneumonia
Frequency	Uncommon; 15% of IP cases
HRCT findings	Subpleural, basilar predominant Ground glass opacity Cysts or emphysema Fibrosis may develop over time
Idiopathic syndrome	Idiopathic DIP (rare)
Associated diseases	Cigarette smoking Connective tissue disease (rare) Drug toxicity (rare) Toxic inhalations (rare) Surfactant protein C mutations (rare)
Related diseases	RB and RB-ILD

IP, interstitial pneumonia; DIP, desquamative interstitial pneumonia; RB, respiratory bronchiolitis; ILD, interstitial lung disease.

FIGURE 9.25 · **Fibrotic nonspecific interstitial pneumonia (NSIP) versus usual interstitial pneumonia (UIP). A.** Prone HRCT shows mild honeycombing (*arrow*) in a patient with NSIP. This finding is not uncommon with fibrotic NSIP, but it is typically limited in severity compared with UIP. **B.** Prone HRCT shows peripheral and basilar predominant traction bronchiectasis (*arrow*) and irregular reticulation in a patient with idiopathic pulmonary fibrosis. The lack of honeycombing favors NSIP, but UIP can present with severe fibrosis in the absence of honeycombing. If the patient has a history of connective tissue disease, this appearance is assumed to represent NSIP, otherwise a biopsy is required for diagnosis.

and as an idiopathic disorder. The name DIP is a misnomer, as the primary pathologic abnormality is the presence of numerous alveolar macrophages. DIP presents in younger patients (peak age 30 to 40 years) than NSIP or UIP and is typically more responsive to treatment (70 to 95% 5-year survival).

DIP and respiratory bronchiolitis (RB) are both histologic patterns associated with smoking and represent different points on a spectrum of the same alveolar macrophage abnormality. In RB, the macrophage infiltrate predominates around small airways, whereas in DIP, the abnormalities are more diffuse. RB is a common incidental histologic abnormality in smokers. If a patient shows RB on histologic examination and is symptomatic, the disease is termed RB-ILD.

HRCT Findings
On HRCT, typical examples of DIP show a distribution similar to that of UIP and NSIP, being peripheral and basilar predominant (Fig. 9.26A–D). GGO is the predominant finding (Fig. 9.27). GGO may be diffuse or have a basal predominance. Findings of fibrosis (reticulation, traction bronchiectasis, and honeycombing) tend to be absent or mild in severity, although DIP may progress to a fibrotic pattern in occasional cases. Scattered cysts and/or emphysema may be seen in affected regions (Fig. 9.28). These cysts can be a clue to diagnosis.

In RB or RB-ILD, HRCT usually shows centrilobular nodules of GGO. The nodules are usually most severe in the central portions of the upper lungs. Mosaic perfusion and/or air trapping may also be present, although this tends to be mild.

As RB and DIP are part of the spectrum of the same disease, an overlap of findings may be present. Thus, DIP may show centrilobular

9

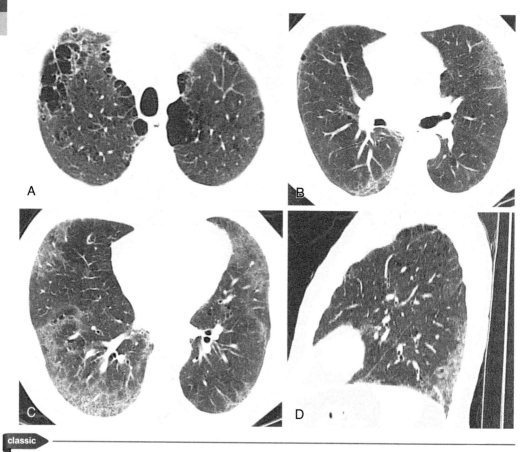

classic

FIGURE 9.26 · **Desquamative interstitial pneumonia (DIP), distribution: Classic appearance.** HRCT through the upper **(A)**, mid- **(B)**, and lower **(C)** lungs shows a peripheral and basilar distribution of ground glass opacity. This is also shown on a sagittal reformatted image **(D)**. Note emphysema in the upper lobes **(A)** in this patient with a history of smoking.

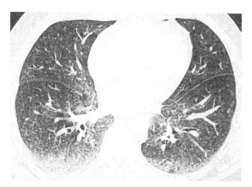

FIGURE 9.27 · **Desquamative interstitial pneumonia (DIP).** HRCT shows peripheral ground glass opacity as an isolated abnormality. This is a nonspecific finding, but in a smoker with chronic symptoms, desquamative interstitial pneumonia is the favored diagnosis.

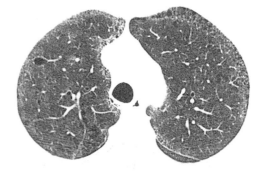

FIGURE 9.28 · **Desquamative interstitial pneumonia (DIP).** The combination of ground glass opacity and cysts or emphysema in the same lung regions suggests DIP. When present in a patient with a smoking history, this combination is usually taken as sufficient evidence for DIP without the need for a biopsy.

GGO nodules, mosaic perfusion, and air trapping, and distribution may be diffuse or predominantly in the upper lobe or lower lobe.

ORGANIZING PNEUMONIA

OP (Table 9.6) is a noninfectious, inflammatory abnormality associated with a wide variety of etiologies and diseases. It is a relatively common pattern seen both pathologically and on HRCT. It was previously known as bronchiolitis obliterans with organizing pneumonia (BOOP), but this term has been dropped for several reasons. First, "OP" is a more accurate reflection of the pathologic appearance of this disorder. Second, this term avoids confusion with airways diseases, namely bronchiolitis obliterans.

On pathology, the predominant finding of OP is that of branching or rounded, polypoid, intra-alveolar granulation tissue in the distal airspaces (Fig. 9.29). This granulation tissue also involves the respiratory bronchioles, which may be the site of initiation of the repair response. These findings are associated with a mild interstitial infiltrate; however, the granulation tissue is the predominant pathologic feature.

Patients with OP commonly present with subacute or chronic symptoms of low-grade fever, dyspnea, and cough, but an acute presentation is also possible. Symptoms are usually less severe than those of UIP, and the disease is responsive to steroids, although not uncommonly it recurs after treatment.

HRCT Findings

The most typical HRCT finding of OP is that of focal areas of consolidation, often nodular or mass-like and often irregular in shape or spiculated, that predominate in the peribronchovascular and subpleural regions (Fig. 9.30). The areas of consolidation are intermixed with regions of normal lung. These findings are often most severe in the lower lobes (Fig. 9.31).

GGO is rarely a predominant abnormality but may be seen as the primary manifestation of OP in immunocompromised patients (Fig. 9.32) or in combination with consolidation. Centrilobular nodules are an infrequent finding in OP but may be seen. Although OP may eventually lead to lung scarring, significant fibrosis is not a common feature.

A finding that is highly suggestive of OP is the *atoll sign* or *reversed halo sign*. This

TABLE 9.6	Features of organizing pneumonia
Frequency	**10% of IP cases**
HRCT findings	Peribronchovascular and subpleural predominant
	Consolidation (often nodular or mass-like)
	Irregular borders
	Small centrilobular nodules (rare)
	Lower lobe predominance
	Development of fibrosis after treatment
	Atoll or reversed halo sign
Idiopathic syndrome	COP
Associated diseases	Connective tissue disease
	Drug toxicity
	Infection
	Toxic inhalations
	Immunologic disorders
	Graft vs. host disease
	Secondary reaction to another disorder (chronic eosinophilic pneumonia, hypersensitivity pneumonitis, granulomatosis with polyangiitis, diffuse alveolar damage)

IP, interstitial pneumonia; NSIP, nonspecific interstitial pneumonia; COP, cryptogenic organizing pneumonia.

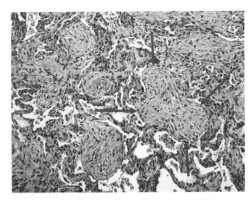

FIGURE 9.29 • **Pathology of organizing pneumonia.** Rounded plugs of granulation tissue (*arrows*) are present in the alveolar spaces corresponding to consolidation on HRCT.

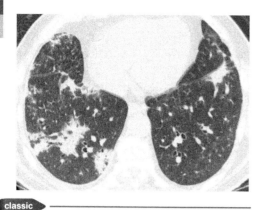

FIGURE 9.30 · Organizing pneumonia (OP): Classic appearance. The classic HRCT findings of OP are depicted in this patient. Peripheral and peribronchovascular consolidation, often with a nodular or mass-like appearance and irregular margins, is seen bilaterally. Note significant unaffected lung intermixed with areas of OP.

manifests as a ring or partial ring of consolidation surrounding a central region of clearing or GGO (Fig. 9.33).

In a small proportion of cases, the atoll or reversed halo sign can reflect the presence of an alternative diagnosis, such as pulmonary infarct, infection (e.g., paracoccidioidomycosis or invasive fungal infection), sarcoidosis, and vasculitis (granulomatosis with polyangiitis [GPA]). When the atoll sign is seen in association with one of these diseases, there are usually clinical or additional radiologic findings to suggest the diagnosis is not OP. For instance, the presence of the atoll sign in a patient with neutropenia should prompt an investigation for invasive fungal infection, specifically mucormycosis. When the atoll sign is present in the absence of these clinical or additional imaging findings, one can be quite confident that OP is present, either as

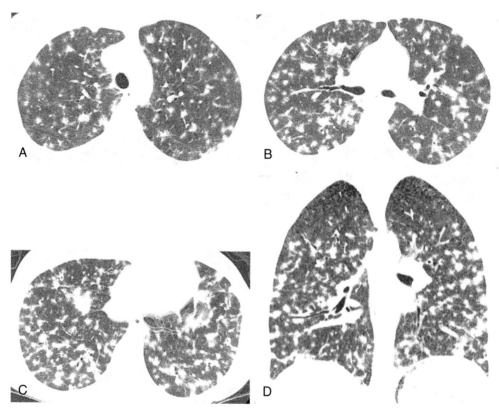

FIGURE 9.31 · Organizing pneumonia, distribution. HRCT images through the upper **(A)**, mid-**(B)**, and lower **(C)** lungs show nodular areas of subpleural and peribronchovascular consolidation. Coronal reformatted image **(D)** shows the lower lobe predominance of disease.

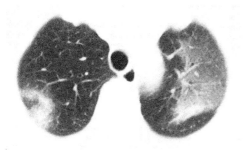

FIGURE 9.32 · **Organizing pneumonia, ground glass opacity.** Organizing pneumonia typically presents with consolidation as the predominant abnormality. Rarely, ground glass opacity is the predominant HRCT finding, particularly in patients with a history of immunosuppression.

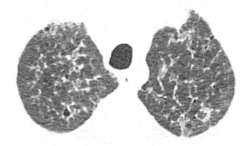

FIGURE 9.34 · **Perilobular opacities.** Interconnecting linear opacities are seen forming polygonal structures that resemble pulmonary lobules. These lines are thicker and more ill-defined than interlobular septa. This patient has cryptogenic organizing pneumonia.

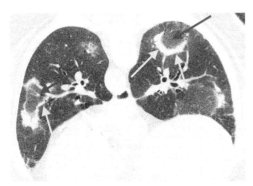

FIGURE 9.33 · **"Atoll sign" or "reversed halo sign" in organizing pneumonia (OP).** A peripheral rim of consolidation (*yellow arrows*) surrounding a central area of clearing or ground glass opacity (*red arrows*) is called the atoll or reversed halo sign. This finding is highly suggestive of OP but is not specific with respect to the cause of OP.

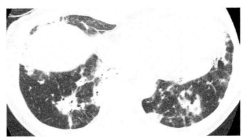

FIGURE 9.35 · **Organizing pneumonia, amiodarone toxicity.** Patchy subpleural and peribronchovascular mass-like regions of irregular consolidation are present. This combination of findings is most suggestive of organizing pneumonia. There are multiple possible causes of organizing pneumonia, one of which is drug toxicity.

the predominant abnormality or as a secondary reaction to a diffuse lung disease.

Another finding that is thought to be specific for OP is the presence of perilobular opacities. On HRCT, this abnormality manifests as interconnecting linear opacities that form polygonal shapes similar to interlobular septa (Fig. 9.34). Perilobular opacities differ from interlobular septal thickening in that they are thicker and much less sharply defined. It is thought that perilobular opacities are due to abnormalities at the periphery of the pulmonary lobule directly adjacent to the interlobular septa.

The multiple causes of OP include connective tissue disease, infection, drugs (Fig. 9.35), toxic inhalations, immunologic disorders, and graft-versus-host disease. OP may also be seen as a secondary process in association with other diseases including infections, chronic eosinophilic pneumonia (Fig. 9.36), HP, GPA (Wegener's granulomatosis) (Fig. 9.37), and DAD. The HRCT in these cases may be indistinguishable from those in which OP is the predominant abnormality. Approximately 50% of cases of OP are idiopathic; this is termed cryptogenic organizing pneumonia (COP) (Fig. 9.38).

The differential diagnosis of OP includes other causes of patchy and chronic

9

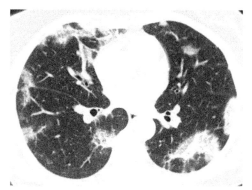

FIGURE 9.36 · **Chronic eosinophilic pneumonia with organizing pneumonia (OP).** Patchy bilateral focal areas of consolidation are seen, which is most suggestive of OP. OP may be seen as a primary abnormality or as a secondary reaction to another diffuse lung disease, such as chronic eosinophilic pneumonia.

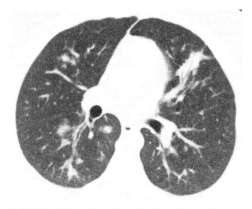

FIGURE 9.37 · **Granulomatosis with polyangiitis with organizing pneumonia (OP).** There are several diseases that may be associated with an OP pattern on pathology and HRCT. These include chronic eosinophilic pneumonia, infection, hypersensitivity pneumonitis, and granulomatosis with polyangiitis. Focal patchy peribronchovascular consolidation in this patient with granulomatosis with polyangiitis corresponded to OP seen on pathology.

consolidation, including chronic eosinophilic pneumonia, invasive mucinous adenocarcinoma, lymphoma, sarcoidosis, and lipoid pneumonia. Note that chronic eosinophilic pneumonia may result in histologic and HRCT findings virtually

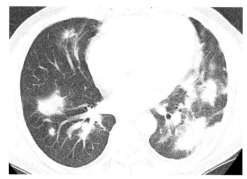

FIGURE 9.38 · **Cryptogenic organizing pneumonia (COP).** Patchy, bilateral mass-like regions of consolidation and ground glass opacity are seen in a patient with chronic symptoms and no contributing history or exposures. COP accounts for approximately 50% of cases of organizing pneumonia.

TABLE 9.7	Features of acute interstitial pneumonia
Frequency	Rare; <2% of IP cases
Histologic pattern	DAD
HRCT findings	Diffuse
	Ground glass opacity and consolidation
	Fibrosis may develop over time (anterior distribution)
Differential diagnosis	Other causes of DAD and ARDS

DAD, diffuse alveolar damage; ARDS, acute respiratory distress syndrome.

indistinguishable from OP; these entities are likely related, differing only in the prevalence of eosinophils.

ACUTE INTERSTITIAL PNEUMONIA

AIP (Table 9.7) is an IIP associated with the histologic pattern of DAD. It usually presents as acute respiratory distress syndrome (ARDS) without an identifiable cause. It has also been called Hamman–Rich syndrome. The clinical presentation is similar to that of known causes of ARDS. Early mortality is high, similar to other causes of ARDS.

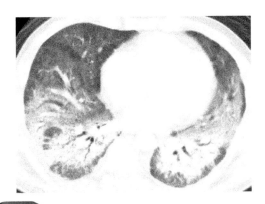

classic ▶

FIGURE 9.39 · **Acute interstitial pneumonia: Classic appearance.** Extensive bilateral ground glass opacity and consolidation in a patient with acute symptoms may represent edema, diffuse alveolar damage, infection, and/or hemorrhage. This patient had a clinical diagnosis of acute respiratory distress syndrome (ARDS) and lung biopsy showed diffuse alveolar damage. No cause for ARDS was identified, and a diagnosis of acute interstitial pneumonia was made.

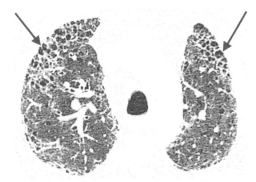

FIGURE 9.40 · **Acute interstitial pneumonia, fibrosis.** One year after a diagnosis of acute interstitial pneumonia (AIP), this patient showed subpleural fibrosis with honeycombing (*arrows*) that has a striking anterior distribution. This is a typical appearance of post-AIP fibrosis.

HRCT Findings

The HRCT findings of AIP are usually indistinguishable from other causes of DAD and ARDS (see Chapter 8). Extensive or diffuse GGO and consolidation are present (Fig. 9.39). If imaged early in its course, the abnormalities may have a peripheral distribution but then quickly become diffuse in nature. Over time, the HRCT of patients who survive shows interval decrease in GGO and consolidation. Often irregular reticulation and other signs of fibrosis develop. Eventually, fibrosis may be the only sequela of AIP. This fibrosis commonly has a peripheral and anterior distribution (Fig. 9.40).

LYMPHOID INTERSTITIAL PNEUMONIA

LIP is a lymphoproliferative disorder associated with connective tissue disease and immunodeficiency disorders such as human immunodeficiency virus infection or common variable immunodeficiency. Rarely it is idiopathic. It will be discussed in more detail in Chapter 17.

The clinical presentation of LIP is usually that of the underlying systemic disorder,

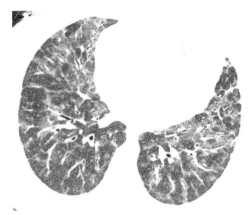

FIGURE 9.41 · **Lymphocytic interstitial pneumonia.** HRCT shows patchy bilateral ground glass opacity in a patient with connective tissue disease. Although this appearance is nonspecific, in this clinical setting, lymphocytic interstitial pneumonia is a possible diagnosis.

although chronic dyspnea and dry cough may be present. LIP tends to be steroid responsive, although up to a third of patients may progress to fibrosis.

HRCT Findings

The most common HRCT finding of LIP is patchy GGO (Fig. 9.41). Consolidation may also be present. These findings are quite nonspecific, and thus, the clinical history is important in diagnosis. Nodules, when present, may be suggestive of LIP in the appropriate clinical setting and are usually centrilobular or perilymphatic in distribution. Centrilobular nodules in LIP reflect the presence of follicular bronchiolitis. Cysts may be present in association with other abnormalities or may be the only manifestation of LIP, particularly in the setting of Sjögren's disease or other connective tissue diseases.

PLEUROPARENCHYMAL FIBROELASTOSIS

PPFE is a recently described pattern of lung injury. On histopathology, an apical predominance of lung fibrosis with elastosis is present and is associated with fibrosis of visceral pleura. It may be idiopathic or due to known diseases including chronic infection, drugs, connective tissue disease, and bone marrow transplantation. PPFE may also manifest as a form of chronic rejection in lung transplant recipients. When idiopathic, the peak age of onset for PPFE is 50 to 60 years. Progression is typical, and the prognosis is poor.

Characteristic HRCT findings include an apical and subpleural distribution of consolidation with architectural distortion, irregular reticulation, traction bronchiectasis, and honeycombing (Fig. 9.42). Fibrosis is associated with pleural thickening, often with extrapleural fat deposition. Progression on HRCT over time is typical.

The differential diagnosis of PPFE on HRCT includes other causes of upper lobe fibrosis. An "apical fibrous cap," an incidental finding that should not be associated with symptoms, will also manifest as apical-predominant fibrosis; however, the degree of fibrosis is less severe, and it should remain stable in extent and severity on serial imaging. Sarcoidosis, scarring from prior granulomatous infection, and pneumoconioses also demonstrate an upper lobe distribution of fibrosis; however, they tend to be peribronchovascular in distribution in distinction to the subpleural predominance in PPFE. These diseases also usually remain stable over time or progress at a rate that is slower than PPFE.

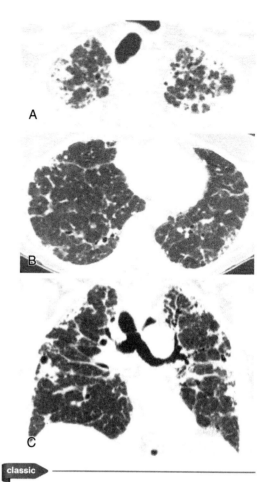

classic

FIGURE 9.42 · A–C. Pleuroparenchymal fibroelastosis: Classic appearance. Axial HRCT image through the upper lung **(A)** demonstrates subpleural consolidation with architectural distortion and bronchiectasis. There is involvement in the mid-lung **(B)**; however, this is much less severe. The subpleural and apical distribution is well demonstrated on a coronal reformatted image **(C)**.

FURTHER READING

Akira M, Yamamoto S, Sakatani M. Bronchiolitis obliterans organizing pneumonia manifesting as multiple large nodules or masses. *AJR Am J Roentgenol.* 1998;170:291-295.

American Thoracic Society/European Respiratory Society International Multidisciplinary Consensus Classification of the Idiopathic Interstitial Pneumonias. *Am J Respir Crit Care Med.* 2002;165:277-304.

Colby TV, Myers JL. The clinical and histologic spectrum of bronchiolitis obliterans including bronchiolitis obliterans organizing pneumonia (BOOP). *Semin Respir Dis*. 1992;13:119-133.

Hartman TE, Primack SL, Swensen SJ, et al. Desquamative interstitial pneumonia: thin-section CT findings in 22 patients. *Radiology*. 1993;187:787-790.

Hartman TE, Swensen SJ, Hansell DM, et al. Nonspecific interstitial pneumonia: variable appearance at high-resolution chest CT. *Radiology*. 2000;217:701-705.

Heyneman LE, Ward S, Lynch DA, et al. Respiratory bronchiolitis, respiratory bronchiolitis-associated interstitial lung disease, and desquamative interstitial pneumonia: different entities or part of the spectrum of the same disease process? *AJR Am J Roentgenol*. 1999;173:1617-1622.

Johkoh T, Müller NL, Cartier Y, et al. Idiopathic interstitial pneumonias: diagnostic accuracy of thin-section CT in 129 patients. *Radiology*. 1999;211:555-560.

Johkoh T, Müller NL, Colby TV, et al. Nonspecific interstitial pneumonia: correlation between thin-section CT findings and pathologic subgroups in 55 patients. *Radiology*. 2002;225:199-204.

Johkoh T, Müller NL, Pickford HA, et al. Lymphocytic interstitial pneumonia: thin-section CT findings in 22 patients. *Radiology*. 1999;212:567-572.

Johkoh T, Müller NL, Taniguchi H, et al. Acute interstitial pneumonia: thin-section CT findings in 36 patients. *Radiology*. 1999; 211:859-863.

Katzenstein AL, Myers JL. Idiopathic pulmonary fibrosis: clinical relevance of pathologic classification. *Am J Respir Crit Care Med*. 1998;157:1301-1315.

Kim SJ, Lee KS, Ryu YH, et al. Reversed halo sign on high-resolution CT of cryptogenic organizing pneumonia: diagnostic implications. *AJR Am J Roentgenol*. 2003;180:1251-1254.

Lee KS, Kullnig P, Hartman TE, Müller NL. Cryptogenic organizing pneumonia: CT findings in 43 patients. *AJR Am J Roentgenol*. 1994;162:543-546.

Lynch DA, Sverzellati N, Travis WD, et al. Diagnostic criteria for idiopathic pulmonary fibrosis: a Fleischner Society white paper. *Lancet Respir Med*. 2018;6:138-153.

Lynch DA, Travis WD, Müller NL, et al. Idiopathic interstitial pneumonias: CT features. *Radiology*. 2005;236:10-21.

Müller NL, Colby TV. Idiopathic interstitial pneumonias: high-resolution CT and histologic findings. *Radiographics*. 1997;17:1016-1022.

Park JS, Lee KS, Kim JS, et al. Nonspecific interstitial pneumonia with fibrosis: radiographic and CT findings in seven patients. *Radiology*. 1995;195:645-648.

Primack SL, Hartman TE, Ikezoe J, et al. Acute interstitial pneumonia: radiographic and CT findings in nine patients. *Radiology*. 1993;188:817-820.

Raghu G, Collard HR, Egan JJ, et al. An official ATS/ERS/JRS/ALAT statement: idiopathic pulmonary fibrosis: evidence-based guidelines for diagnosis and management. *Am J Respir Crit Care Med*. 2011;183:788-824.

Travis WD, Hunninghake G, King TE, et al. Idiopathic nonspecific interstitial pneumonia: report of an American Thoracic Society project. *Am J Respir Crit Care Med*. 2008;177:1338-1347.

9

Connective Tissue Diseases

INTRODUCTION

Connective tissue diseases (CTDs) may have a variety of manifestations including diffuse or focal lung disease, pleural or pericardial abnormalities, vascular abnormalities, and esophageal disease. Most patients with CTD have extra-pulmonary manifestations, but in some cases, lung abnormalities are seen in isolation or as the first manifestation of disease.

This chapter provides an overview of the approach to diagnosis of lung disease in these patients, followed by a discussion of the most common lung manifestations of specific CTDs.

A GENERAL APPROACH TO DIAGNOSIS

CTDs may result in a number of pulmonary abnormalities that reflect the various ways the lung reacts to injury (Table 10.1). The interstitial pneumonias (IPs) are common in patients with CTD, including usual interstitial pneumonia (UIP), nonspecific interstitial pneumonia (NSIP), lymphoid interstitial pneumonia (LIP) and follicular bronchiolitis, organizing pneumonia (OP), and diffuse alveolar damage (DAD). Although patients tend to present with a single pattern, an overlap of more than one pattern is sometimes seen. The IPs are described in detail in the preceding chapter.

In addition, patients with CTD may show intrathoracic abnormalities not related to an IP. These may be specific to the individual CTD. These include pulmonary edema, vasculitis, pulmonary hypertension, pulmonary hemorrhage, pleural or pericardial effusion, lung nodules, bronchiectasis, constrictive bronchiolitis, and esophageal dilatation.

The initial presentation of diffuse lung disease may precede the diagnosis of CTD. High-resolution computed tomography (HRCT) plays a major role in suggesting the presence of a pattern of lung disease (e.g., NSIP) consistent with CTD and excluding alternative diagnoses. In some patients, HRCT findings precipitate a workup for CTD.

Role of HRCT in CTD

The role of HRCT in patients with known or suspected CTD is different than in those with many other diffuse lung diseases. The main roles of HRCT include the following.

Diagnosis

Diagnostic criteria exist for each of the CTDs. These criteria include clinical symptoms, physical examination findings, and serologic abnormalities. With the exception of scleroderma, lung disease is not part of any of these criteria.

Serologic tests are often obtained as a screening test in patients with lung disease of unclear etiology; if positive, a more intensive search for CTD will be undertaken. The most useful serological indices are those relatively specific for a particular CTD (e.g., Scl-70 in scleroderma), although no serology is diagnostic of a single disease.

HRCT plays little role in the diagnosis of a patient who meets criteria for a specific CTD, although it may indicate associated lung disease is present. However, HRCT can be helpful when a CTD is suspected, but the diagnostic criteria are not met. It is estimated that as many as 20% of patients who are determined to have idiopathic lung disease at initial presentation are subsequently diagnosed as having CTD

TABLE 10.1	Abnormalities that may be seen in patients with connective tissue disease

Usual interstitial pneumonia
Nonspecific interstitial pneumonia
Lymphoid interstitial pneumonia
Follicular bronchiolitis
Organizing pneumonia
Diffuse alveolar damage
Constrictive bronchiolitis
Pulmonary edema
Pulmonary hemorrhage
Pulmonary hypertension
Serositis (pleural or pericardial effusion)
Miscellaneous (nodules, bronchiectasis, esophageal dilatation)

TABLE 10.2	HRCT findings of usual and nonspecific interstitial pneumonia
Usual interstitial pneumonia	Subpleural, basilar predominant Honeycombing Other signs of fibrosis (traction bronchiectasis, irregular reticulation)
Nonspecific interstitial pneumonia	Subpleural, basilar predominant Ground glass opacity Fibrosis (traction bronchiectasis, irregular reticulation) No or mild honeycombing Subpleural sparing

10

on interval clinical follow-up. Several findings on HRCT suggest CTD as an etiology. In any patient with an NSIP pattern on HRCT, an underlying CTD should be sought, as this is one of the most common causes of NSIP. If a patient has multicompartmental disease (more than one of the following; lung, pleura or pericardium, pulmonary vasculature, or esophagus), CTD should be suspected.

Determining the Pattern of Lung Disease

Because the diagnosis of CTD is made predominantly using clinical and serologic findings, lung biopsy is not commonly obtained in patients with a CTD and lung abnormalities. However, HRCT provides an evaluation of the nature of the lung disease and the pattern of injury present. Determining the pattern of injury has important implications for treatment and prognosis.

Evaluating Progression over Time and Response to Treatment

Although pulmonary function tests (PFTs) are the primary diagnostic tool used in the serial follow-up of CTD patients with known lung disease, HRCT plays an important complementary role. HRCT is more accurate than PFTs in patients with early lung disease or multicompartmental disease. HRCT may also be helpful in distinguishing the reversible versus irreversible components to the lung disease that are seen on initial imaging. This is particularly helpful when NSIP is the predominant pattern.

PATTERNS OF DIFFUSE LUNG DISEASE

As HRCT is the primary method of characterizing diffuse lung disease in patients with CTD, a knowledge of their manifestations and distinguishing features is important.

UIP and NSIP

UIP and NSIP are the most common patterns of diffuse lung disease and fibrosis in patients with CTD. Typical findings (Table 10.2) include honeycombing, traction bronchiectasis, and irregular reticulation. Ground glass opacity (GGO) is less common, except in NSIP, particularly the cellular subtype. Fibrosis is only rarely seen with LIP and follicular bronchiolitis, OP, and constrictive bronchiolitis.

In general, NSIP is the most common pattern seen in patients with CTD. It is most typical of scleroderma, polymyositis, dermatomyositis, and mixed CTD. UIP is seen most frequently in patients with rheumatoid lung disease. It is similar in appearance to UIP in patients with IPF, but honeycombing often has an anterior predominance or appears "bubbly" in appearance, and without other findings of fibrosis, such as traction bronchiectasis. NSIP most commonly results in peripheral, lower lobe GGO with subpleural sparing, or reticulation with traction bronchiectasis having the same distribution.

Although often having different appearances, in some patients, UIP and NSIP may be difficult to differentiate using HRCT. In particular, the fibrotic subtype of NSIP can closely resemble UIP, although the clinical significance of this distinction in CTD patients is uncertain. In UIP, honeycombing is a significant finding (Fig. 10.1), whereas in NSIP, it is either absent or minimal in extent (Fig. 10.2). The greater the severity of fibrosis in the absence of honeycombing, the more likely NSIP becomes. Subpleural sparing strongly suggests NSIP over UIP (Fig. 10.3). While the presence of GGO is more common with NSIP, it is not specific in distinguishing NSIP from UIP. Keep in mind that in patients with CTD, findings typical of both NSIP and UIP may coexist.

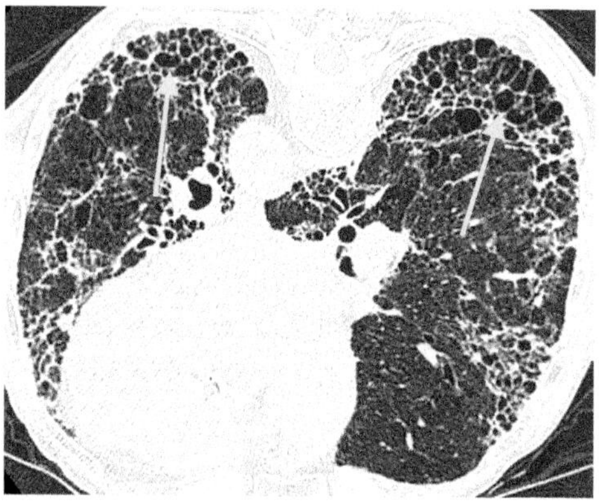

LIP and Follicular Bronchiolitis

LIP and follicular bronchiolitis are thought to represent different points on a spectrum of the lymphoid lung infiltration; thus, their findings may overlap. The typical findings of LIP (Table 10.3) include patchy GGO, centrilobular or perilymphatic nodules, and, to a lesser extent, consolidation. Lung cysts in LIP may be seen in association with other findings (Fig. 10.4) or as an isolated abnormality. Cysts are typically thin walled and limited in number, and vessels may be seen in association with their walls.

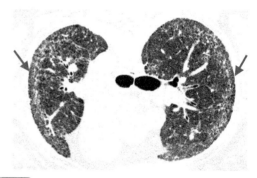

classic

FIGURE 10.3 · Nonspecific interstitial pneumonia (NSIP) with subpleural sparing: Classic appearance. Prone HRCT shows irregular reticulation and traction bronchiolectasis in the peripheral lung, without significant honeycombing. Sparing of the immediate subpleural lung (*arrows*) is highly suggestive of NSIP. While the irregular reticulation likely represents irreversible disease (fibrotic NSIP), some of these abnormalities may resolve with treatment.

classic

FIGURE 10.1 · Usual interstitial pneumonia in rheumatoid arthritis: Classic appearance. Prone HRCT shows peripheral and basilar fibrosis with extensive honeycombing (*arrows*) typical of usual interstitial pneumonia. Although this may be seen with any connective tissue disease, it is most common with rheumatoid lung disease.

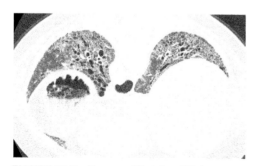

FIGURE 10.2 · Nonspecific interstitial pneumonia (NSIP) in scleroderma. Basilar predominant fibrosis is present with irregular reticulation and traction bronchiectasis. No honeycombing is seen. In the setting of known connective tissue disease, this is compatible with fibrotic NSIP, and a biopsy is not usually required for diagnosis.

TABLE 10.3	HRCT findings of lymphoid interstitial pneumonia and follicular bronchiolitis

Centrilobular nodules of ground glass opacity
Perilymphatic nodules
Patchy, bilateral ground glass opacity
Patchy, bilateral consolidation
Lung cysts (thin walled, limited in number)

Follicular bronchiolitis represents localized lymphoid infiltration of bronchioles. On HRCT, it commonly presents with centrilobular nodules of GGO (Fig. 10.5). Air trapping and mosaic perfusion may also be present.

Lung cysts may occur and are thought to reflect the presence of air trapping associated with follicular bronchiolitis. These are typically thin walled, limited in number to a dozen or a few dozen, predominate in the lung bases, and typically show vessels in, or adjacent to, their walls.

Among the CTDs, LIP and follicular bronchiolitis are most commonly seen in patients with Sjögren's disease and to a lesser extent rheumatoid arthritis (RA). Isolated lung cysts in the setting of Sjögren's disease are highly suggestive of LIP. LIP and follicular bronchiolitis may also be seen in combination with other patterns of lung disease. For instance, patients with NSIP may have centrilobular nodules in the peripheral lung representing follicular bronchiolitis.

GGO, in the absence of other signs of fibrosis, is not commonly seen with the other patterns of chronic lung disease in CTD, with the exception of NSIP. NSIP is typically peripheral and basilar in distribution, whereas LIP and follicular bronchiolitis usually show involvement of the central lung regions. Chronic ground glass and centrilobular nodules may be seen with diseases unrelated to CTD such as hypersensitivity pneumonitis and smoking-related lung disease.

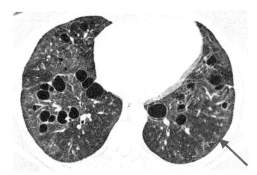

FIGURE 10.4 · Lymphoid interstitial pneumonia. Cysts are seen in association with ground glass opacity in a patient with polymyositis. Small areas of ground glass opacity appear to have a centrilobular distribution (*arrow*).

Organizing Pneumonia

OP typically presents with focal areas of consolidation with irregular borders that often appear nodular or mass-like (Table 10.4). The distribution of consolidation is typically peribronchovascular and/or subpleural (Fig. 10.6A, B). GGO is less common and is more common in immunosuppressed patients. Centrilobular nodules are a rare finding. Architectural distortion and mild bronchial dilatation may be seen associated with these opacities. After treatment, OP may result in mild scarring or may result in fibrosis resembling NSIP.

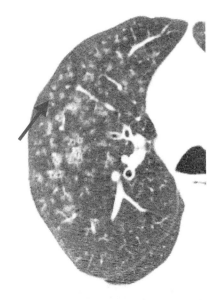

FIGURE 10.5 · Follicular bronchiolitis. Centrilobular nodules of ground glass opacity are noted, associated with mild bronchial dilatation. Note that the nodules are located at a distance from the pleural surfaces (*arrow*) and are evenly spaced from one another. This is typical of a centrilobular distribution.

TABLE 10.4	HRCT findings of organizing pneumonia

Consolidation, focal, irregular borders, often nodular or mass-like
Ground glass opacity (uncommon)
Centrilobular nodules (rare)
Peribronchovascular/subpleural predominant
Atoll or reversed halo sign

OP as an isolated abnormality is one of the least common patterns seen in CTD, but it is most closely associated with polymyositis and dermatomyositis and is particularly common in antisynthetase syndrome. Although it may be seen as the primary abnormality, it is commonly associated with other patterns such as NSIP.

Consolidation is uncommon with other causes of chronic CTD-related diffuse lung disease, although it may occasionally be seen with LIP. Patients on immunosuppressive medications are predisposed to developing infections that may closely resemble OP, particularly fungal and mycobacterial disease (Fig. 10.7). Patients with fibrotic lung disease are at increased risk for malignancies whose findings occasionally overlap with those of OP.

Pulmonary Edema, Pulmonary Hemorrhage, and DAD

Pulmonary edema, pulmonary hemorrhage, and DAD are uncommon patterns in CTD. They are most closely associated with systemic lupus erythematosus (SLE). Patients present with a single or multiple acute episodes.

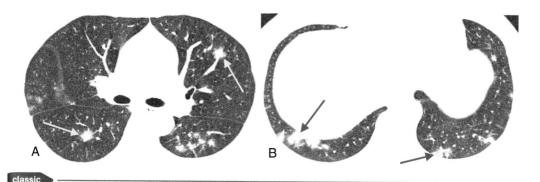

classic

FIGURE 10.6 · Organizing pneumonia: Classic appearance. Patchy peribronchovascular (**A**, *arrows*) and subpleural (**B**, *arrows*) consolidation is seen in a patient with organizing pneumonia due to systemic lupus erythematosus–associated lung disease.

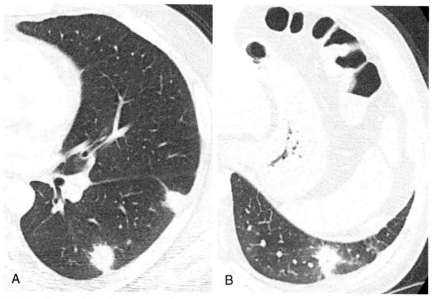

FIGURE 10.7 · Fungal infection resembling organizing pneumonia in a patient with connective tissue disease. HRCT images through the mid-lung (**A**) and lung base (**B**) show large ill-defined nodules from fungal infection that have an appearance similar to organizing pneumonia.

These three patterns share many HRCT features. They all commonly present with diffuse or symmetric GGO. Consolidation may also be present. Smooth interlobular septal thickening as an isolated finding suggests pulmonary edema. The combination of GGO and interlobular septal thickening, the crazy paving pattern, may be seen with any of these patterns.

Constrictive Bronchiolitis

Constrictive bronchiolitis (Table 10.5) is associated with mosaic perfusion and/or air trapping on HRCT, with or without associated bronchiectasis (Fig. 10.8). The severity of constrictive bronchiolitis may vary from patchy and lobular to diffuse lung involvement. Consolidation, GGO, nodules, and tree-in-bud opacities are typically absent. Constrictive bronchiolitis is not a common manifestation of CTD. It is most commonly associated with RA, SLE, and rarely scleroderma.

In the setting of CTD, mosaic perfusion may also be related to chronic vascular disease and with pulmonary arterial hypertension and/or pulmonary arterial thromboembolic disease. Airways and vascular causes of mosaic perfusion are often distinguishable by their morphology (Fig. 10.9). The mosaic perfusion associated with airways disease often involves smaller lung regions, is patchy in distribution, and may show lobular regions of decreased lung attenuation. Mosaic perfusion from vascular disease is typically more extensive, peripheral, and nonlobular in appearance. The presence of air trapping confirms airways disease.

Isolated mosaic perfusion on HRCT may also be seen with asthma, hypersensitivity pneumonitis, and chronic vascular diseases.

Bronchiectasis

Bronchiectasis in the absence of fibrosis is most commonly seen in patients with RA and Sjögren's disease. This finding may be due to chronic infection or constrictive bronchiolitis. Bronchiectasis may be seen as an isolated finding or in association with bronchial wall thickening, mosaic perfusion, or air trapping. When infection is present, it is usually associated with centrilobular nodules, tree-in-bud opacities, and/or consolidation.

Pulmonary Hypertension

Pulmonary hypertension is a relatively common manifestation of collagen vascular disease. It is most closely associated with scleroderma, SLE, and mixed CTD. Pulmonary hypertension may be due to parenchymal lung fibrosis

TABLE 10.5	HRCT findings of constrictive bronchiolitis

Mosaic perfusion
Air trapping
Bronchiectasis
Absence of nodules, tree-in-bud unless complicated by infection

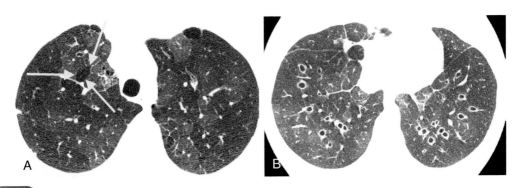

classic

FIGURE 10.8 • **Constrictive bronchiolitis in rheumatoid arthritis: Classic appearance.** HRCT image through the apex **(A)** demonstrates patchy mosaic perfusion with sharply demarcated lobules of decreased attenuation (*arrows*). Image through the lung bases **(B)** shows bronchiectasis in association with mosaic perfusion.

10

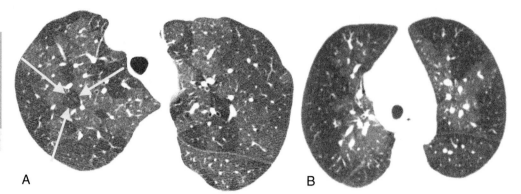

FIGURE 10.9 · **Mosaic perfusion from airways versus vascular disease.** Mosaic perfusion from airways disease **(A)** appears as sharply demarcated, lobular areas of decreased lung attenuation (*arrows*). Vascular disease, such as chronic pulmonary embolism **(B)** appears as larger, peripheral, nonlobular areas of decreased lung attenuation.

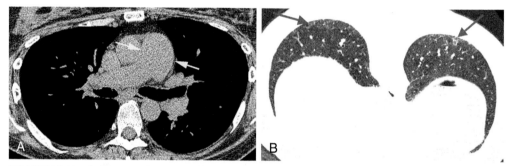

FIGURE 10.10 · **Pulmonary hypertension with mild lung fibrosis. A.** Enlargement of the main pulmonary artery (*yellow arrows*) is present in a scleroderma patient with pulmonary hypertension. **B.** Prone HRCT shows minimal subpleural reticulation and ground glass opacity (*red arrows*) likely due to nonspecific interstitial pneumonia. The degree of pulmonary hypertension is out of proportion to the severity of lung findings, suggesting vasculitis.

or pulmonary vascular disease. The vascular disease may be due to vasculitis, arterial fibrosis, chronic pulmonary emboli, or in situ thrombus. Primary vascular disease should be considered when the HRCT shows main pulmonary artery or right heart dilatation in the presence of mild or no parenchymal lung disease (Fig. 10.10).

Serositis

Inflammation of the pleura and pericardium is a common occurrence in patients with CTD. This may be manifested as pleural/pericardial effusions or thickening on CT. These effusions are commonly exudative; thus, pleural thickening and enhancement may be present. Effusions are not typical of other causes of diffuse lung disease such as idiopathic pulmonary

fibrosis and hypersensitivity pneumonitis. The combination of diffuse lung disease and pleural or pericardial abnormalities increases the likelihood of CTD as a cause. Serositis is most closely associated with SLE and RA.

Overlap of Patterns

Although one of the above patterns often predominates in patients with CTD, it is not uncommon for two or more of these patterns to be present at the same time. In fact, an overlap of patterns is suggestive of CTD, compared with other causes of diffuse lung disease. In this context, HRCT in a patient with CTD may show findings typical of more than one pattern (Fig. 10.11). The most common patterns to overlap include NSIP, LIP/follicular bronchiolitis, and OP.

HRCT FINDINGS IN SPECIFIC CTDS

Any type of CTD may present with any of the abnormalities listed above, but specific diseases tend to be associated with specific abnormalities (Table 10.6). It is important for the radiologist to be able to recognize the pattern present on HRCT and the connective tissues with which it is most commonly associated. This is particularly true during the initial presentation of a patient with diffuse lung disease. Initially, patients may not meet all the criteria for a specific CTD, and imaging may be helpful in elucidating the nature of the patient's systemic disorder.

Progressive Systemic Sclerosis (Scleroderma)

Progressive systemic sclerosis, or scleroderma, is a systemic disorder with primary manifestations of skin thickening and tightening. Other common abnormalities include Raynaud's phenomenon, and esophageal dysmotility. Lung disease is present in up to 80% of patients. Scl-70 and Anti-U3 RNP antibodies are specific for scleroderma.

The majority of patients with scleroderma-related lung disease show an NSIP pattern on HRCT (Fig. 10.12A–D), manifested as subpleural and basilar predominant traction bronchiectasis, irregular reticulation, and/or GGO. Sparing of the immediate subpleural lung is not uncommon and supports a diagnosis of NSIP.

When significant honeycombing is present, UIP is more likely, the second most common pattern seen with scleroderma (Fig. 10.13). Pulmonary hypertension may also be seen in scleroderma patients because of either the parenchymal lung disease or vascular disease.

CREST

The CREST syndrome is a form of limited cutaneous scleroderma. CREST is an acronym for calcinosis, Raynaud's phenomena, esophageal dysmotility, sclerodactyly, and telangiectasia. Patients with CREST show a higher incidence of pulmonary vascular disease and a lower incidence of fibrotic lung disease than other patients with scleroderma.

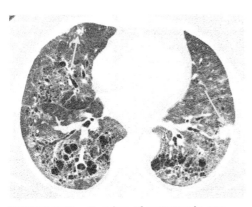

FIGURE 10.11 · **Overlap of patterns in connective tissue disease.** Pathologically this patient with mixed connective tissue disease had more than one interstitial pneumonia pattern present. Patchy, bilateral ground glass opacity and cysts correspond to lymphoid interstitial pneumonia. Focal areas of nodular consolidation (*arrows*) correspond to organizing pneumonia.

TABLE 10.6	Common patterns associated with specific connective tissue diseases
Scleroderma	NSIP
	UIP
	Pulmonary hypertension (particularly in CREST)
Rheumatoid arthritis	UIP
	NSIP
	LIP
	Bronchiectasis
Systemic lupus erythematosus	Diffuse alveolar damage
	Hemorrhage
	Edema
	Pleural/pericardial effusions
Poly/ dermatomyositis	NSIP
	OP
	Diffuse alveolar damage
Sjögren's syndrome	NSIP
	LIP
Mixed connective tissue disease	NSIP
	UIP

NSIP, nonspecific interstitial pneumonia; UIP, usual interstitial pneumonia; OP, organizing pneumonia; LIP, lymphoid interstitial pneumonia; CREST, calcinosis, Raynaud's phenomena, esophageal dysmotility, sclerodactyly, and telangiectasia.

10

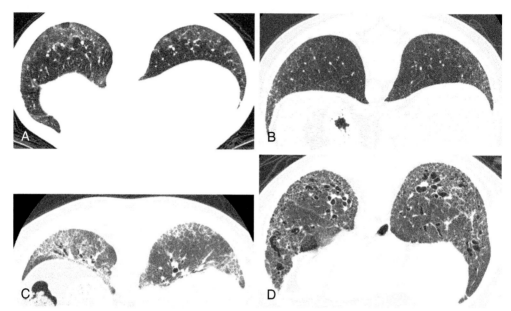

FIGURE 10.12 · **Spectrum of nonspecific interstitial pneumonia (NSIP) abnormalities in scleroderma.** Four patients with scleroderma-related NSIP are shown on prone HRCT. **A.** Prone HRCT shows peripheral and basilar ground glass opacity without evidence of fibrosis in a patient with cellular NSIP. **B.** Prone HRCT shows very early irregular reticulation without traction bronchiectasis or honeycombing. This could represent either fibrotic or cellular NSIP. **C.** The irregular reticulation in this case is more severe and associated with traction bronchiectasis, compatible with fibrotic NSIP. **D.** Late disease with severe fibrosis shows extensive traction bronchiectasis and irregular reticulation.

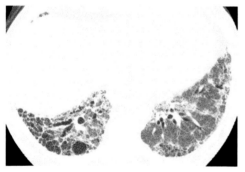

FIGURE 10.13 · **Usual interstitial pneumonia (UIP) in scleroderma.** Peripheral, basilar fibrosis with honeycombing is compatible with a pattern of UIP in a patient with scleroderma. This appearance is indistinguishable from idiopathic pulmonary fibrosis and other causes of a UIP pattern.

Rheumatoid Arthritis

RA is characterized by an arthritis that has a predilection for the hands, particularly the proximal interphalangeal and metacarpophalangeal joints. Rheumatoid factor is commonly positive in patients with RA. Approximately 40% of patients with RA will have lung disease.

The most common patterns seen in RA are UIP and NSIP. UIP demonstrates a peripheral and basilar predominance of fibrosis with honeycombing, indistinguishable from idiopathic pulmonary fibrosis (Fig. 10.14A, B). NSIP demonstrates a basilar predominance of GGO, traction bronchiectasis, and/or reticulation with or without subpleural sparing. Uncommon patterns seen in patients with RA include follicular bronchiolitis/LIP and OP.

Bronchiectasis is a frequent finding on HRCT in patients with RA, including those without fibrotic lung disease. Bronchiolitis may be due to chronic infection or constrictive bronchiolitis.

Rheumatoid nodules visible on CT are a rare manifestation and patients are typically asymptomatic. They may be single or multiple, can become large, and may cavitate. As with any cause of cavitary nodules, rheumatoid nodules may be complicated by bronchopleural fistula.

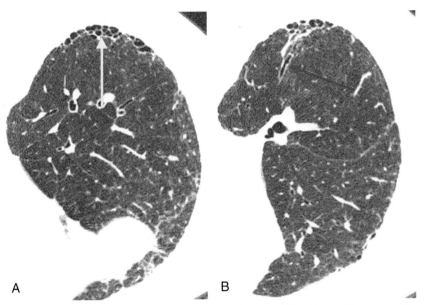

FIGURE 10.14 · **Usual interstitial pneumonia (UIP) in rheumatoid arthritis.** Honeycombing (**A**, *yellow arrow*) and mild traction bronchiectasis (**B**, *red arrow*) are seen in the subpleural lung regions. UIP is the most common pattern seen in patients with rheumatoid arthritis–related interstitial lung disease.

Systemic Lupus Erythematosus

SLE has a variety of possible clinical manifestations including rash, oral ulcers, photosensitivity, arthritis, and serositis. Disorders involving the renal, neurologic, and hematologic systems are common as well. Multiple serologies may be positive, including antinuclear antibody, antiphospholipid antibodies, anti–double-stranded DNA antibodies, and anti-Smith antibodies. Anti–double-stranded DNA antibodies are specific for SLE.

The lung disease associated with SLE differs somewhat from that of other CTDs. DAD, diffuse alveolar hemorrhage, and pulmonary edema are the most common manifestations (Fig. 10.15). A combination of these is seen in patients with so-called *lupus pneumonitis*. These have similar appearances on HRCT, with extensive or diffuse areas of GGO and/or consolidation. Patients with multiple episodes of pulmonary hemorrhage may eventually develop fibrosis.

Serositis is common in SLE. Pleural or pericardial effusions may be seen in isolation or associated with lung disease. Pleural/pericardial thickening or enhancement may also be present, reflecting the presence of an

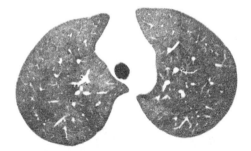

FIGURE 10.15 · **Pulmonary hemorrhage in systemic lupus erythematosus.** Symmetric bilateral ground glass opacity in the setting of systemic lupus erythematosus is a nonspecific finding and could represent edema, diffuse alveolar damage, atypical infection, or hemorrhage.

exudative effusion. Constrictive bronchiolitis or bronchiectasis may also be seen.

Vanishing or *shrinking lung syndrome* is a rare manifestation of SLE, in which patients present with dyspnea and restrictive defects on PFTs but have no evidence of parenchymal lung disease on HRCT. The primary radiographic finding is elevation of the hemidiaphragms. This may be due to muscular weakness or phrenic nerve dysfunction.

IPs and pulmonary fibrosis are uncommon manifestations of SLE, but UIP, NSIP, and OP may be seen.

Polymyositis and Dermatomyositis

The features of myositis include muscle weakness, arthritis, and constitutional symptoms. Dermatomyositis also shows skin changes. Anti-Jo-1 antibodies are frequently positive and specific for an inflammatory myositis. Pulmonary symptoms are often due to chronic interstitial lung disease, but weakness of the respiratory muscles and recurrent aspiration from pharyngeal muscle weakness may also be responsible.

NSIP is the most common diffuse lung disease associated with myositis (Fig. 10.16). HRCT often shows basilar, subpleural predominant ground glass, irregular reticulation, and/or traction bronchiectasis with or without subpleural sparing. OP is another common pattern, manifesting by patchy consolidation. An overlap of NSIP and OP may be present with consolidation involving the subpleural and basilar lung regions (Fig. 10.17).

An acute presentation of DAD is not uncommon with a rapid development of extensive GGO on HRCT. UIP is an uncommon manifestation of myositis. Rare associated patterns include LIP.

Sjögren's Disease

Sjögren's disease is a CTD that shows prominent ocular and oral involvement. Dysfunction of the lacrimal and salivary glands produces dry eyes and dry mouth. Patients often show the positive autoantibodies anti-SSA and anti-SSB.

The most common patterns of lung disease in patients with Sjögren's disease are NSIP and LIP. The HRCT findings of NSIP are similar to those of scleroderma. OP and UIP may be seen in Sjögren's disease but are relatively uncommon.

LIP commonly shows multiple lung cysts as an isolated abnormality (Fig. 10.18). Cysts are usually round and thin walled. They involve all lung regions and are less numerous than cysts seen in lymphangioleiomyomatosis and Langerhans cell histiocytosis; usually cysts number a few dozen or less. GGO and centrilobular GGO nodules may also be associated with LIP or follicular bronchiolitis, but this is less common than isolated cysts.

Other lymphoproliferative diseases may be present in patients with Sjögren's disease.

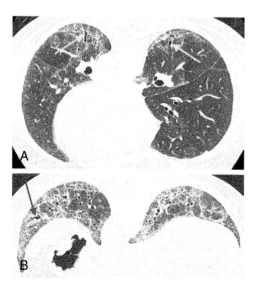

FIGURE 10.16 · **Polymyositis with nonspecific interstitial pneumonia.** Prone HRCT through the mid- **(A)** and lower **(B)** lungs demonstrates peripheral and basilar predominant irregular reticulation and traction bronchiectasis (*arrows*). There is relative sparing of the immediate subpleural interstitium.

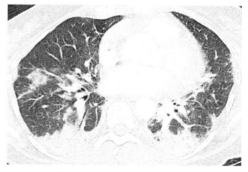

FIGURE 10.17 · **Polymyositis with overlap of nonspecific interstitial pneumonia (NSIP) and organizing pneumonia.** HRCT shows subpleural and posterior consolidation. The distribution is typical of NSIP, but consolidation is not a typical NSIP finding. Pathologically there were components of both NSIP and organizing pneumonia present. Consolidation on HRCT is more typical of organizing pneumonia.

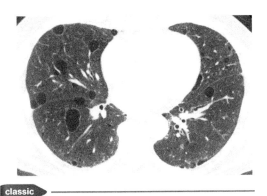

classic

FIGURE 10.18 · Lymphoid interstitial pneumonia in Sjögren's disease: Classic appearance. Lung cysts may be seen as an isolated abnormality in lymphoid interstitial pneumonia, particularly in the setting of Sjögren's disease. They are round and thin walled and limited in number.

Focal lymphoid hyperplasia represents a benign, reactive collection of lymphoid cells. Its most common HRCT manifestation is a solitary pulmonary nodule or focal region of consolidation. Multiple nodules have also been described. Lymphoma is seen with a much greater incidence in patients with Sjögren's disease compared with the population as a whole and may resemble focal lymphoid hyperplasia. Biopsy of suspicious abnormalities is generally performed to distinguish these two entities.

Mixed CTD

As the name suggests, mixed CTD shows overlapping features of other CTDs, primarily scleroderma, SLE, and myositis. Anti-RNP antibodies are often present and may precede the development of symptoms. Lung disease is present in approximately 60% of patients.

NSIP and UIP are the most common patterns seen. Other less common patterns include LIP, OP, and pulmonary vascular disease.

Interstitial Pneumonia with Autoimmune Features

Interstitial pneumonia with autoimmune features (IPAF) is a designation given to patients with some features of CTD, but who do not meet all of the criteria for any specific one.

Multiple other terms have also been used in the past to describe this entity including undifferentiated CTD, lung-dominant CTD, and autoimmune featured interstitial lung disease. To make a diagnosis of IPAF, patients must have evidence of an IP on HRCT or pathology and alternative causes of an IP (e.g., drug toxicity) must be excluded.

The criteria for IPAF are divided into three domains: (1) clinical, (2) serologic, and (3) morphologic. Patients must have at least one positive finding in two of the three domains. Both HRCT and pathology are included as part of the morphologic domain. HRCT features that are included are as follows:

1. HRCT patterns of lung disease
   a. NSIP
   b. OP
   c. NSIP and OP overlap
   d. LIP
2. Multicompartment disease (in addition to an IP)
   a. Pleural effusion and/or thickening
   b. Pericardial effusion and/or thickening
   c. Airways disease
   d. Pulmonary vasculopathy

As an example, in a patient presenting with shortness of breath, HRCT shows peripheral and basilar GGO with subpleural sparing, suggestive of NSIP. The patient has a positive rheumatoid factor but no clinical manifestations of connective tissue disease. Hand radiographs demonstrate normal findings. This patient could be classified as IPAF with one positive feature in both the serologic and morphologic domain.

FURTHER READING

Aquino SL, Webb WR, Golden J. Bronchiolitis obliterans associated with rheumatoid arthritis: findings on HRCT and dynamic expiratory CT. *J Comput Assist Tomogr.* 1994;18:555-558.

Bankier AA, Kiener HP, Wiesmayr MN, et al. Discrete lung involvement in systemic lupus erythematosus: CT assessment. *Radiology.* 1995;196:835-840.

Bhalla M, Silver RM, Shepard JO, McLoud TC. Chest CT in patients with scleroderma: prevalence of asymptomatic esophageal dilatation and mediastinal lymphadenopathy. *AJR Am J Roentgenol.* 1993;161:269-272.

10

Fenlon HM, Doran M, Sant SM, Breatnach E. High-resolution chest CT in systemic lupus erythematosus. *AJR Am J Roentgenol.* 1996;166:301-307.

Fischer A, Antoniou KM, Brown KK, et al. An official European Respiratory Society/American Thoracic Society research statement: interstitial pneumonia with autoimmune features. *Eur Respir J.* 2015;46:976-987.

Franquet T, Giménez A, Monill JM, et al. Primary Sjögren's syndrome and associated lung disease: CT findings in 50 patients. *AJR Am J Roentgenol.* 1997;169:655-658.

Fujii M, Adachi S, Shimizu T, et al. Interstitial lung disease in rheumatoid arthritis: assessment with high-resolution computed tomography. *J Thorac Imaging.* 1993;8:54-62.

Kim JS, Lee KS, Koh EM, et al. Thoracic involvement of systemic lupus erythematosus: clinical, pathologic, and radiologic findings. *J Comput Assist Tomogr.* 2000;24:9-18.

Kim EJ, Elicker BM, Maldonado F, et al. Usual interstitial pneumonia in rheumatoid arthritis-associated interstitial lung disease. *Eur Respir J.* 2010;35:1322-1328.

Lee HK, Kim DS, Yoo B, et al. Histopathologic pattern and clinical features of rheumatoid arthritis-associated interstitial lung disease. *Chest.* 2005;127:2019-2027.

Mino M, Noma S, Taguchi Y, et al. Pulmonary involvement in polymyositis and dermatomyositis: sequential evaluation with CT. *AJR Am J Roentgenol.* 1997;169:83-87.

Primack SL, Müller NL. Radiologic manifestations of the systemic autoimmune diseases. *Clin Chest Med.* 1998;19:573-586.

Remy-Jardin M, Remy J, Wallaert B, et al. Pulmonary involvement in progressive systemic sclerosis: sequential evaluation with CT, pulmonary function tests, and bronchoalveolar lavage. *Radiology.* 1993;188:499-506.

Remy-Jardin M, Remy J, Cortet B, et al. Lung changes in rheumatoid arthritis: CT findings. *Radiology.* 1994;193:375-382.

Schurawitzki H, Stiglbauer R, Graninger W, et al. Interstitial lung disease in progressive systemic sclerosis: high-resolution CT versus radiography. *Radiology.* 1990;176:755-759.

Souza AS Jr, Müller NL, Marchiori E, Soares-Souza LV, de Souza Rocha M. Pulmonary abnormalities in ankylosing spondylitis: inspiratory and expiratory high-resolution CT findings in 17 patients. *J Thorac Imaging.* 2004;19:259-263.

Tanaka N, Kim JS, Newell JD, et al. Rheumatoid arthritis-related lung diseases: CT findings. *Radiology.* 2004;232:81-91.

Tanaka N, Newell JD, Brown KK. Collagen vascular disease-related lung disease: high-resolution computed tomography findings based on the pathologic classification. *J Comput Assist Tomogr.* 2004;28:351-360.

Tanoue LT. Pulmonary involvement in collage vascular disease: a review of the pulmonary manifestations of the Marfan syndrome, ankylosing spondylitis, Sjögren's syndrome, and relapsing polychondritis. *J Thorac Imaging.* 1992;7:62-77.

Taorimina VJ, Miller WT, Gefter WB. Progressive systemic sclerosis subgroups: variable pulmonary features. *AJR Am J Roentgenol.* 1981;137:277-285.

Tazelaar HD, Viggiano RW, Pickersgill J. Interstitial lung disease in polymyositis and dermatomyositis. clinical features and prognosis as correlated with histologic findings. *Am Rev Respir Dis.* 1990;141:727-733.

Smoking-Related Lung Disease

INTRODUCTION

Cigarette smoking is well known for its association with lung cancer, but diffuse lung disease is also an established cause of smoking-related morbidity. There are a variety of different manifestations of smoking-related diffuse lung disease with different treatments and prognoses. This chapter focuses on respiratory bronchiolitis (RB), desquamative interstitial pneumonia (DIP), emphysema, Langerhans cell histiocytosis (LCH), acute eosinophilic pneumonia, and smoking-related fibrosis as the primary manifestations of diffuse lung disease related to cigarette smoke inhalation.

RB AND DIP

RB and *DIP* represent a similar reaction of lung to inhaled cigarette smoke, although they differ in their incidence, the severity of the specific abnormality present, and their association with symptoms. In the case of RB, cigarette smoke inhalation induces reactive changes in and around small airways, characterized by focal areas of alveolar macrophage infiltrate and mild interstitial inflammation. In DIP, there is more generalized intra-alveolar macrophage accumulation and inflammation. DIP is more commonly symptomatic than RB.

Pathologically, RB is seen in virtually all smokers, but it is responsible for symptoms in only a small minority of patients. RB is thought to represent a factor in the development of centrilobular emphysema. It is hypothesized that chronic cellular infiltration and inflammation associated with RB eventually leads to lung destruction and emphysema.

When RB is a cause of symptoms, the disease is termed *respiratory bronchiolitis interstitial lung disease (RB-ILD)*.

Both RB-ILD and DIP typically present in young patients (peak age 30 to 40 years) and have a significantly better prognosis than most other interstitial lung diseases, with a good response to smoking cessation and/or treatment with steroids. Up to 25% of patients with DIP may eventually develop lung fibrosis in the absence of appropriate treatment.

HRCT Findings in RB and DIP

The high-resolution computed tomography (HRCT) findings of RB and DIP differ (Tables 11.1 and 11.2) but commonly coexist, given the overlap between these two entities. Typically, HRCT in RB/RB-ILD shows centrilobular ground glass opacity (GGO) nodules, reflecting the bronchiolar and peribronchiolar macrophage infiltrate typical of this disease (Fig. 11.1A, B). These nodules tend to predominate in the upper lobes and in central lung regions, similar to the distribution of centrilobular emphysema. There may be associated mosaic perfusion or air trapping, but this tends to be mild (Fig. 11.2A, B).

DIP almost always presents with GGO as the predominant finding. The GGO is typically subpleural and basal in distribution (Fig. 11.3; also see Figs. 9.26 to 9.28), similar to the distribution of usual interstitial pneumonia and nonspecific interstitial pneumonia (NSIP). Scattered cysts or patchy emphysema may be associated with the areas of GGO (Fig. 11.4). The combination of GGO with associated cysts or emphysema in a smoker is strongly suggestive of this diagnosis. In a minority of patients, fibrosis develops in areas previously affected by GGO. This is manifested by irregular reticulation and traction bronchiectasis (Fig. 11.5). Honeycombing is rare, although the cysts of DIP may occasionally resemble honeycombing.

As RB and DIP represent a spectrum of abnormalities, an overlap of their typical findings may be present on HRCT in smokers (Fig. 11.6A, B). GGO may have a variable distribution from subpleural/basilar predominant to central/upper lobe predominant. Patchy GGO may be seen in combination with GGO centrilobular nodules. Cysts or emphysema, mosaic perfusion, and air trapping may be associated with any of these abnormalities. RB and DIP may show the headcheese sign, a combination of GGO and mosaic perfusion on inspiratory HRCT or air trapping on expiratory HRCT.

Differential Diagnosis

The differential diagnosis of RB and DIP in a patient with chronic symptoms includes other disorders that produce GGO, ground glass centrilobular nodules, cysts, and mosaic perfusion. Hypersensitivity pneumonitis (HP) is a common cause of these findings (Fig. 11.7). Although it is thought that there is a reduced likelihood of HP in cigarette smokers, smoking does not preclude a diagnosis of HP. The presence of fibrosis in association with GGO or centrilobular nodules favors HP because fibrosis is uncommon with RB/DIP (Fig. 11.8). Moreover, mosaic perfusion and air trapping tend to be more severe in HP.

TABLE 11.1	HRCT findings of respiratory bronchiolitis

HRCT finding

Centrilobular nodules of ground glass opacity
Mild mosaic perfusion/air trapping
Central, upper lobe distribution

TABLE 11.2	HRCT findings of desquamative interstitial pneumonia

HRCT finding

Ground glass opacity
Focal air-density lucencies (cysts or emphysema)
Subpleural and basilar distribution

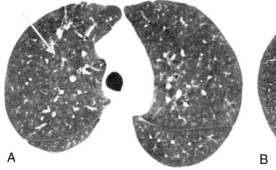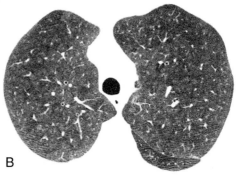

A   B

classic

FIGURE 11.1 · Respiratory bronchiolitis and respiratory bronchiolitis interstitial lung disease: Classic appearance. A. An asymptomatic smoker shows centrilobular nodules of ground glass opacity (*arrow*) on HRCT, typical of the peribronchiolar cellular infiltration and inflammation seen in respiratory bronchiolitis (RB). **B.** HRCT in a patient with mild dyspnea shows more extensive and larger centrilobular nodules of ground glass opacity, reflecting respiratory bronchiolitis. Because RB is associated with symptoms in this patient, it is termed respiratory bronchiolitis interstitial lung disease.

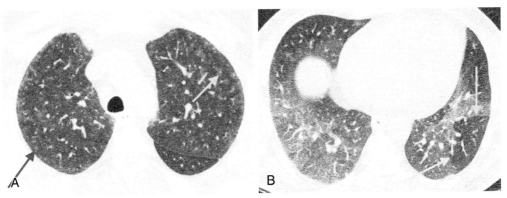

FIGURE 11.2 · **Respiratory bronchiolitis with mild air trapping.** HRCT through the upper lobes **(A)** shows centrilobular nodules of ground glass opacity (*arrows*). Expiratory HRCT through the lower lungs **(B)** shows patchy air trapping (*arrows*).

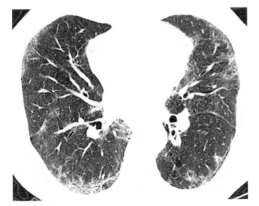

FIGURE 11.3 · **Desquamative interstitial pneumonia.** HRCT shows peripheral areas of ground glass opacity in this smoker with desquamative interstitial pneumonia.

Follicular bronchiolitis/lymphoid interstitial pneumonia (FB/LIP) is another abnormality that may show centrilobular ground glass nodules, GGO, and mild mosaic perfusion/air trapping. Patients with FB/LIP typically have a history of connective tissue disease or immunocompromise. Other causes of centrilobular ground glass nodules include acute viral infections, rare pneumoconioses, and vascular diseases such as hemorrhage.

NSIP may have a distribution identical to that of DIP, with subpleural and basilar abnormalities (Fig. 11.9). These patients usually have a history of connective tissue disease or an exposure. The presence of fibrosis suggests NSIP.

EMPHYSEMA

Chronic cellular infiltration and inflammation due to smoke inhalation may eventually lead to lung destruction and emphysema. The HRCT appearances are reviewed briefly here (Table 11.3) and described in detail in Chapter 5.

Centrilobular Emphysema

Centrilobular emphysema is most closely associated with smoking. The HRCT findings of centrilobular emphysema are usually diagnostic and do not require lung biopsy. HRCT may be more sensitive than pulmonary function tests in patients with early disease.

The HRCT findings of centrilobular emphysema include focal air-attenuation lucencies without well-defined walls (i.e., black holes), which involve the central and upper lung regions (Fig. 11.7). Small vessels, representing the centrilobular artery or arteries, may be seen in the center of these focal lucencies. Bullae may be seen.

Paraseptal Emphysema

Paraseptal emphysema may be seen in association with centrilobular emphysema. It is related to smoking in many patients. This form of emphysema appears as a single layer of subpleural air-attenuation cysts with paper-thin walls. When large, areas of paraseptal emphysema represent bullae.

11

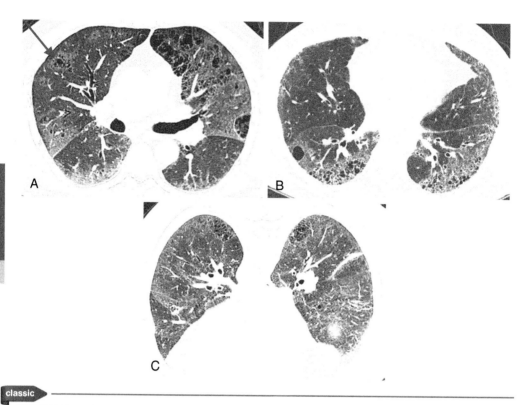

A

B

C

classic

FIGURE 11.4 · Desquamative interstitial pneumonia: Classic appearance. A. Patchy ground glass opacity is present with a subpleural predominance. Note focal emphysema or cysts within the areas of ground glass opacity (*arrow*). This combination is particularly suggestive of desquamative interstitial pneumonia (DIP). **B.** Subpleural ground glass opacity is associated with air-density cystic lucencies. The cystic lucencies can be distinguished from honeycombing by the fact that many are not subpleural and there is no evidence of fibrosis such as traction bronchiectasis. **C.** Prone computed tomography shows predominantly peripheral ground glass opacity and cystic lucencies in a smoker with DIP.

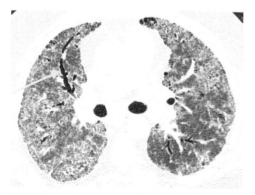

FIGURE 11.5 · Desquamative interstitial pneumonia with fibrosis. Fibrosis is an uncommon sequela of desquamative interstitial pneumonia and typically is manifested by traction bronchiectasis (*arrow*) and/or irregular reticulation superimposed on ground glass opacity. Honeycombing is distinctly rare.

Panlobular Emphysema

Panlobular emphysema is often associated with alpha-1-antitrypsin deficiency but may also be seen in severe cases of smoking-related emphysema (Fig. 11.8). Panlobular emphysema on HRCT shows diffuse lung lucency with attenuated vessels. The distribution is usually lower lobe predominant in alpha-1-antitrypsin deficiency. In smokers, it may be more severe in the upper lobes.

LANGERHANS CELL HISTIOCYTOSIS

In adults, pulmonary LCH occurs primarily in smokers. As with RB and DIP, the peak age at presentation for adult LCH is approximately

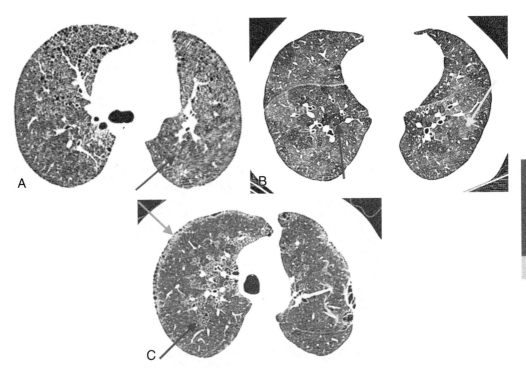

FIGURE 11.6 · **Respiratory bronchiolitis and desquamative interstitial pneumonia overlap in three patients. A.** A combination of centrilobular nodules of ground glass opacity (*arrow*) and more diffuse patchy ground glass opacity and emphysema are present. **B.** High-resolution computed tomography shows a combination of ground glass opacity (*yellow arrow*) and lobular mosaic perfusion (*red arrow*). This represents the "headcheese" sign. **C.** Patchy glass opacity is associated with cystic lucencies. The more peripheral areas of ground glass (*blue arrow*) are more typical of desquamative interstitial pneumonia, whereas the central lobular areas of ground glass (*red arrow*) are more typical of respiratory bronchiolitis.

30 to 40 years. Symptoms vary widely. Patients may be asymptomatic or may have severe dyspnea. Lung transplantation may be necessary in some patients. As with any cystic lung disease, the initial clinical presentation may be the development of a pneumothorax.

HRCT Findings

On HRCT, the appearance of LCH (Table 11.4) varies with the stage of disease. In early cases, small scattered lung nodules are typically seen; over time, these may cavitate (Fig. 11.9A, B). Nodules in LCH are commonly of soft tissue attenuation, although rarely centrilobular ground glass nodules may be the primary manifestation.

With further progression, thick-walled lung cysts develop, and a combination of nodules, cavitary nodules, and cysts may be seen. Cysts tend to be irregular, having bizarre,

branching, and cloverleaf shapes (Fig. 11.10). Late disease may present with cysts that nearly replace the normal lung (Fig. 11.11). Cysts eventually become thin walled, and differentiation from centrilobular emphysema may be difficult.

Abnormalities in LCH show a distinct upper lobe predominance, with relative sparing of the lung bases and costophrenic angles. Associated pleural effusions are uncommon.

Differential Diagnosis

The differential diagnosis of LCH includes other cystic lung diseases (Fig. 11.12A, B), particularly lymphangioleiomyomatosis (LAM). Both of these diseases may produce extensive cystic lung disease. However, differentiation is often possible. In LCH, cysts have bizarre shapes and upper lobe predominance and may be thick walled. The cysts of LAM, in contrast, are usually round, thin walled, and diffuse in distribution. Furthermore, LAM occurs almost entirely in women. A man with cystic lung disease is not likely to have LAM. Other cystic lung diseases, such as LIP, usually show fewer cysts.

The presence of nodules favors LCH, whereas the presence of pleural effusions favors LAM. Other causes of cavitary nodules, such as septic emboli, fungal infection, Wegener's granulomatosis, cystic metastases (e.g., endometrial carcinoma), and tracheobronchial papillomatosis, may resemble LCH, but nodules in these diseases are often larger.

ACUTE EOSINOPHILIC PNEUMONIA

Acute eosinophilic pneumonia (AEP) is usually classified with the other eosinophilic lung diseases; however, there is evidence that the majority of patients with AEP are smokers and,

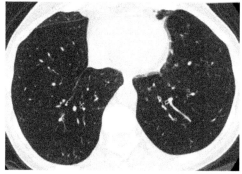

classic

FIGURE 11.7 · Centrilobular emphysema: Classic appearance. HRCT of the left lung shows the typical morphology of centrilobular emphysema. Focal air-attenuation lucencies are present in the central lung regions without visible walls. A centrilobular artery is seen in the center of some of these lucencies (*arrows*).

FIGURE 11.8 · Panlobular emphysema associated with smoking. When extensive, smoking-related emphysema may be panlobular in distribution. This manifests as diffuse lung lucency associated with small vessels.

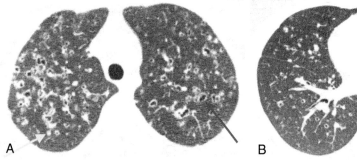

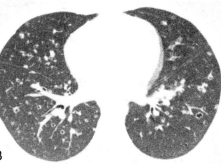

classic

FIGURE 11.9 · Langerhans cell histiocytosis, early stage: Classic appearance. HRCT shows a combination of soft tissue attenuation nodules (*yellow arrow*) and cavitary nodules or cysts (*red arrow*). The cysts are irregularly shaped and have variable thickness of their walls. These show much greater involvement of the upper lungs **(A)** compared with the lower lungs **(B)**. Nodules are typical of early disease.

TABLE 11.3	HRCT findings of emphysema
Centrilobular	Upper, central lung distribution Focal air-density lucencies Walls not typically seen Centrilobular arteries (ie. dots) at the center of the lucencies
Paraseptal	Subpleural distribution Focal air-density lucencies Lucencies have discrete, thin walls Cysts in single layer Associated centrilobular emphysema may be present
Panlobular	Lower lung, diffuse distribution Increased lung lucency, abnormality not usually focal Small vessels in affected regions

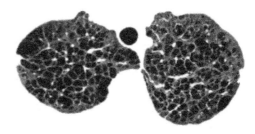

FIGURE 11.11 · **A Langerhans cell histiocytosis, cysts.** When severe, the cysts of Langerhans cell histiocytosis are extensive and may show near-complete replacement of the lung parenchyma. Usually nodules are not present at this stage. This pattern may be difficult to distinguish from extensive emphysema.

TABLE 11.4	HRCT findings of Langerhans cell histiocytosis

Centrilobular nodules of soft tissue attenuation
Cavitation of nodules with progression to thick-walled cysts
Irregular, bizarre-shaped cysts
Upper lobe predominance; sparing of the costophrenic angles
Spontaneous pneumothorax

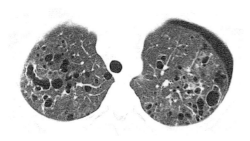

classic ▶

FIGURE 11.10 · **Langerhans cell histiocytosis, late stage with cysts: Classic appearance.** There is a predominance of cysts in this smoker. The cysts are irregular in shape. Some have thin walls and others are thick walled. A left pneumothorax is also present. Except for acute symptoms associated with the pneumothorax, the patient was asymptomatic.

in particular, smokers who have changed their smoking habits (e.g., increased the number of cigarettes smoked per day) in the month leading up to the onset of acute symptoms. Patients present with acute symptoms similar to pulmonary edema, infection, or diffuse alveolar damage. The most typical HRCT appearance is a combination of diffuse GGO and smooth interlobular septal thickening, resembling pulmonary edema. Diagnosis is important in AEP because of its responsiveness to corticosteroids. This entity is discussed further in Chapter 13.

FIBROTIC LUNG DISEASE

Lung fibrosis is a common pathologic finding in smokers and is often seen in asymptomatic patients. Two pathologic terms have been used to describe the presence of fibrosis in smokers; these are smoking-related interstitial fibrosis and air space enlargement with fibrosis. These may represent the fibrotic sequela of subclinical RB and DIP, although the HRCT in most patients with smoking-related interstitial fibrosis is normal, and the pathologic findings are below the resolution of HRCT. In other cases, typical findings of RB and DIP may be present. It is important to note that GGO is not uncommonly a sign of microscopic fibrosis in this setting; thus, more typical HRCT signs of fibrosis (reticulation, traction bronchiectasis, and honeycombing) are often lacking.

Patients with *combined pulmonary fibrosis and emphysema (CPFE)* (Fig. 11.13) are unique in that their lung volumes on pulmonary function tests may appear relatively normal given the presence of both a restrictive and obstructive abnormality. Diffusing capacity for carbon monoxide, however, is

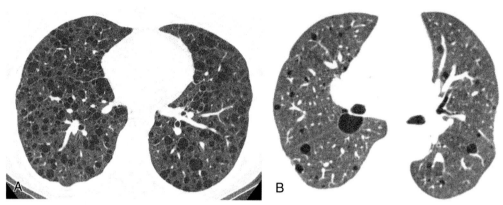

FIGURE 11.12 · **Differential diagnosis of Langerhans cell histiocytosis (LCH).** Both LCH and lymphangioleiomyomatosis (LAM) can produce extensive cystic lung disease. **A.** The cysts of LAM differ from those of LCH in that they have a round and regular shape. Nodules are not common in LAM, and the disease does not show sparing of the lung bases. **B.** Lung cysts in neurofibromatosis. Cysts are less numerous than in LCH and are round in shape.

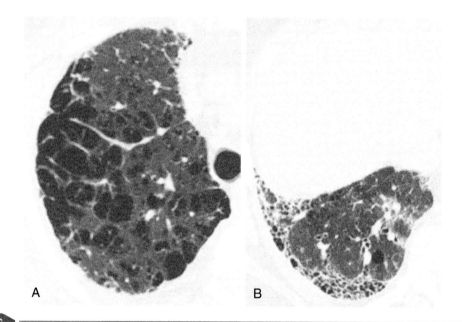

classic

FIGURE 11.13 · **Combined pulmonary fibrosis and emphysema: Classic appearance. A.** Centrilobular emphysema is seen in the upper lobes. **B.** Fibrosis is present in the lower lobes, resulting in peripheral honeycombing, compatible with usual interstitial pneumonia. This combination is associated with relatively normal lung volumes on pulmonary function tests and a higher incidence of pulmonary hypertension.

often abnormal even when the other metrics are near normal. These patients have a higher risk of developing pulmonary hypertension.

Smokers have a greater risk of developing idiopathic pulmonary fibrosis (IPF). Of the patients with IPF, 40 to 80% have a smoking history. The presence of emphysema can complicate the diagnosis of fibrotic lung disease on HRCT. Centrilobular or paraseptal emphysema in the peripheral lung may be mistaken for honeycombing, particularly when there is adjacent GGO or reticulation. In such cases, abnormalities in the lower lungs on HRCT may be more diagnostic of fibrosis, as emphysema tends to be an upper lobe process. There should be a higher threshold for describing the pattern of usual interstitial pneumonia on HRCT when significant emphysema is present.

FURTHER READING

Abbott GF, Rosado-de-Christenson ML, Franks TJ, et al. Pulmonary Langerhans cell histiocytosis. *Radiographics.* 2004;24:821-841.

Brauner MW, Grenier P, Tijani K, et al. Pulmonary Langerhans cell histiocytosis: evolution of lesions on CT scans. *Radiology.* 1997;204:497-502.

Foster WL Jr, Gimenez EI, Roubidoux MA, et al. The emp-hysemas: radiologic-pathologic correlations. *Radiographics.* 1993;13:311-328.

Goldin JG. Imaging the lungs in patients with pulmonary emphysema. *J Thorac Imaging.* 2009;24:163-170.

Hartman TE, Primack SL, Swensen SJ, et al. Desquamative interstitial pneumonia: thin-section CT findings in 22 patients. *Radiology.* 1993;187:787-790.

Heyneman LE, Ward S, Lynch DA, et al. Respiratory bronchiolitis-associated interstitial lung disease, and desquamative interstitial pneumonia: different entities or part of the spectrum of the same disease process? *AJR Am J Roentgenol.* 1999;173:1617-1622.

Hidalgo A, Franquet T, Gimenez A, et al. Smoking-related interstitial lung disease: radiologic-pathologic correlation. *Eur Radiol.* 2006;16:2463-2470.

Nakanishi M, Demura Y, Mizuno S, et al. Changes in HRCT findings in patients with respiratory bronchiolitis-associated interstitial lung disease after smoking cessation. *Eur Respir J.* 2007;29:453-461.

Park JS, Brown KK, Tuder RM, Hale VA, King TE Jr, Lynch DA. Respiratory bronchiolitis-associated interstitial lung disease: radiologic features with clinical and pathologic correlation. *J Comput Assist Tomogr.* 2002;26:13-20.

Remy-Jardin M, Remy J, Gosselin B, Becette V, Edme JL. Lung parenchymal changes secondary to cigarette smoking: pathologic-CT correlations. *Radiology.* 1993;186:643-651.

Remy-Jardin M, Edme JL, Boulenguez C, Remy J, Mastora I, Sobaszek A. Longitudinal follow-up study of smoker's lung with thin-section CT in correlation with pulmonary function tests. *Radiology.* 2002;222:261-270.

Ryu JH, Myers JL, Capizzi SA, Douglas WW, Vassallo R, Decker PA. Desquamative interstitial pneumonia and respiratory bronchiolitis-associated interstitial lung disease. *Chest.* 2005;127:178-184.

Tazi A, Soler P, Hance AJ. Adult pulmonary Langerhans cell histiocytosis. *Thorax.* 2000;55:405-416.

Thurlbeck WM, Müller NL. Emphysema: definition, imaging, and quantification. *AJR Am J Roentgenol.* 1994;163:1017-1025.

11

INTRODUCTION

Sarcoidosis is an immune-mediated disorder characterized by the presence of noncaseating granulomas. Its cause in unknown, but infectious or noninfectious environmental agents, along with genetic and host factors, are likely involved. Sarcoidosis is typically diagnosed in patients less than 50 years of age, but it may present in older patients.

Sarcoidosis affects the thorax in at least 90% of cases, and approximately 25% of patients have respiratory symptoms at diagnosis, usually dyspnea. For this reason, HRCT is often the initial diagnostic examination obtained in patients suspected of having sarcoidosis. Up to one-half of patients with sarcoidosis are asymptomatic and diagnosed by incidental findings on radiological examinations performed for other purposes.

Sarcoidosis demonstrates striking demographic differences, with the highest prevalence seen in people of Scandinavian descent and African-Americans. It is much less common in Asia and in countries close to the equator than in the United States. Mortality from sarcoidosis, approximately 1 to 5%, is low compared with other diffuse lung diseases.

STAGING OF SARCOIDOSIS

Staging of sarcoidosis is based on plain radiography and has not been validated using HRCT. Subtle parenchymal lung changes or lymphadenopathy on HRCT may not be seen on chest radiographs.

The stages based on chest radiographs are as follows:

Stage 0: normal
Stage I: hilar lymphadenopathy only
Stage II: hilar lymphadenopathy + parenchymal lung disease
Stage III: parenchymal lung disease only
Stage IV: fibrosis

This staging system is of some value in determining prognosis and predicting the likelihood of spontaneous regression of findings without treatment. 60 to 90% of patients with Stage I disease show spontaneous regression, whereas only 10 to 20% of patients with Stage III disease will show spontaneous regression.

LUNG ABNORMALITIES IN SARCOIDOSIS

Pulmonary abnormalities in sarcoidosis are a manifestation of interstitial or airway granulomas and the subsequent development of pulmonary fibrosis or airway obstruction. The variety of abnormalities that may be seen on HRCT include perilymphatic nodules, consolidation and masses, ground glass opacity, mosaic perfusion, air trapping, irregular reticulation, traction bronchiectasis, cysts, and honeycombing (Table 12.1). Abnormalities typically have an upper lobe predominance, although this is not always the case.

TABLE 12.1	Characteristic HRCT findings of sarcoidosis
Nodules	Perilymphatic distribution
	Peribronchovascular and subpleural predominance
	Nodules well defined
	Satellite nodules and the galaxy sign
Consolidation	Patchy, bilateral
	Peribronchovascular and subpleural distribution
Airways disease	Bronchostenosis or obstruction
	Atelectasis
	Mosaic perfusion
	Air trapping
Fibrosis	Irregular reticulation
	Traction bronchiectasis
	Parahilar fibrotic masses
	Cystic disease
	Honeycombing (rare)
	Upper lobe, peribronchovascular distribution

Perilymphatic Nodules

The granulomas of sarcoidosis involve or occur in relation to pulmonary lymphatics. Clusters of microscopic granulomas appear as small nodules having a *perilymphatic distribution*, which is described in detail in Chapter 3. Nodules tend to involve the lung in a patchy fashion, with some areas of lung appearing abnormal and some areas appearing unaffected.

The following structures are typically involved by perilymphatic nodules in sarcoidosis:

1. Parahilar peribronchovascular interstitium
2. Centrilobular (peribronchovascular) interstitium
3. Subpleural interstitium
4. Interlobular septa

Nodules in sarcoidosis are typically well defined and have a preference for the parahilar peribronchovascular and subpleural interstitium (Figs. 12.1 to 12.3). Frequently, there are clusters of nodules surrounding central bronchi and pulmonary arteries. Mass-like conglomerates of nodules may be present in these locations. Nodules and clusters of nodules are also frequently seen

in the subpleural interstitium, including the interstitium adjacent to fissures. Often in patients with sarcoidosis, nodules are limited to the peribronchovascular and subpleural regions, although the severity of involvement in these two locations may vary greatly (Figs. 12.1 to 12.3).

When peribronchovascular nodules are numerous, or when they involve the airway wall, they may cause narrowing or obstruction of central bronchi, occasionally producing lobar collapse (Fig. 12.4).

Rarely, the nodules of sarcoidosis show a centrilobular (Fig. 12.5) or interlobular septal predominance (Fig. 12.6). In such cases, nodules are usually also seen in the subpleural and peribronchovascular interstitium.

Sarcoidosis may occasionally have an appearance that mimics a random distribution of nodules (see Chapter 3). However, in such cases, there is often some evidence that the pattern is perilymphatic. Nodules in these cases are not usually uniform, with a greater number of peribronchovascular or subpleural nodules than would be expected with a random distribution (Fig. 12.7).

Because the nodules in sarcoidosis involve the interstitium around the central and peripheral airways, transbronchial biopsy is frequently able to provide histologic confirmation of the disease. However, the biopsy results in these cases must be interpreted in the context of the HRCT findings and clinical presentation. Noncaseating granulomas, typical of sarcoidosis, may be seen in other disorders as well. Thus the final diagnosis reflects a compilation of the pathology, radiology, and clinical factors.

Differential Diagnosis

Although the large majority (>90%) of patients showing perilymphatic nodules on HRCT have sarcoidosis, the differential diagnosis (Table 12.2) includes lymphangitic spread of malignancy, lymphoid interstitial pneumonia (LIP), pneumoconioses such as silicosis and coal worker's pneumoconiosis, and amyloidosis. Clinical history is important in suggesting one of these alternative diagnoses. For instance, patients

12

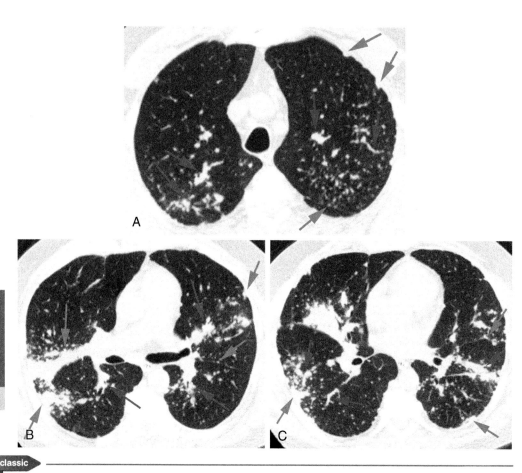

classic

FIGURE 12.1 · Sarcoidosis: Classic appearances. A–C. In a patient with extensive lung involvement, HRCT shows clusters and masses of nodules that predominate in relation to the peribronchovascular interstitium surrounding parahilar arteries and bronchi (*red arrows*, **B**), more peripheral artery and bronchial branches (*red arrows* **A** and **C**), and the subpleural interstitium in the peripheral lung and adjacent to fissures (*blue arrows*). This patient has extensive lung involvement.

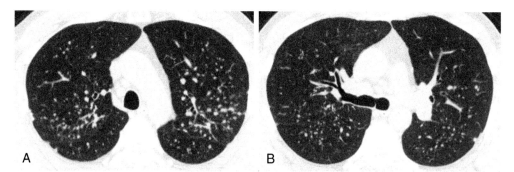

FIGURE 12.2 · Typical sarcoidosis with peribronchovascular and subpleural nodules. A. HRCT shows scattered nodules in the parahilar regions, although a clear-cut relationship to airways and bronchi is more difficult to identify than in Fig. 12.1. Subpleural nodules are easily seen. **B.** At a lower level, the nodules are less numerous. An upper lobe predominance is typical of sarcoidosis.

with LIP usually have a history of connective tissue disease or immunocompromise. Lymphangitic spread of malignancy typically occurs in patients with a known tumor. Patients with pneumoconiosis have an extensive exposure history. Sarcoidosis tends to occur in a younger patient population than the other causes of perilymphatic nodules.

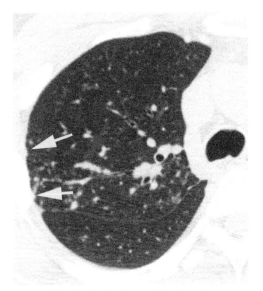

FIGURE 12.3 · **Typical sarcoidosis with peribronchovascular and subpleural nodules.** In this patient with limited involvement of the right upper lobe, peribronchovascular (*red arrow*) and subpleural (*yellow arrows*) nodules are visible.

The morphology and distribution of nodules may also be helpful in suggesting sarcoidosis as the likely cause of perilymphatic nodules. Nodules in sarcoidosis often predominate in the peribronchovascular and subpleural interstitium. The nodules of lymphangitic spread of malignancy, the second most frequent cause of perilymphatic nodules, often predominate in relation to interlobular septa. Also lymphangitic spread of malignancy may be unilateral or basilar predominant, whereas sarcoidosis is typically bilateral, symmetric, and upper lobe predominant. Peribronchovascular nodules in lymphangitic spread of malignancy are usually associated with other evidence of tumor within the chest. Pneumoconioses may have a predominance of nodules in the centrilobular regions and typically involve the posterior upper lobes.

Consolidation and Masses

Sarcoidosis may present with mass-like consolidation representing confluent granulomatous disease. Because the masses of granulomas are often peribronchial, air bronchograms may be visible (Figs. 12.8 to 12.10). This appearance is sometimes termed "alveolar sarcoid," despite the fact that the granulomas do not involve the alveolar spaces.

Consolidation in sarcoidosis is often patchy, upper lobe predominant, and peribronchovascular in distribution. It may be mass-like in appearance. Discrete small nodules ("satellite nodules") may be seen at

12

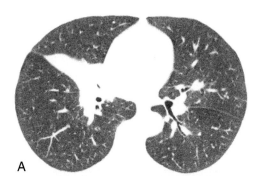

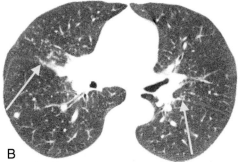

A   B

FIGURE 12.4 · **Sarcoidosis with right middle lobe collapse.** Extensive peribronchovascular granulomas or endobronchial granulomas may cause bronchial narrowing or obstruction. **A.** In this patient, right middle lobe collapse is the result of bronchial involvement. **B.** At a different level, this patient shows scattered nodules with involvement of the fissures (*arrows*).

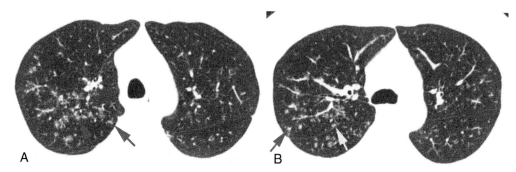

FIGURE 12.5 · **Centrilobular nodules in sarcoidosis. A** and **B.** In this patient, nodules predominate in relation to centrilobular structures and appear ill-defined (*red arrows*). A few scattered subpleural nodules are also visible (*yellow arrow*, **B**). The peribronchovascular interstitium extends into the peripheral lung, in relation to centrilobular bronchioles and arteries. In some patients, granulomas in sarcoidosis predominate in relation to these structures, resulting in well-defined or ill-defined centrilobular nodules.

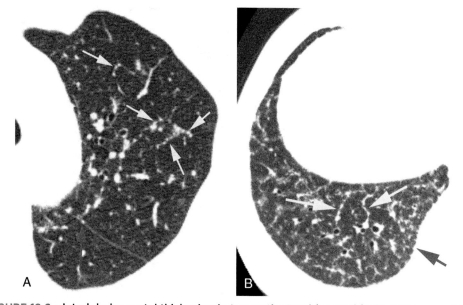

FIGURE 12.6 · **Interlobular septal thickening in two patients with sarcoidosis.** Rarely sarcoidosis presents with nodular interlobular septal thickening as a predominant abnormality. **A.** In a patient with limited lung involvement, nodular septal thickening (*yellow arrows*) is visible in the left upper lobe. A few subpleural nodules are also seen (*red arrow*). **B.** In a different patient, nodular interlobular septal thickening predominates (*yellow arrows*) in the right lower lobe, and subpleural nodules are also visible (*red arrow*).

the periphery of areas of consolidation (Figs. 12.8 to 12.10), which is evidence that consolidation represents confluent granulomatous disease as opposed to an alveolar process. An area of mass-like consolidation with individual nodules at the periphery has been termed the *galaxy sign* and is most commonly seen with sarcoidosis.

In distinction to pneumonia, consolidation in sarcoidosis is chronic and persistent over time. The differential diagnosis of chronic consolidation includes organizing pneumonia, chronic eosinophilic pneumonia, invasive mucinous adenocarcinoma, lymphoma, and lipoid pneumonia. The reversed halo sign or atoll sign (see Chapter 4)

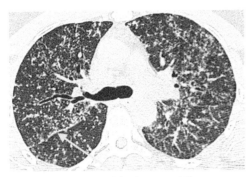

FIGURE 12.7 · **Sarcoidosis resembling a random distribution of nodules.** Superficially, the nodules appear random in distribution, with uniform lung involvement. A more detailed inspection reveals that the nodules are patchy in distribution, with more nodules along the fissures (*arrow*) than would be expected with a random pattern.

TABLE 12.2	Differential diagnosis of sarcoidosis
Finding	**Differential diagnosis**
Perilymphatic nodules	Lymphangitic spread of malignancy
	Pneumoconioses
	Amyloid
	Lymphoid interstitial pneumonia
Patchy consolidation	Organizing pneumonia
	Chronic eosinophilic pneumonia
	Invasive mucinous adenocarcinoma
	Lymphoma
	Lipoid pneumonia
Upper lobe fibrosis	Hypersensitivity pneumonitis
	Prior tuberculosis/fungal infection
	Pneumoconioses
	Radiation
	Ankylosing spondylitis
Symmetric hilar lymphadenopathy	Pneumoconioses
	Metastases
	Amyloid
	Castleman's disease

is very suggestive of organizing pneumonia and only very rarely seen with sarcoidosis. Although the galaxy sign is common in sarcoidosis, it may also be seen in silicosis and coal worker's pneumoconiosis, talcosis, other granulomatous diseases, and invasive mucinous adenocarcinoma.

Ground Glass Opacity

Rarely sarcoidosis may present with patchy ground glass opacity as the predominant finding (Fig. 12.11). Ground glass opacity in sarcoidosis reflects the presence of numerous microscopic granulomas. Even when ground glass opacity is the predominant abnormality, small discreet nodules are often seen in association. When these nodules are absent, the HRCT is nonspecific. As the lung findings in these cases are not particularly suggestive of sarcoidosis, lymphadenopathy, if present, may be the only clue as to the diagnosis.

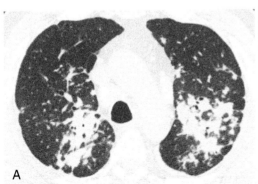

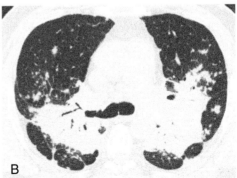

A

B

classic

FIGURE 12.8 · **"Alveolar" sarcoidosis and the galaxy sign: Classic appearance. A and B.** Confluent peribronchovascular granulomas result in mass-like parahilar consolidation. Air bronchograms are visible within the areas of consolidation. Small nodules adjacent to the large masses are satellite nodules. The combination of the large mass and surrounding satellites is termed the "galaxy sign."

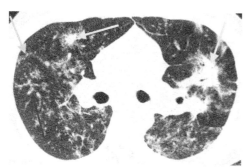

FIGURE 12.9 · Consolidation in sarcoidosis. A combination of consolidation (*yellow arrows*) in association with more discrete peribronchovascular (*red arrow*) and subpleural (*blue arrow*) nodules may be seen in sarcoidosis. The consolidation represents confluent granulomatous disease.

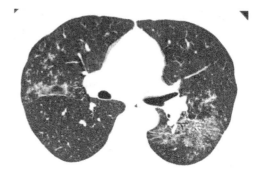

FIGURE 12.11 · Sarcoidosis with ground glass opacity (GGO). Patchy GGO is present in the left lung, but even within areas of GGO, small discrete nodules can be appreciated. GGO as an isolated finding is a rare manifestation of sarcoidosis.

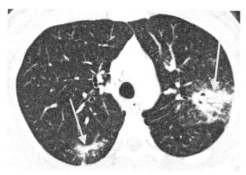

FIGURE 12.10 · Consolidation in sarcoidosis. Patchy consolidation is seen adjacent to bronchi and fissures (*yellow arrows*), with an air bronchogram visible in the left upper lobe. Small nodules are present at the edges of the areas of consolidation (satellite nodules). This feature may help distinguish sarcoidosis from other causes of chronic consolidation and is termed the galaxy sign.

Airway Abnormalities

Occasionally, HRCT in sarcoidosis shows nodular thickening of the walls of large airways. The nodules, a few millimeters in diameter and similar in size to lung nodules seen in this disease, project into the airway lumen.

Mosaic perfusion and/or air trapping may be seen in association with obstruction or narrowing of small airways by granulomas (Fig. 12.12). Depending on the level of bronchial/bronchiolar obstruction, the distribution of these findings may be lobular, segmental, or lobar (Fig. 12.4).

Mosaic perfusion and air trapping are not usually isolated abnormalities in patients with sarcoidosis. At presentation, airway abnormalities are almost always associated with other findings, such as nodules (Fig. 12.12). However, after treatment, the airways disease may persist, even after the nodules resolve.

A combination of air trapping and nodules may be seen with several other diffuse lung diseases such as hypersensitivity pneumonitis, respiratory bronchiolitis, follicular bronchiolitis, and atypical infections. The nodules in these cases differ from sarcoidosis in that they are of ground glass opacity, whereas the nodules in sarcoidosis tend to be dense and well defined. Pneumoconioses and LIP may show perilymphatic nodules and associated mild mosaic perfusion and air trapping. It is unusual for lymphangitic spread of tumor and amyloidosis to produce mosaic perfusion and air trapping.

Fibrosis

Fibrosis occurs in approximately 20% of patients with sarcoidosis and is associated with a poor outcome. The fibrosis is usually upper lobe, central, and peribronchovascular in distribution. Irregular reticulation is common (Fig. 12.13). Fibrotic masses may be seen in some patients (Fig. 12.14). Masses are often associated with traction bronchiectasis and irregular air bronchograms. Honeycombing may also be present (Fig. 12.15), but the overall distribution of fibrosis differs from idiopathic pulmonary

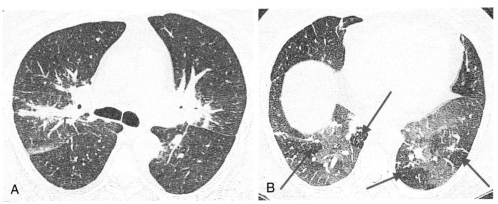

FIGURE 12.12 · Sarcoidosis with air trapping. A. Typical peribronchovascular interstitial thickening is present in the upper lobes in this patient with sarcoidosis. **B.** On a postexpiratory image, patchy areas of air trapping (*arrows*) at the lung bases reflect small airway stenosis or occlusion by granulomas or associated fibrosis.

classic

FIGURE 12.13 · Sarcoidosis with fibrosis: Classic appearance. Irregular reticular opacities predominate in the parahilar and peribronchovascular regions of the upper lobes. There is distortion of the fissures and subpleural areas of fibrosis are also visible.

12

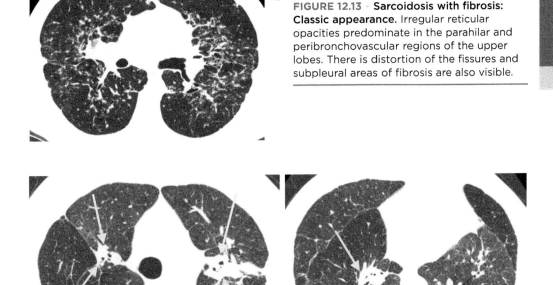

FIGURE 12.14 · Sarcoidosis with fibrotic masses. A. Lung fibrosis associated with sarcoidosis typically predominates in the upper lobes and peribronchovascular regions (*arrows*). Masses of fibrous tissue may result. As in this case, there is associated volume loss and architectural distortion, and dilated bronchi (i.e., traction bronchiectasis) may be visible within the masses. **B.** In some patients, similar masses of fibrosis (*arrows*) are seen in the lower lobes.

fibrosis (IPF). IPF usually presents with a basilar and peripheral distribution of fibrosis.

Confluent areas of fibrosis may be manifested as mass-like areas of consolidation with architectural distortion, usually surrounding central bronchi (Fig. 12.16). This may be termed *progressive massive fibrosis (PMF)*, although PMF is usually used to refer to similar abnormalities occurring in silicosis. Consolidative areas of fibrosis can be distinguished from "alveolar sarcoidosis" by the presence of associated traction bronchiectasis and architectural distortion. Given the upper lobe predominance of disease, the hila are often retracted superiorly.

Large cysts may be seen in areas of fibrosis in patients with sarcoidosis. These may represent dilated bronchi (traction bronchiectasis) or areas of emphysema (Fig. 12.17). Traction bronchiectasis is common in end-stage sarcoidosis. Mycetoma is a common complication of cystic sarcoidosis.

The differential diagnosis of sarcoidosis with fibrosis includes other chronic lung diseases that are upper lobe predominant including many pneumoconioses, most specifically silicosis or coal worker's pneumoconiosis, prior tuberculosis or fungal infection, radiation fibrosis, and ankylosing spondylitis. Although hypersensitivity pneumonitis is typically mid-lung predominant, an upper lobe distribution of fibrosis is not uncommon and findings may overlap those typical of sarcoidosis. PMF is most commonly seen with sarcoidosis, pneumoconioses, or prior granulomatous infections.

LYMPHADENOPATHY

Hilar and mediastinal lymphadenopathy are common manifestations of sarcoidosis and may be seen as an isolated abnormality or in conjunction with parenchymal lung disease. The lymphadenopathy is typically symmetric in distribution, with involvement of the hilar, paratracheal, aortopulmonary window, and/or subcarinal regions (Fig. 12.18). Hilar involvement is most characteristic.

Although the presence of typical lymph node enlargement on CT can be helpful in supporting a diagnosis of sarcoidosis, keep in mind that many patients with HRCT findings diagnostic or strongly suggestive of

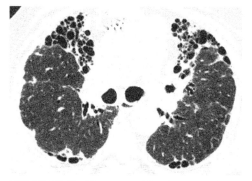

FIGURE 12.15 · **Honeycombing in sarcoidosis.** Honeycombing may be seen as a manifestation of end-stage sarcoidosis. The distribution differs from idiopathic pulmonary fibrosis by being predominant in the upper lobes and/or having significant involvement of the central lung regions.

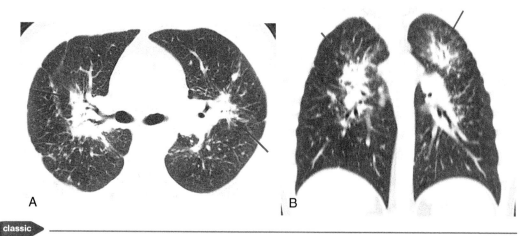

A   B

classic ▶

FIGURE 12.16 · **Sarcoidosis resembling progressive massive fibrosis: Classic appearance.** Axial **(A)** and coronal **(B)** images show masses of consolidative fibrosis (*arrows*) and traction bronchiectasis within the central lung regions in a patient with sarcoidosis. These findings resemble progressive massive fibrosis seen in patients with silicosis.

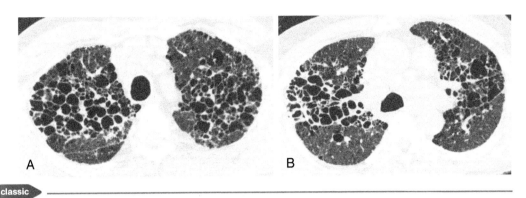

classic

FIGURE 12.17 · **End-stage sarcoidosis traction bronchiectasis and cyst formation: Classic appearance.** Images through the upper **(A)** and mid- **(B)** lungs show extensive parahilar and upper lobe cystic disease may be seen with end-stage sarcoidosis. Differentiating dilated bronchi from cysts or emphysema may be difficult. Mycetoma is common in patients with this manifestation of fibrosis in sarcoidosis.

12

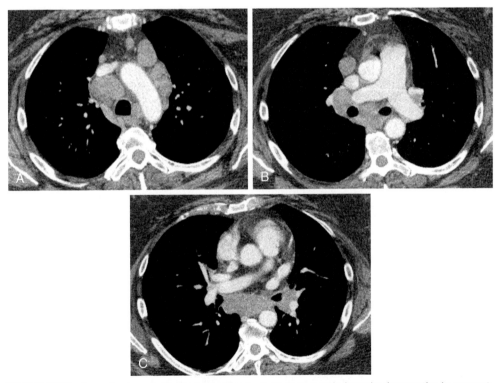

FIGURE 12.18 · **Lymphadenopathy in sarcoidosis. A–C.** Symmetric lymphadenopathy is present in the paratracheal, aortopulmonary, subcarinal, and hilar regions. The combination of symmetric and hilar involvement is strongly suggestive of sarcoidosis. However, lymph node enlargement is not necessary for the HRCT diagnosis of this disease.

sarcoidosis have no evidence of lymph node enlargement. A diagnosis of sarcoidosis can be made based on the presence of typical lung abnormalities alone.

Lymphadenopathy in sarcoidosis may be hypermetabolic on positron emission tomography with standard uptake values that overlap with malignancy (Fig. 12.19). A symmetric distribution of mediastinal and hilar lymphadenopathy in a patient of the appropriate demographic is very suggestive of sarcoidosis. Lymph nodes may be calcified or noncalcified. The morphology of calcification may be diffuse, hazy, and central; may have an eggshell pattern (Fig. 12.20); or may be heterogeneous. Necrosis in lymph nodes is rare.

The differential diagnosis (Table 12.3) includes other causes of symmetrical lymphadenopathy including pneumoconioses, amyloidosis, and Castleman's disease. Metastases are an uncommon cause of symmetrical disease, but this pattern is occasionally seen with gastrointestinal tumors, genitourinary tumors, lung cancer, breast cancer, and leukemia. Granulomatous infections, such as mycobacterial and fungal disease, are typically asymmetric. Lymphoma is often a concern in patients with suspected sarcoidosis; however, the majority of cases of lymphoma are asymmetric.

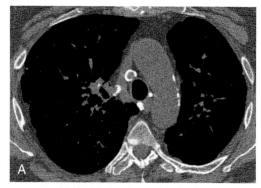

FIGURE 12.19 · **Positron emission tomography (PET) in sarcoidosis.** The distribution of lymph node activity on PET scanning is the same as on CT, with paratracheal (*yellow arrow*), subcarinal (*red arrow*), and hilar (*blue arrows*) involvement. The PET avidity of these nodes may be in the same range as malignancy.

TABLE 12.3	Differential diagnosis of lymphadenopathy in sarcoidosis
Commonly symmetric	Pneumoconioses
	Amyloidosis
	Castleman's disease
Rarely symmetric	Metastases
	Lymphoma
	Mycobacterial/fungal infection

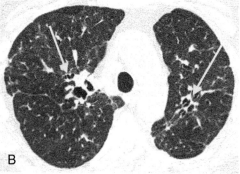

FIGURE 12.20 · **Eggshell calcification of mediastinal lymph nodes in sarcoidosis.** The nodes of sarcoidosis may be calcified. The pattern of calcification is variable but may be peripheral/eggshell in distribution, dense, or hazy. In this patient, eggshell calcification **(A)** is associated with parahilar fibrosis and traction bronchiectasis (*arrows*, **B**).

FURTHER READING

Brauner MW, Grenier P, Mompoint D, et al. Pulmonary sarcoidosis: evaluation with high-resolution CT. *Radiology.* 1989;172:467-471.

Brauner MW, Lenoir S, Grenier P, et al. Pulmonary sarcoidosis: CT assessment of lesion reversibility. *Radiology.* 1992;182:349-354.

Criado E, Sánchez M, Ramírez J, et al. Pulmonary sarcoidosis: typical and atypical manifestations at high-resolution CT with pathologic correlation. *Radiographics.* 2010;30:1567-1586.

Gleeson FV, Traill ZC, Hansell DM. Evidence of expiratory CT scans of small-airway obstruction in sarcoidosis. *AJR Am J Roentgenol.* 1996;166: 1052-1054.

Hamper UM, Fishman EK, Khouri NF, et al. Typical and atypical CT manifestations of pulmonary sarcoidosis. *J Comput Assist Tomogr.* 1986;10:928-936.

Hansell DM, Milne DG, Wilsher ML, Wells AU. Pulmonary sarcoidosis: morphologic associations of airflow obstruction at thin-section CT. *Radiology.* 1998;209:697-704.

Lee KS, Kim TS, Han J, et al. Diffuse micronodular lung disease: HRCT and pathologic findings. *J Comput Assist Tomogr.* 1999;23:99-106.

Lenique F, Brauner MW, Grenier P, et al. CT assessment of bronchi in sarcoidosis: endoscopic and pathologic correlations. *Radiology.* 1995;194:419-423.

Lynch DA, Webb WR, Gamsu G, et al. Computed tomography in pulmonary sarcoidosis. *J Comput Assist Tomogr.* 1989;13:405-410.

Miller BH, Rosado-de-Christenson ML, McAdams HP, Fishback NF. Thoracic sarcoidosis: radiologic-pathologic correlation. *Radiographics.* 1995;15:421-437.

Müller NL, Kullnig P, Miller RR. The CT findings of pulmonary sarcoidosis: analysis of 25 patients. *AJR Am J Roentgenol.* 1989;152:1179-1182.

Müller NL, Mawson JB, Mathieson JR, et al. Sarcoidosis: correlation of extent of disease at CT with clinical, functional, and radiographic findings. *Radiology.* 1989;171:613-618.

Nakatsu M, Hatabu H, Morkawa K, et al. Large coalescent parenchymal nodules in pulmonary sarcoidosis: "Sarcoid Galaxy" sign. *AJR Am J Roentgenol.* 2002;178:1389-1393.

Nishimura K, Itoh H, Kitaichi M, et al. Pulmonary sarcoidosis: correlation of CT and histopathologic findings. *Radiology.* 1993;189:105-109.

Padley SP, Padhani AR, Nicholson A, Hansell DM. Pulmonary sarcoidosis mimicking cryptogenic fibrosing alveolitis on CT. *Clin Radiol.* 1996;51:807-810.

Patil SN, Levin DL. Distribution of thoracic lymphadenopathy in sarcoidosis using computed tomography. *J Thorac Imaging.* 1999; 14:114-117.

Remy-Jardin M, Beuscart R, Sault MC, et al. Subpleural micronodules in diffuse infiltrative lung diseases: evaluation with thin-section CT scans. *Radiology.* 1990;177:133-139.

Remy-Jardin M, Giraud F, Remy J, et al. Pulmonary sarcoidosis: role of CT in the evaluation of disease activity and functional impairment and in prognosis assessment. *Radiology.* 1994;191:675-680.

Traill ZC, Maskell GF, Gleeson FV. High-resolution CT findings of pulmonary sarcoidosis. *AJR Am J Roentgenol.* 1997;168:1557-1560.

12

Hypersensitivity Pneumonitis and Eosinophilic Lung Disease

HYPERSENSITIVITY PNEUMONITIS

Hypersensitivity pneumonitis (HP) represents an exaggerated immune reaction to inhaled organic antigens. The possible sources of these antigens are diverse and include microbes, animals, plant material, and various chemicals. Although different schemes have been proposed; HP is typically considered in three stages or categories (acute, subacute, and chronic). These provide a useful framework with which to discuss the clinical, pathologic, and radiologic spectrum of findings.

Acute HP is rare and involves a large antigen exposure leading to the rapid onset of cough, dyspnea, and fever. Exposure to moldy hay in farmer's lung is the most typical example of acute HP.

Subacute HP is common and demonstrates symptoms that are similar to, but less severe than acute HP. Exposures leading to the development of symptoms are more prolonged, extending over weeks to months.

Chronic HP is also common and involves long-term exposure to low levels of antigen over a period of years. It is typically associated with lung fibrosis.

There are striking differences in the prevalence of HP based on the antigen exposure. For instance, up to 15% of pigeon breeders will develop HP. However, only 50% of patients with known HP will have an identifiable exposure, even with careful history taking and examination of the patients' environments.

Smoking is thought to be relatively protective against the development of HP, but smoking does not preclude this disease.

Histopathology

A wide spectrum of pathologic findings may be present. The subacute stage is characterized by interstitial inflammation and cellular infiltration. In the chronic stage, fibrosis is the predominant finding. Regardless of the predominant feature, the findings tend to be bronchiolocentric (Fig. 13.1), reflecting the airway-centric nature of the disease. Poorly formed granulomas (Fig. 13.2) are a characteristic finding. These differ from the discreet and well-formed granulomas in sarcoidosis. Organizing pneumonia is also a common pathologic feature of HP. Pathologic findings indistinguishable from idiopathic nonspecific interstitial pneumonia (NSIP) or usual interstitial pneumonia (UIP) may be present. In these cases, the presence of an exposure or HRCT findings may suggest the correct diagnosis.

HRCT Findings

The HRCT findings of HP vary depending on the clinical presentation.

Acute HP

The findings of acute HP have not been extensively documented, as most patients are not imaged in this stage. The HRCT findings are likely similar to those of subacute HP but may be more extensive (Fig. 13.3) and demonstrate an increased incidence of consolidation.

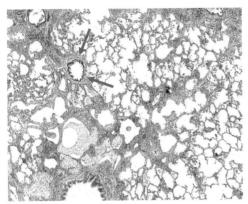

FIGURE 13.1 · **Pathology of hypersensitivity pneumonitis.** On low power, there is diffuse interstitial inflammation and fibrosis that is more severe around the airways (*arrows*).

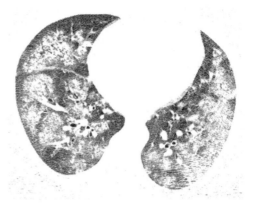

FIGURE 13.3 · **Acute hypersensitivity pneumonitis (HP).** Extensive bilateral ground glass opacity is seen in a patient with acute HP secondary to mold exposure. These abnormalities are nonspecific and more severe than that typically present with subacute HP.

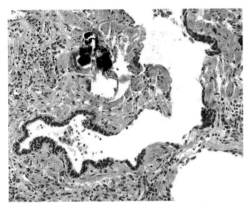

FIGURE 13.2 · **On high power, a poorly formed granuloma (*arrows*) is noted, composed of a multinucleated giant cell and histiocytes.** A calcified Schaumann body, commonly seen in granulomas, is noted.

TABLE 13.1	HRCT findings of subacute hypersensitivity pneumonitis

Patchy GGO
Centrilobular nodules of GGO
Mosaic perfusion and air trapping
Headcheese sign (combination of GGO and
   mosaic perfusion/air trapping)
Mid–lower lung distribution, spares costophrenic
   angles

GGO, ground glass opacity.

Subacute HP

The diagnosis of subacute HP is usually based on the presence of a combination or constellation of abnormalities, including ground glass opacity (GGO), centrilobular nodules of GGO, mosaic perfusion or air trapping, and the *headcheese sign* (Table 13.1).

Ground Glass Opacity

GGO in HP is often patchy and bilateral in distribution. It may be seen in isolation, in which case it is a nonspecific finding (Fig. 13.4). Isolated GGO may be seen with a variety of acute diseases (infections, edema, diffuse alveolar damage, and hemorrhage) and chronic diseases (invasive mucinous adenocarcinoma, interstitial pneumonias, organizing pneumonia, eosinophilic pneumonia, lipoid pneumonia, and alveolar proteinosis). When associated with other findings of subacute HP, such as air trapping, the specificity of GGO for a diagnosis of HP increases significantly.

Centrilobular Nodules of GGO

This is a common finding in subacute HP and reflects peribronchiolar inflammation, cellular infiltration, and poorly marginated granulomas. HP is the most common cause of centrilobular GGO nodules in association with subacute and chronic symptoms. The nodules are often diffuse or symmetric (Fig. 13.5). In the setting of an identifiable exposure to an organic antigen, a pattern of diffuse centrilobular GGO nodules are considered diagnostic of subacute HP. The differential diagnosis of centrilobular GGO nodules includes respiratory bronchiolitis, follicular bronchiolitis, atypical infections, and vascular diseases, including pulmonary hemorrhage.

Mosaic Perfusion, Air Trapping, and the Headcheese Sign

Mosaic perfusion and air trapping on expiratory scans may be seen in association with other abnormalities (Figs. 13.5B and 13.6) or may be an isolated abnormality (Fig. 13.7). Mosaic perfusion appears as one or more focal areas of decreased lung attenuation associated with a reduction in size of vessels within

the lucent region (see Chapter 5). It reflects the presence of bronchiolitis and bronchiolar obstruction occurring as a result of bronchiolar inflammation, with decreased vessel size and lung attenuation due to reflex vasoconstriction. Often areas of mosaic perfusion and air trapping appear lobular (i.e., they represent secondary pulmonary lobules), and multiple lobules in multiple lobes are typically involved. It may persist after treatment of HP and following resolution of GGO or nodules. When seen as an isolated abnormality, the differential diagnosis includes asthma and constrictive bronchiolitis.

The combination of patchy mosaic perfusion and GGO has been termed the *headcheese sign*; it is highly suggestive of HP (Fig. 13.8). Both GGO and mosaic perfusion must be present. GGO reflects the cellular infiltration typical of HP, whereas the mosaic perfusion reflects bronchiolar obstruction. It is called the headcheese sign because of its resemblance to a sausage of the same name (see Chapter 5).

The differential diagnosis of the headcheese sign includes desquamative interstitial pneumonia (DIP)/respiratory bronchiolitis, follicular bronchiolitis/lymphoid interstitial pneumonia, sarcoidosis, and atypical infections.

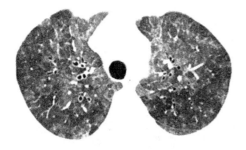

FIGURE 13.4 · Subacute hypersensitivity pneumonitis (HP) with ground glass opacity. Patchy ground glass opacity is a nonspecific finding that may be seen in a variety of disorders. It may be the only manifestation of subacute HP but more commonly is associated with other findings such as mosaic perfusion and centrilobular nodules.

Consolidation

The presence of consolidation is rare in HP. However, it may be the predominant feature

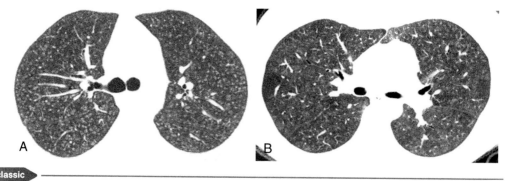

A   B

`classic`

FIGURE 13.5 · Subacute hypersensitivity pneumonitis (HP) with centrilobular ground glass opacity nodules: Classic appearances. A and B. HP is the most common cause of diffuse centrilobular nodules of ground glass opacity. In the setting of an appropriate exposure, such as this patient with a chronic mold exposure, the HRCT should be considered diagnostic of HP. In the absence of an exposure, biopsy is required for diagnosis. In another patient **(B)**, note that the centrilobular nodules are associated with areas of low-attenuation mosaic perfusion.

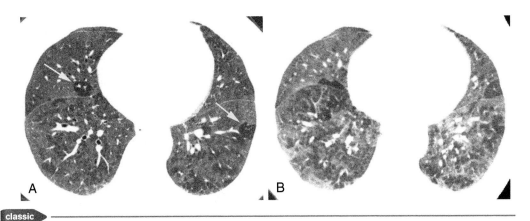

classic

FIGURE 13.6 · **Subacute hypersensitivity pneumonitis (HP) with mosaic perfusion and air trapping: Classic appearance. A.** HRCT in a 66-year-old bird fancier shows patchy and lobular areas of decreased lung attenuation (*arrows*) representing mosaic perfusion. Ground glass opacity is also present. **B.** Air trapping within the regions of mosaic perfusion is seen on a dynamic expiratory scan. Mosaic perfusion and/or air trapping may be seen in combination with other abnormalities or as an isolated finding in patients with HP, either at initial presentation or after treatment. Not uncommonly, these are the only abnormalities that persist after treatment of subacute HP.

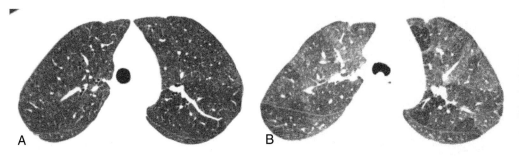

13

FIGURE 13.7 · **Subacute hypersensitivity pneumonitis (HP) with isolated mosaic perfusion and air trapping. A.** Other than subtle mosaic perfusion, the inspiratory scan appears nearly normal. **B.** On expiration, air trapping is clearly seen. This appearance may be seen in patients with subacute HP before or after treatment.

in cases of acute HP or in subacute HP in which secondary organizing pneumonia is also present (Fig. 13.9). On HRCT, patchy consolidation in HP may be indistinguishable from cryptogenic organizing pneumonia, eosinophilic pneumonia, invasive mucinous adenocarcinoma, and other causes of chronic consolidation.

Distribution of Abnormalities
In patients with HP, abnormalities typically predominate in the mid-lungs, with sparing of the inferior costophrenic angles (Fig. 13.10). However, an upper lobe distribution is not uncommon, and only a small percentage of cases

predominate in the lower lobes. Distribution may help distinguish HP from the interstitial pneumonias that typically predominate in the lung bases (UIP, NSIP, and DIP), with involvement of the costophrenic angles. Also, in the axial plane, HP is usually diffuse or central in distribution, whereas the interstitial pneumonias are typically peripheral and subpleural.

Chronic HP
The cardinal finding of chronic HP is fibrosis. The pattern of fibrosis and associated abnormalities may be used to distinguish HP from other fibrotic lung diseases (Table 13.2). The most common findings of fibrosis seen with

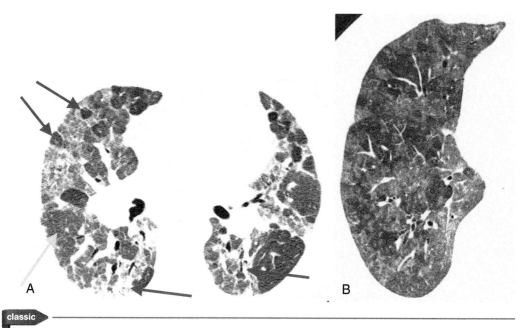

FIGURE 13.8 · **Subacute hypersensitivity pneumonitis (HP) with the "headcheese" sign in two patients: Classic appearances. A.** The combination of lobular mosaic perfusion (*dark blue arrows*), geographic areas of ground glass opacity (*red arrows*), and normal lung (*light blue arrow*) constitutes the headcheese sign and is highly suggestive of HP. **B.** In a different patient with HP, geographic areas of mosaic perfusion and ground glass opacity are well demonstrated. Air trapping was visible on expiratory scans.

13

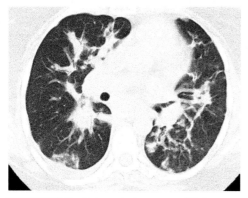

FIGURE 13.9 · **Subacute hypersensitivity pneumonitis (HP) with organizing pneumonia.** Patchy peribronchovascular consolidation is present in a patient with HP, typical of organizing pneumonia. Although organizing pneumonia is commonly seen pathologically in patients with HP, it is only rarely seen as the predominant abnormality on HRCT.

HP are traction bronchiectasis and irregular reticulation (Fig. 13.10). Honeycombing may also be present (Fig. 13.11). The distribution of fibrosis is the same as the distribution of abnormalities in subacute HP, often involving

the central lung regions and the mid- or upper lungs (Figs. 13.10 and 13.11). This helps distinguish chronic HP from fibrosis in UIP or NSIP.

The combination of lung fibrosis with mosaic perfusion or air trapping, similar to the *headcheese sign,* but with fibrosis replacing GGO, is suggestive of chronic HP (Figs. 13.11 and 13.12). The presence of significant mosaic perfusion or air trapping (multiple lobules in three or more lobes) is considered "inconsistent with a diagnosis of UIP."

There may be an overlap of the findings of chronic and subacute HP. Fibrosis typical of chronic HP may be present in association with GGO and/or centrilobular nodules typical of subacute HP (Fig. 13.13).

Atypical HRCT manifestations of HP include findings resembling NSIP or rarely UIP.

EOSINOPHILIC LUNG DISEASES

Eosinophilic lung diseases (Table 13.3) represent a heterogeneous group of disorders that are characterized by the presence of a lung

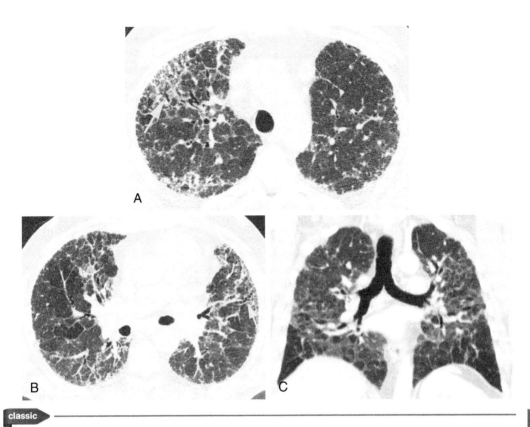

classic

FIGURE 13.10 · Chronic hypersensitivity pneumonitis (HP): Classic appearance. A and **B.** In a patient with chronic HP, fibrosis, reticulation, and traction bronchiectasis (*yellow arrows*) involve the entire cross section of the lung, both central and subpleural regions. **C.** Coronal reformatted image shows the mid-lung predominance typical of HP. Lucency at the lung bases is due to mosaic perfusion.

13

TABLE 13.2	HRCT findings of chronic hypersensitivity pneumonitis

HRCT findings
Irregular reticulation
Traction bronchiectasis
Honeycombing
Associated findings of subacute HP (centrilobular nodules, mosaic perfusion, air trapping)
Mid–lower lung distribution, spares costophrenic angles
Diffuse or central distribution in the axial plane

HP, hypersensitivity pneumonitis.

abnormality and increased eosinophils in the lung and/or blood. Of note, many "non-eo-sinophilic" lung diseases may show a mild increase in eosinophils. For example, asthma may show mild elevations of serum eosino-phils and eosinophils on lung biopsy, but it

is not a disease whose primary abnormality is eosinophilic infiltration. Peripheral eosino-philia is present in the majority of eosinophilic lung diseases, with the exception of acute eosinophilic pneumonia (AEP).

Eosinophilic lung diseases can be clas-sified by whether their cause is known or unknown (idiopathic). Those with a known cause include allergic bronchopulmonary aspergillosis (ABPA), bronchocentric gran-ulomatosis, drug treatment, and parasitic infections.

Those with an unknown cause include simple pulmonary eosinophilia, chronic eosinophilic pneumonia (CEP), hypereo-sinophilic syndrome, and Churg–Strauss syndrome (also known as eosinophilic gran-ulomatosis with polyangiitis; see Chapter 7). Although AEP was previously classified as

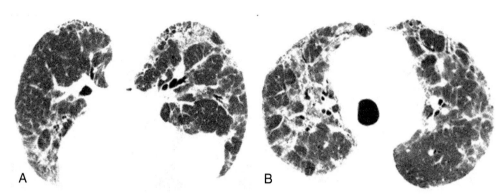

A   B

FIGURE 13.11 · **Chronic hypersensitivity pneumonitis with honeycombing. A.** Honeycombing is visible posteriorly at the lung base. **B.** A scan through the upper lobes shows more extensive fibrosis, involving the entire cross section of the lung. Lobular areas of sparing likely reflect mosaic perfusion. As opposed to idiopathic pulmonary fibrosis, the distribution of fibrosis in this patient shows significant involvement of the central lung and upper lobes.

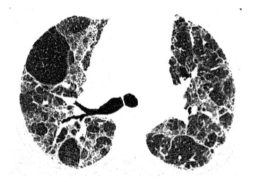

FIGURE 13.12 · **Chronic hypersensitivity pneumonitis with fibrosis and mosaic perfusion.** Reticulation and traction bronchiectasis involve the upper lobes. Multiple lobular and multilobular lucencies reflect mosaic perfusion.

an idiopathic disorder, recent data suggest that the majority of cases are related to cigarette smoking. The idiopathic diseases may be further subclassified by whether they have an acute or chronic presentation. Acute presentations are seen with simple pulmonary eosinophilia and AEP. Chronic symptoms are seen with CEP and hypereosinophilic syndrome.

Idiopathic Eosinophilic Disorders
Simple Pulmonary Eosinophilia (Loeffler Syndrome)

Loeffler syndrome is a rare disease of unknown cause that is characterized by an acute presentation followed by spontaneous regression, usually within 1 month. Patients have mild or absent symptoms in the presence of chest X-ray or CT abnormalities.

The most typical HRCT finding is migratory, nonsegmental consolidation (Fig. 13.14). This is often peripheral and involves the mid- or upper lungs. While new areas of consolidation appear, others resolve, and complete regression within 1 month is typical. GGO, nodules, and bronchial wall thickening may be associated with the consolidation but are not particularly suggestive of this disease.

Acute Eosinophilic Pneumonia

AEP is characterized by a rapid onset of symptoms, usually less than 1 week before presentation. AEP presents with a single episode that does not recur after treatment; however, progression to acute respiratory distress syndrome and death may occur. Although previously classified as an idiopathic disorder, the majority of cases of AEP are seen in cigarette smokers, particularly in those who have changed their smoking habits (e.g., increased number of cigarettes smoked per day) in the month leading up to the acute presentation. As opposed to other eosinophilic lung diseases, AEP often does not show a peripheral eosinophilia, although increased eosinophils on bronchoalveolar lavage is typical.

Typical HRCT findings include diffuse or extensive GGO (Fig. 13.15) or consolidation.

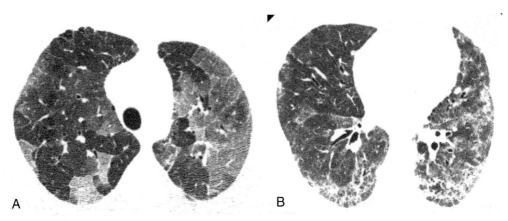

A   B

FIGURE 13.13 · **Overlap of subacute and chronic hypersensitivity pneumonitis. A.** HRCT through the upper lobes shows findings typical of subacute hypersensitivity pneumonitis, with patchy ground glass opacity (GGO) and mosaic perfusion, the headcheese sign. **B.** HRCT through the lung bases shows GGO with extensive reticulation indicative of fibrosis. Hypersensitivity pneumonitis not uncommonly presents with a combination of findings of subacute and chronic disease on the same HRCT.

TABLE 13.3	Features of eosinophilic disorders	
Disease	**Features**	**HRCT findings**
Idiopathic eosinophilic disorders		
Simple pulmonary eosinophilia	Acute, spontaneous regression within 1 mo, mild symptoms	Migratory, peripheral upper lung consolidation
Acute eosinophilic pneumonia	Acute, single episode, absence of peripheral eosinophilia, may progress to ARDS	Diffuse GGO and consolidation
CEP	Chronic, most common idiopathic eosinophilic disease, asthma in 50%	Peripheral and peribronchovascular consolidation
Hypereosinophilic syndrome	Multiorgan involvement, nervous systemic and cardiac most common, men in third or fourth decade	Diffuse/consolidation and interlobular septal thickening
Eosinophilic granulomatosis with polyangiitis (Churg–Strauss)	Involvement of the lungs, central nervous system, and skin	Nonsegmental consolidation or GGO often in a peripheral distribution, and resembling CEP
Known eosinophilic disorders		
Allergic bronchopulmonary aspergillosis	Hypersensitivity reaction to *Aspergillus* in airways, asthma, or cystic fibrosis history	Upper-mid-lung bronchiectasis (often cystic), other evidence of airways disease
Bronchocentric granulomatosis	Idiopathic or due to asthma, immunosuppression, or connective tissue disease	Masses, lobular consolidation, airway impaction
Drugs	Most common drugs: bleomycin, amiodarone, nitrofurantoin, phenytoin, and methotrexate	Resembles idiopathic eosinophilic disorders
Parasitic infections	Rare in developed countries, travel to endemic regions	Variable: nodules, consolidation, CEP

ARDS, acute respiratory distress syndrome; GGO, ground glass opacity; CEP, chronic eosinophilic pneumonia.

Pathologically, this corresponds to eosinophilic infiltration and diffuse alveolar damage. Associated findings may include smooth interlobular septal thickening and nodules.

These findings are usually indistinguishable from other causes of diffuse lung disease in the acute setting such as pulmonary edema, acute respiratory distress syndrome, atypical

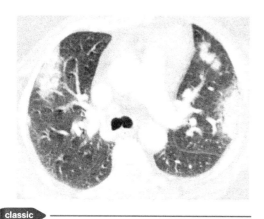

`classic`

FIGURE 13.14 · Simple pulmonary eosinophilia (Loeffler syndrome): Classic appearance. Peripheral nonsegmental consolidation is seen in the upper lobes bilaterally in a patient presenting with 2 weeks of cough. On sequential chest X-rays, this was migratory. This appearance is typical of simple pulmonary eosinophilia; however, correlation with increased serum and lung eosinophils is necessary.

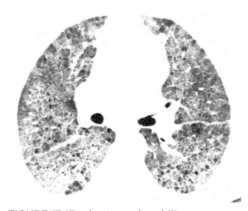

FIGURE 13.15 · Acute eosinophilic pneumonia. Diffuse ground glass opacity and interlobular septal thickening are present. These findings are nonspecific but most often seen with edema, infection, diffuse alveolar damage, and hemorrhage. There was no clinical evidence of any of these diseases, and lung biopsy was performed. Acute eosinophilic pneumonia was proven pathologically.

infection, and hemorrhage. AEP is, in general, highly responsive to corticosteroids, showing rapid improvement in symptoms and clearing within days to weeks.

Chronic Eosinophilic Pneumonia

CEP is the most common of the idiopathic eosinophilic disorders. Patients present with chronic symptoms, often of several months duration. Asthma is a commonly associated disorder, seen in approximately half the patients. Blood eosinophilia is typically present. Treatment with steroids often leads to prompt resolution. It is important to note that CEP may be seen as a reaction to drugs, parasitic infections, and other lung insults. Idiopathic CEP is, thus, a diagnosis of exclusion in which other possible causes are ruled out.

Consolidation is the most frequent HRCT finding (Fig. 13.16). Classically, it is peripheral and upper lobe in distribution (Fig. 13.17A–C), often described as the "photographic negative" of pulmonary edema. More commonly, however, consolidation is patchy, bilateral, and both peribronchovascular and subpleural in distribution. The *atoll* or *reversed halo sign* (see Chapter 4) may be present (Fig. 13.18). Less typical findings include small nodules, GGO, and reticulation. After treatment, complete resolution is typical, but linear areas of atelectasis or scar, which may parallel the pleural surface, may persist.

These findings are very similar to those of organizing pneumonia, and in fact, these two entities may be indistinguishable. Pathologically, organizing pneumonia is often seen in association with CEP, and significant overlap between these two entities exists. An upper lobe predominance of abnormalities is more typical of CEP (Fig. 13.19), whereas organizing pneumonia often has a lower lobe predominance. Other causes of chronic consolidation that may resemble CEP include sarcoidosis, mucinous adenocarcinoma, lymphoma, and lipoid pneumonia.

Hypereosinophilic Syndrome

Hypereosinophilic syndrome is a systemic disorder that has a course that is prolonged, usually more than 6 months, and is characterized by eosinophilic tissue infiltration of multiple organs. Central nervous system and cardiac involvement are most common, but lung disease occurs in approximately 40% of patients. A typical patient is male and aged 20 to 40 years.

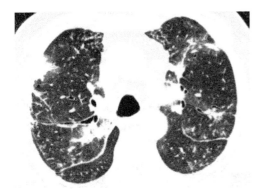

FIGURE 13.16 · Chronic eosinophilic pneumonia (CEP). Patchy, peripheral, nonsegmental consolidation is seen in the upper lobes in this patient with 4 months of dyspnea and cough. Although this finding is nonspecific by itself, the presence of increased eosinophils in the lung or serum in association with these findings is highly suggestive of CEP.

HRCT abnormalities are usually a reflection of pulmonary edema related to cardiac involvement, rather than pulmonary disease. Findings include diffuse or symmetric GGO (Fig. 13.20) and/or consolidation. Smooth interlobular septal thickening is also a common finding. When eosinophilic infiltration is present, nodules are most characteristic. These tend to be 1 cm or less in diameter, often with an associated halo of GGO.

Eosinophilic Granulomatosis with Polyangiitis (Churg–Strauss Syndrome)

Eosinophilic granulomatosis with polyangiitis, previously known as Churg–Strauss syndrome, is a disease that has features of both an eosinophilic disorder and vasculitis. It is seen predominantly in patients with a history of asthma or allergy but often presents in patients who are significantly older than the usual initial onset of asthma. It is a systemic disorder with predominant involvement of the lungs, central

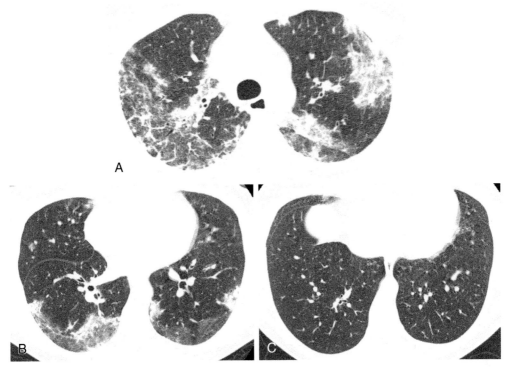

FIGURE 13.17 · Chronic eosinophilic pneumonia. Images through the upper **(A)**, mid- **(B)**, and lower **(C)** lungs show peripheral and upper lobe predominant consolidation and ground glass opacity. These findings are typical of chronic eosinophilic pneumonia.

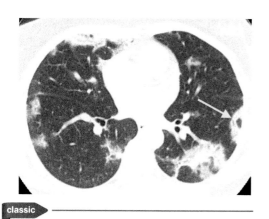

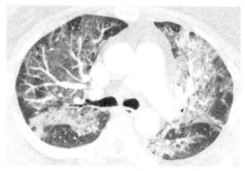

FIGURE 13.20 · Hypereosinophilic syndrome. Diffuse nonspecific ground glass opacity is present in a patient with 8 months of dyspnea. This finding may be seen in a variety of disorders, but in the setting of hypereosinophilic syndrome, it is due to either eosinophilic infiltration of the lung or pulmonary edema from cardiac disease.

classic

FIGURE 13.18 · Chronic eosinophilic pneumonia (CEP): Classic appearance. Patchy bilateral, predominantly peripheral consolidation is present. A ring of consolidation surrounding an area of central clearing (*arrow*), the "atoll sign," is compatible with organizing pneumonia and CEP.

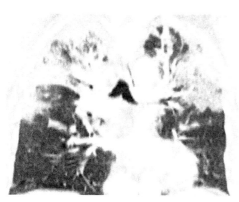

FIGURE 13.19 · Chronic eosinophilic pneumonia (CEP) with upper lobe distribution. Coronal CT shows extensive, peripherally predominant consolidation in a patient with chronic dyspnea. This is a typical appearance and distribution of CEP. Organizing pneumonia, which may closely resemble CEP, usually has a lower lobe predominance.

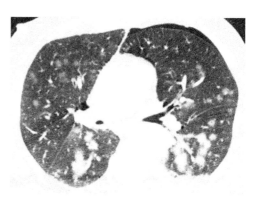

FIGURE 13.21 · Churg–Strauss syndrome. Centrilobular, lobular, and nodular areas of consolidation and ground glass opacity are present in a patient with a history of asthma. In a patient with suspected eosinophilic disease, the lobular nature of abnormalities may suggest Churg–Strauss syndrome.

nervous system, and skin. Other typical features include eosinophilia, greater than 10% of the white blood cell count, neuropathy, transient or migratory pulmonary opacities, sinus abnormalities, and increased tissue eosinophils.

Typical HRCT findings include nonsegmental consolidation or GGO often in a peripheral distribution, and resembling CEP. These abnormalities may have a lobular distribution (Fig. 13.21). This finding may help in distinguishing this disease from other eosinophilic lung diseases such as CEP. Other findings include centrilobular nodules, interlobular septal thickening, and bronchial wall thickening.

13

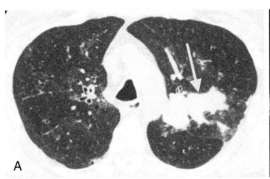 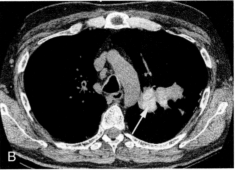

FIGURE 13.22 · **Allergic bronchopulmonary aspergillosis. A.** Focal bronchiectasis with mucoid impaction (*arrow*) is seen in the left upper lobe. **B.** The mucoid impaction (*arrow*) is of high attenuation. This is highly suggestive of allergic bronchopulmonary aspergillosis.

Eosinophilic Disorders with a Known Etiology

Allergic Bronchopulmonary Aspergillosis

ABPA is a disease predominantly seen in asthmatics or patients with cystic fibrosis (see Chapter 6). The diagnosis is usually clinical and based on peripheral eosinophilia, increased serum IgE levels, and reactivity to *Aspergillus fumigatus* on skin tests in a patient with symptoms unresponsive to traditional asthma treatments. This disease is characterized by a hypersensitivity reaction to *Aspergillus* that colonizes the airways. The *Aspergillus* does not invade the lung itself but induces inflammation within the airway lumen.

The minimum criteria for ABPA include the following:

1. Asthma
2. Immediate cutaneous reactivity to aspergillus
3. Total serum IgE >1000 ng/mL
4. Elevated specific IgE/IgA for aspergillus
5. Central bronchiectasis in the absence of distal bronchiectasis

The most characteristic HRCT finding of ABPA is bronchiectasis involving the central mid- or upper lungs. The lack of distal airways involvement in the effected regions is particularly suggestive of ABPA. The bronchiectasis is usually unilateral or asymmetric, as opposed to the symmetric diseases such as cystic fibrosis. The bronchiectasis may be cylindrical, varicose, or cystic (Fig. 13.22). Bronchial wall thickening and mucoid impaction are usually associated with the bronchial dilatation. The mucoid impaction may be high in attenuation because *Aspergillus* accumulates calcium and metal ions.

The combination of central bronchiectasis with high-density mucoid impaction is particularly suggestive of this diagnosis. There may be signs of small airways inflammation (centrilobular nodules, tree-in-bud opacities, and bronchiolectasis), but the large airways findings usually predominate.

Bronchocentric Granulomatosis

This is a rare disease characterized pathologically by necrotizing granulomatosis inflammation around bronchioles and small bronchi. It is commonly seen in asthmatics and is associated with *Aspergillus* organisms and thus shares similarities with ABPA. It may be seen in nonasthmatic patients and, in that case, is either idiopathic or associated with disorders such as immunosuppression or connective tissue disease. The HRCT findings have not been well documented. Described findings include masses, lobular consolidation, and airway impaction.

Drug Treatment

Drug reactions involving the lungs are described in greater detail in Chapter 15.

13

These reactions may be associated with one of several different patterns. Eosinophilic lung disease is a rare manifestation of a drug reaction; it may closely resemble any of the idiopathic eosinophilic disorders. Thus, before making the diagnosis of an idiopathic eosinophilic disorder, an examination of drug history is important. The most common drugs to present with this pattern include chemotherapeutic agents such as bleomycin, amiodarone, nitrofurantoin, phenytoin, and methotrexate.

Parasitic Infections

Parasitic infections are uncommon in the United States but are often seen in tropical and subtropical regions such as Africa, South America, and southern Asia. Lung abnormalities may be due to direct invasion by parasites or a secondary allergic reaction to infections elsewhere within the body. Peripheral eosinophilia is typically present.

The HRCT findings of parasitic infections are variable and depend on the offending organism, but the findings are usually nonspecific, and correlation with travel to endemic regions is most important for diagnosis. Nodules are common and often more than 1 cm in size, with irregular borders or adjacent GGO. These may be migratory and are most characteristic of *Ascaris lumbricoides*, *Clonorchis sinensis*, *Paragonimus westermani*, and schistosomiasis. Extensive infection with *Strongyloides stercoralis* may result in diffuse ground glass or consolidation as a manifestation of diffuse lung dissemination of the organism. Allergic reactions to the organisms or antigens released during their treatment can result in eosinophilic pneumonia or other reactions described above.

FURTHER READING

Adler BD, Padley SP, Müller NL, et al. Chronic hypersensitivity pneumonitis: high-resolution CT and radiographic features in 16 patients. *Radiology*. 1992;185:91-95.

Arakawa H, Webb WR. Air trapping on expiratory high-resolution CT scans in the absence of inspiratory scan abnormalities: correlation with pulmonary function tests and differential diagnosis. *AJR Am J Roentgenol*. 1998;170:1349-1353.

Bain GA, Flower CD. Pulmonary eosinophilia. *Eur J Radiol*. 1996;23:3-8.

Buschman DL, Waldron JA Jr, King TE Jr. Churg-Strauss pulmonary vasculitis. High-resolution computed tomography scanning and pathologic findings. *Am Rev Respir Dis*. 1990;142:458-461.

Cheon JE, Lee KS, Jung GS, et al. Acute eosinophilic pneumonia: radiographic and CT findings in six patients. *AJR Am J Roentgenol*. 1996;167:1195-1199.

Ebara H, Ikezoe J, Johkoh T, et al. Chronic eosinophilic pneumonia: evolution of chest radiograms and CT features. *J Comput Assist Tomogr*. 1994;18:737-744.

Glazer CS, Rose CS, Lynch DA. Clinical and radiologic manifestations of hypersensitivity pneumonitis. *J Thorac Imaging*. 2002;17:261-272.

Greenberger PA. Allergic bronchopulmonary aspergillosis. *J Allergy Clin Immunol*. Elsevier. 2002;110:685-692.

Hansell DM, Moskovic E. High-resolution computed tomography in extrinsic allergic alveolitis. *Clin Radiol*. 1991;43:8-12.

Hansell DM, Wells AU, Padley SP, Müller NL. Hypersensitivity pneumonitis: correlation of individual CT patterns with functional abnormalities. *Radiology*. 1996;199:123-128.

Hewitt MG, Miller WT Jr, Reilly TJ, Simpson S. The relative frequencies of causes of widespread ground-glass opacity: a retrospective cohort. *Eur J Radiol*. 2014;10:1970-1976.

Hirschmann JV, Pipavath SNJ, Godwin JD. Hypersensitivity pneumonitis: a historical, clinical, and radiologic review. *Radiographics*. 2009;29:1921-1938.

Jeong YJ, Kim KI, Seo IJ, et al. Eosinophilic lung diseases: a clinical, radiologic, and pathologic overview. *Radiographics*. 2007;27:617-639.

Kang EY, Shim JJ, Kim JS, Kim KI. Pulmonary involvement of idiopathic hypereosinophilic syndrome: CT findings in five patients. *J Comput Assist Tomogr*. 1997;21:612-615.

Kim Y, Lee KS, Choi DC, et al. The spectrum of eosinophilic lung disease: radiologic findings. *J Comput Assist Tomogr*. 1997;21:920-930.

King MA, Pope-Harman AL, Allen JN, et al. Acute eosinophilic pneumonia: radiologic and clinical features. *Radiology*. 1997;203:715-719.

Lynch DA, Newell JD, Logan PM, et al. Can CT distinguish hypersensitivity pneumonitis from idiopathic pulmonary fibrosis? *AJR Am J Roentgenol*. 1995;165:807-811.

Remy Jardin M, Remy J, Wallaert B, Müller NL. Subacute and chronic bird breeder hypersensitivity pneumonitis: sequential evaluation with CT and correlation with lung function tests and bronchoalveolar lavage. *Radiology*. 1993;198:111-118.

Rossi SE, Erasmus JJ, McAdams HP, et al. Pulmonary drug toxicity: radiologic and pathologic manifestations. *Radiographics*. 2000;20:1245-1259.

Silva CIS, Müller NL, Lynch DA, et al. Chronic hypersensitivity pneumonitis: differentiation from idiopathic pulmonary fibrosis and nonspecific interstitial pneumonia by using thin-section CT. *Radiology*. 2008;246:288-297.

Silver SF, Müller NL, Miller RR, Lefcoe MS. Hypersensitivity pneumonitis: evaluation with CT. *Radiology*. 1989;173:441-445.

Webb WR. Thin-section CT of the secondary pulmonary lobule: anatomy and the image—the 2004 Fleischner lecture. *Radiology.* 2006;239:322-338.

Winn RE, Kollef MH, Meyer JI. Pulmonary involvement in the hypereosinophilic syndrome. *Chest.* 1994;105:656-660.

Worthy SA, Müller NL, Hansell DM, Flower CD. Churg-Strauss syndrome: the spectrum of pulmonary CT findings in 17 patients. *AJR Am J Roentgenol.* 1998;170:297-300.

13

Pulmonary Infections

INTRODUCTION

Infection is a common cause of lung disease in both immunocompromised patients and those with a normal immune status. This chapter focuses on a general approach to suspected infection, the role of high-resolution computed tomography (IIRCT), and typical HRCT findings and provides a discussion of different patterns of infection based on the type of organism.

ROLE OF HRCT IN INFECTION

HRCT has several uses in patients with suspected infection. These include the detection of abnormalities, differentiating infections from noninfectious lung disease, determining the most likely organism or organisms to be involved, and the follow-up of treated infection.

Detection of Abnormalities

HRCT is highly sensitive in the detection of pulmonary infections. However, viral infections that only involve the upper respiratory tract may be difficult to recognize using CT. Detection of disease is particularly important in patients with immune deficiencies in which significant pulmonary infection may be present with minimal or absent symptoms or in the presence of a normal chest radiograph. A normal HRCT essentially rules out pulmonary infection from most organisms.

Differentiating Infectious versus Noninfectious Lung Disease

Understanding the common HRCT findings of infection, and their specificity, is important in the interpretation of HRCT. It is also important to be aware of noninfectious causes of lung abnormalities that may mimic infection. As infection is common, it is often assumed to be a cause of lung abnormalities in the acute setting, but this is not always the case. Abnormalities such as aspiration, pulmonary edema, diffuse alveolar damage, and pulmonary hemorrhage may present with symptoms similar to infection. Additionally, certain inflammatory, noninfectious diffuse lung diseases may present with acute symptoms such as hypersensitivity pneumonitis, organizing pneumonia, and acute eosinophilic pneumonia.

Determining the Most Likely Organism(s)

Once infection is determined to be a likely cause of lung abnormalities, the most likely offending organism(s) should be considered. This determination is fundamentally based on the recognition of specific HRCT findings. It is important to keep in mind that there may be significant overlap between HRCT patterns resulting from different infections or more than one organism may be responsible for abnormalities; a differential diagnosis is almost always required in interpreting HRCT in patients with suspected infection.

HRCT is most helpful in distinguishing infections caused by atypical organisms (i.e., viral organisms, atypical bacterial organisms such as *Chlamydia* and *Mycoplasma pneumoniae*, and *Pneumocystis jiroveci*) from those caused by more common organisms (typical bacteria, mycobacteria, and fungi).

Atypical organisms tend to present with diffuse, symmetric, or extensive bilateral abnormalities. Ground glass opacity is often a significant component of the HRCT findings. Other organisms usually present with unilateral or asymmetric and patchy abnormalities. Consolidation is often a significant finding with these organisms.

For example, a single focal region of consolidation in a patient with human immunodeficiency virus (HIV) infection or acquired immunodeficiency syndrome (AIDS) is more likely a common bacterial infection than *P. jiroveci* infection. This has important implications in terms of diagnostic evaluation and treatment.

Follow-up of Treated Infection

After treatment for infection has been initiated, follow-up is often obtained using clinical symptoms and chest radiographs. HRCT is an alternative when the clinical symptoms are ambiguous or when the chest radiographs do not demonstrate the disease clearly. It is important to note that a temporary worsening of the imaging findings may occur after the initiation of treatment. This often occurs in the first two weeks after the start of treatment and should not necessarily be interpreted as worsening of the infection. A paradoxical worsening of abnormalities on imaging may also occur during a period of time in which a patient regains immune function. Examples include a rebound of the white blood cell count in a previously neutropenic patient or the increase of lymphocytes in a patient with AIDS being treated with antiretroviral therapy. This phenomenon is called *immune reconstitution inflammatory syndrome*.

CLINICAL CONSIDERATIONS

Immune Status

Knowledge of the patient's immune status plays a major role in determining the most likely infectious cause of HRCT abnormalities.

Infections that occur in patients with normal immune status include bacteria (*Streptococcus*, *Chlamydia*, *Haemophilus*, and *Mycoplasma*), viruses (Influenza and Adenovirus), environmental fungi (coccidioidomycosis, histoplasmosis, blastomycosis),

and mycobacterial (tuberculous and nontuberculous) diseases.

Infections in immunocompromised patients vary depending on the type of immune suppression. For instance, patients with HIV infection are predisposed to infection by specific organisms, which are rarely seen in immunocompetent hosts, such as *Cryptococcus*, *P. jiroveci*, and Cytomegalovirus. Neutropenic hosts are predisposed to a different group of organisms including *Candida*, *Aspergillus*, fungal species causing mucormycosis, and *Escherichia coli*.

Bacterial infections are common regardless of a patient's immune status. Moreover, keep in mind that immunocompromised patients may be infected by more than one organism at a time, resulting in a mix of HRCT manifestations. An immunocompromised patient may also become superinfected with a second organism during treatment of the initial infection.

Geographic Considerations

Certain infections show significant geographic or regional variability based on environmental differences. For instance, coccidioidomycosis is a relatively common infection in the Southwest United States but is only rarely encountered in the Midwest and Eastern states. Histoplasmosis and blastomycosis have other geographic distributions. Parasitic infections are more commonly encountered in underdeveloped or tropical countries.

HRCT FINDINGS OF INFECTION

In a patient with acute symptoms, infection is almost always considered as a cause of HRCT abnormalities. In a patient with chronic symptoms, infection is less likely, although certain infections, such as atypical mycobacterial and fungal organisms, may have a chronic course, as do diseases with a predisposition to chronic infection, such as cystic fibrosis or immune deficiency. The HRCT findings present will determine the likelihood of infection as the etiology. The most common HRCT findings of infection and their differential diagnosis are shown in Table 14.1.

14

TABLE 14.1	Findings of infection and differential diagnosis	
HRCT finding or pattern	**Most common infections**	**Noninfectious causes**
Diffuse opacities (ground glass > consolidation)	• Viruses • Atypical bacteria • *Pneumocystis jiroveci* pneumonia (PJP)	• Pulmonary edema • Diffuse alveolar damage • Hemorrhage
Focal or asymmetric opacities (consolidation > ground glass)	• Bacteria • Mycobacteria • Fungi	• Aspiration • Invasive mucinous adenocarinoma
Centrilobular nodules (soft tissue attenuation)	• Bacteria • Mycobacterial • Fungal	• Aspiration • Vascular diseases (edema, hemorrhage) • Invasive mucinous adenocarcinoma

Centrilobular nodules (ground glass attenuation)	• Viruses
	• Atypical bacteria
	• PJP
		• Acute setting
		  • Pulmonary edema
		  • Hemorrhage
		  • Hypersensitivity pneumonitis
		• Chronic setting
		  • Hypersensitivity pneumonitis
		  • Respiratory bronchiolitis
		  • Follicular bronchiolitis
		  • Pulmonary hypertension

Tree-in-bud	• Any acute infection • Diseases that predispose to chronic infection (cystic fibrosis, immunodeficiency, etc.)	• Aspiration • Sarcoidosis • Invasive mucinous adenocarcinoma • Follicular bronchiolitis • Talcosis • Intravascular metastases • Panbronchiolitis
Large nodules and cavities	• Septic emboli • Bacterial lung abscess • Fungi • Mycobacteria • Nocardia and actinomyces	• Malignancy • Vasculitis • Tracheobronchial papillomatosis
Random pattern of small nodules	• Tuberculosis • Fungal infection (cocci, histo, blasto)	• Malignancy

Ground Glass Opacity and Consolidation

In patients with ground glass opacity or consolidation resulting from infection, the organism most likely responsible depends on the distribution of abnormalities. When diffuse or symmetric abnormalities are present, atypical organisms (i.e., virus, atypical bacterial organisms such as *Chlamydia*, *M. pneumoniae*, and *P. jiroveci*) are most likely (Fig. 14.1). Moreover, atypical organisms are most likely to present if ground glass opacity is the predominant abnormality. The ground glass opacities may have a lobular distribution.

When patchy, focal, or asymmetrical abnormalities are present, bacterial, fungal, and mycobacterial infections are the primary considerations. These most commonly present with consolidation as the predominant abnormality.

Ground glass opacity and consolidation are nonspecific findings and in the acute setting may be seen with infection, aspiration, pulmonary edema, diffuse alveolar damage, and hemorrhage.

Centrilobular Nodules of Soft Tissue Attenuation

In the acute setting, centrilobular nodules of soft tissue attenuation (Fig. 14.2) are likely due to infection. Endobronchial spread of bacterial, mycobacterial, or fungal organisms is the most

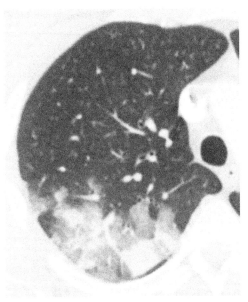

FIGURE 14.1 · **Ground glass opacity and consolidation.** Geographic ground glass opacity and consolidation are seen in a patient with adenoviral infection.

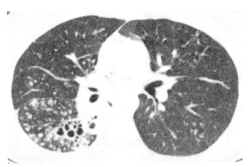

FIGURE 14.2 · **Centrilobular nodules of soft tissue attenuation in tuberculosis.** Soft tissue attenuation centrilobular nodules are seen in the right lower lobe. This centrilobular distribution is compatible with endobronchial spread of infection in this patient with reactivation tuberculosis. Note the cavitary lesions.

common cause. This appearance represents an early manifestation of bronchopneumonia.

Aspiration is also a consideration when findings are in dependent lung regions. Occasionally, vascular diseases, such as pulmonary edema or hemorrhage, may present with centrilobular nodules of soft tissue attenuation. A vascular etiology should be considered when the abnormalities are diffuse or bilateral and symmetric. In the chronic

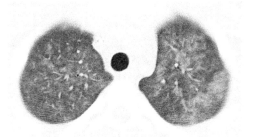

FIGURE 14.3 · **Centrilobular nodules of ground glass opacity (GGO) in cytomegalovirus infection.** Symmetric, evenly spaced GGO nodules are noted in a centrilobular distribution. Among infections, this appearance is most typical of atypical organisms. Possible noninfectious etiologies in the acute setting include pulmonary edema, diffuse alveolar damage, hemorrhage, and hypersensitivity pneumonitis.

setting, chronic or recurrent infection/aspiration and invasive mucinous adenocarcinoma are the most common causes of centrilobular nodules of soft tissue attenuation.

Centrilobular Nodules of Ground Glass Opacity

In a patient with acute symptoms, infection is one of several causes of centrilobular nodules of ground glass opacity (Fig. 14.3). It is most characteristic of infections that produce peribronchiolar inflammation without bronchiolar impaction, such as viral and atypical bacterial infections such as *Chlamydia* and *M. pneumoniae*.

The differential diagnosis includes vascular etiologies such as pulmonary edema and pulmonary hemorrhage, in addition to hypersensitivity pneumonitis. In the chronic setting, nodules of this type are unlikely to represent infection and are most typical of hypersensitivity pneumonitis, respiratory bronchiolitis, follicular bronchiolitis, and pulmonary hypertension.

Tree-in-Bud

Tree-in-bud (TIB) in a patient with acute symptoms (Fig. 14.4) is highly suggestive of infection. It is not specific with regard to the type of infection, but bacterial and mycobacterial infections are most likely. Fungal infections and viral infections are less likely to be associated with this abnormality. Aspiration without infection also occasionally produces TIB with acute symptoms.

14

In patients with chronic symptoms, TIB is also commonly due to infection. This may be due to chronic or recurrent acute infections. A

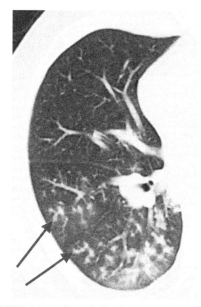

FIGURE 14.4 · Tree-in-bud. Branching tubular opacity with associated nodules (*arrows*) is seen in the peripheral regions of the right lower lobe in a patient with bacterial bronchopneumonia. The tree-in-bud sign is highly suggestive of infection, and the diagnosis can often be made by sputum analysis.

common cause of chronic infection with TIB is atypical mycobacteria. Bronchiectasis of any cause, cystic fibrosis, immunodeficiency, primary ciliary dyskinesia, allergic bronchopulmonary aspergillosis, and disorders of the bronchial cartilage may also lead to chronic infection with TIB, but these also show prominent involvement of the large airways.

Panbronchiolitis is predominantly a small airways disease that presents with chronic TIB; it is uncommon. In the appropriate clinical setting, noninfectious causes of TIB to be considered include sarcoidosis, invasive mucinous adenocarcinoma, follicular bronchiolitis, talcosis, and intravascular metastases.

Airway Wall Thickening and Impaction

Large airway infection, associated with bronchial wall thickening and sometimes luminal impaction (Fig. 14.5A, B), in a patient with suspected infection is often associated with other abnormalities, such as centrilobular nodules, consolidation, or TIB (see Chapter 6). It is occasionally seen as an isolated finding, in which case atypical organisms (viral, *Chlamydia*, *M. pneumoniae*) are the most likely etiologies.

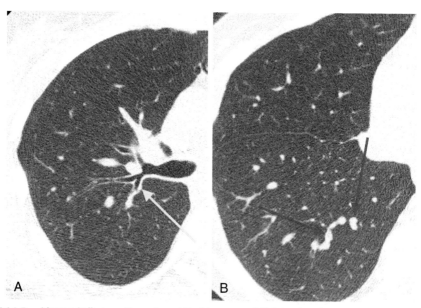

A   B

FIGURE 14.5 · Airway inflammation. A and **B.** Airway wall thickening (*arrow*, **A**) and impaction (*arrows*, **B**) may be the only signs of infection. In isolation, this is most typical of viral infection, such as in this patient with rhinovirus infection.

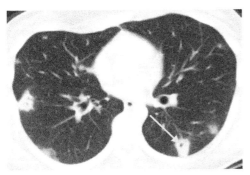

FIGURE 14.6 · **Large nodules and cavities.** Infection is the most common cause of large nodules and cavities (*arrow*). The most common infections to produce this pattern include septic emboli, bacterial abscesses, fungal infection, and mycobacterial infection. This patient was diagnosed with septic emboli from infective endocarditis.

Other common etiologies of isolated airway thickening and impaction include asthma and acute or chronic bronchitis. This finding should be distinguished from thickening of the peribronchovascular interstitium that may be seen with pulmonary edema and lymphangitic spread of tumor.

Large Nodules and Cavities

Large nodules (more than 1 cm in diameter) and cavities are commonly due to infection. The most likely infections to produce these patterns include septic embolism (Fig. 14.6), bacterial lung abscess, and fungal and mycobacterial infections. *Nocardia* and *Actinomyces* are rare infections that commonly present with large nodules and/or cavities. An air-fluid level within a cavitary nodule or mass suggests bacterial infection.

Noninfectious causes of large nodules and cavities include malignancy, vasculitis such as Wegener's granulomatosis, and rare disorders such as tracheobronchial papillomatosis. Clinical history is important in distinguishing infectious versus noninfectious causes of this pattern. The thickness of the cavity wall may also be helpful in making this distinction. A wall thickness less than 5 mm suggests a benign process, whereas a wall thickness greater than 15 mm suggests a malignancy (Fig. 14.7A, B). A wall thickness between 5 and 15 mm is

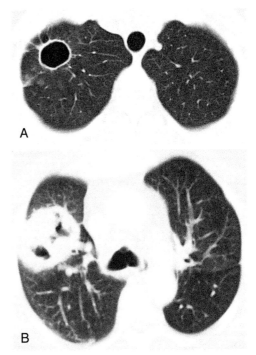

FIGURE 14.7 · **Cavities, thickness of wall.** The thickness of the wall of a cavity helps determine the likelihood of a benign or malignant etiology. A wall thickness <5 mm is likely due to a benign etiology **(A)** such as in this patient with a resolving coccidioidomycosis infection. A wall thickness >15 mm is likely due to a malignant etiology **(B)** such as in this patient with a primary lung squamous cell carcinoma.

not helpful in predicting the likelihood of a benign versus malignant process.

A Random Pattern of Small Nodules (Miliary Infection)

A random pattern of nodules is present when small nodules do not demonstrate a particular distribution with respect to the lung structures or the pulmonary lobule (see Chapter 3). They typically show a diffuse and homogeneous distribution with involvement of the subpleural interstitium. Overall, random nodules are diffuse and uniform in distribution. Random nodules are usually of soft tissue attenuation, sharply marginated, and easily visible when only a few millimeters in size.

The differential diagnosis of random nodules primarily includes miliary tuberculosis

14

TABLE 14.2	HRCT findings of lobar and bronchopneumonia

Lobar pneumonia	Bronchopneumonia
Consolidation, single lobe or multiple lobes, nonsegmental distribution	Consolidation, patchy, asymmetric, segmental distribution
Nodules usually absent	Centrilobular nodules, tree-in-bud
Air bronchograms in regions of consolidation	Airway wall thickening and impaction

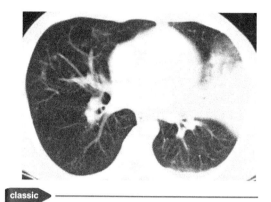

classic

FIGURE 14.8 · Lobar pneumonia: Classic appearance. HRCT shows consolidation in the lingula of a patient with *Streptococcus pneumoniae* infection. Note that the consolidation is limited by the major fissure. Only minimal abnormality is seen elsewhere. Nodules and tree-in-bud are not a feature of this pattern. This is typical of infections centered within the alveolar spaces.

(TB) or other mycobacteria, miliary fungal infection (e.g., histoplasmosis and coccidioidomycosis), and hematogenous spread of malignancy.

BACTERIAL INFECTIONS

Bacterial infections are common and, in general, should be considered the most likely infectious cause of many HRCT abnormalities. They may be hospital or community acquired. The most common hospital-acquired organisms include *Staphylococcus aureus*, *Pseudomonas aeruginosa*, *E. coli*, *Acinetobacter*, *Klebsiella*, and *Haemophilus influenzae*. The most common community-acquired organisms include *Streptococcus pneumoniae*, *H. influenzae*, *S. aureus*, and gram-negative organisms. Atypical bacterial infections such as *Chlamydia* and *M. pneumoniae* are also common bacterial infections acquired in the community but have unique imaging features. These will be discussed later in conjunction with viral organisms and *P. jiroveci*, as these infections all share many features.

Bacterial infections classically result in one of three patterns: lobar pneumonia, bronchopneumonia (Table 14.2), and atypical pneumonia (discussed later in this chapter). Note that there may be significant overlap between these patterns, particularly between bronchopneumonia and lobar pneumonia.

Lobar Pneumonia

In lobar pneumonia, the infection originates in, and is predominantly centered in, the alveolar spaces. Spread to adjacent alveoli occurs through the pores of Kohn, small interalveolar pores, and the canals of Lambert. Associated spread via the airways is typically absent. The infection is limited by fissures.

This pattern is most typical of *Streptococcus*, *H. influenzae*, *Klebsiella*, and *Moraxella catarrhalis*. The HRCT findings (Fig. 14.8) include the following:

1. Consolidation marginated by fissures
2. Prominent air bronchograms
3. Single lobe or multiple lobes affected, nonsegmental distribution

The differential diagnosis of lobar pneumonia includes mycobacterial and fungal infections, both of which can produce an isolated region of consolidation. An upper lobe distribution might suggest one of these, but this is not a constant feature.

Bronchopneumonia

The defining feature of this pattern is endobronchial spread of infection. The infection is centered within airways and is often associated with airway impaction. The process spreads outward from the centrilobular bronchiole, forming a centrilobular

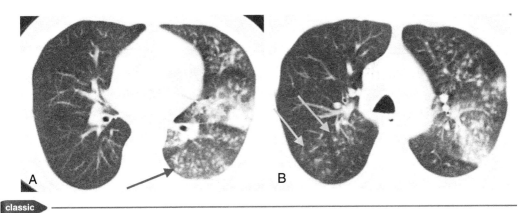

FIGURE 14.9 · **Bronchopneumonia: Classic appearance. A.** Bacterial infections that spread via the airways are characterized by patchy, asymmetric, ill-defined centrilobular nodules of varying sizes (*red arrow*) progressing to areas of confluent consolidation (*yellow arrow*). **B.** Note the segmental distribution of findings in the upper lobes (*arrows*).

nodule, and may continue to spread until the entire pulmonary lobule is involved. Adjacent involved lobules may coalesce to form confluent areas of consolidation. This pattern is typical of *S. aureus*, *P. aeruginosa*, *Klebsiella*, and *E. coli*. The HRCT findings (Fig. 14.9A, B) of this type of spread include the following:

1. Centrilobular nodules of soft tissue attenuation (various sizes, ill-defined borders)
2. TIB opacities
3. Airway wall thickening, impaction, and dilatation
4. Consolidation
5. Patchy, lobular, or segmental distribution

The differential diagnosis of a bronchopneumonia includes mycobacterial and fungal infections. Mycobacterial disease very commonly demonstrates endobronchial spread. In TB, there is often, but not always, a dominant focus of cavitary pneumonia in the upper lobes. Nontuberculous mycobacterial (NTMB) infection such as *Mycobacterium avium-intracellulare* (MAI) often demonstrates extensive inflammation of the airways with little associated consolidation. Except in immunosuppressed patients, fungal diseases do not commonly produce this pattern. Airway-invasive aspergillosis is an example of this type of infection.

Septic Embolism

Septic embolism (embolization of infected clot) most commonly occurs in patients with infective endocarditis; however, other sources, such as catheter induced thrombus, are also possible. Septic emboli involving pulmonary arteries produce infected infarcts. Typical HRCT features include multiple bilateral nodules and masses with cavitation. A vessel may be seen leading up to these nodules or masses; the *feeding vessel sign*. As opposed to bland infarcts, the masses and nodules associated with septic emboli are not necessarily peripheral and wedge-shaped.

RARE BACTERIAL INFECTIONS

Actinomyces Infection

Actinomyces is a normal part of oral flora that, when aspirated, may produce a pneumonia. Predisposing factors for developing infection include alcoholism, poor dental hygiene, and preexisting lung disease such as emphysema or bronchiectasis. On HRCT, Actinomyces usually presents with nodule(s), mass(es), or consolidation. A nodule may be the earliest manifestation. Often only one or a few nodules are present, and widespread nodular disease is not typical. Nodules may have a peripheral rim of ground glass opacity. Over time, the

14

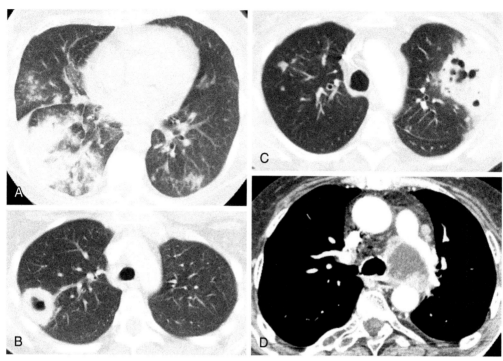

FIGURE 14.10 · **Nocardia pneumonia. A.** Focal consolidation in the right lower lobe is associated with centrilobular nodules. This is most suggestive of typical bacterial bronchopneumonia, but this patient was eventually diagnosed with nocardia. **B.** A solitary cavitary mass is present in the right upper lobe. This is one possible manifestation of nocardia but is more commonly seen in bacterial, fungal, and mycobacterial infections. **C.** Focal left upper lobe consolidation with cavitation is present. The most common etiologies of this abnormality are mycobacterial or fungal infection, but nocardia may present with this finding. **D.** Necrotic mediastinal lymphadenopathy is present in the aortopulmonary window. This was associated with cavitary consolidation in the left lower lobe (not shown).

14

nodule(s) increase in size to produce a mass or focal region of consolidation. The consolidation frequently cavitates, producing low-density, nonenhancing regions. Pleural and chest wall involvement may be seen in advanced infections.

Nocardia Infection

Nocardia is present in soil. Nocardia infection is typically seen in the setting of immunocompromise, such as HIV infection, organ transplantation, leukemia, lymphoma, and chronic immunosuppressive medication. The radiographic features are similar to Actinomyces infection and include nodule(s), mass(es) (Fig. 14.10A–D), and consolidation. These may be associated with lymphadenopathy.

MYCOBACTERIAL INFECTIONS

Mycobacterial infection is usually classified as tuberculous (i.e., TB) and nontuberculous or atypical mycobacterial infection. Although there is overlap in their presentation and HRCT appearances, they often can be differentiated.

Tuberculosis

TB is a common disease worldwide, but its prevalence in the United States and other developed nations is significantly lower than that in Third World countries. Within the United States, there is a higher incidence of TB in patients with HIV infection and other immunocompromised patients than in the general population. It is a major public health

TABLE 14.3	HRCT findings of tuberculosis	
Primary	**Reactivation**	**Miliary**
Consolidation, upper or lower lung	Consolidation, upper lobes or superior segment of lower lobes	Well-defined nodules
Lymphadenopathy	Cavities	Nodules usually <3 mm
Nonspecific nodule	Centrilobular nodules and/or tree-in-bud opacities	Diffuse, homogeneous
Consolidation + lymphadenopathy most suggestive	Pleural effusions/thickening	Random distribution on HRCT

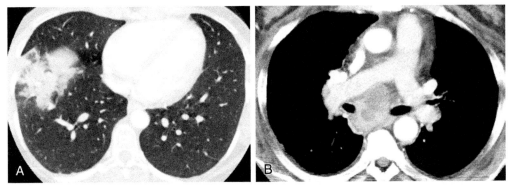

FIGURE 14.11 · **Primary tuberculosis in two different patients. A.** A nonspecific area of consolidation is seen in the anterior segment of the right lower lobe. This appearance is most commonly a manifestation of community-acquired bacterial pneumonia. This patient was diagnosed with tuberculosis via sputum analysis. **B.** Necrotic lymphadenopathy is visible in the subcarinal space. This finding, in isolation, may also be a manifestation of primary tuberculosis. This patient was diagnosed at bronchoscopy using Wang needle biopsy.

problem, and thus rapid diagnosis and treatment is important.

Imaging plays an important role in the detection of TB and its differentiation from other diseases. There are several different patterns of infection with TB (Table 14.3), although overlap between the patterns may occur. TB cannot be excluded based solely on imaging, but the majority of TB cases produce imaging abnormalities that correspond to one of three patterns including: primary, reactivation, and military TB.

Primary TB

The infection associated with an initial exposure to TB usually elicits an inflammatory response that sequesters the bacilli and prevents further progression of disease. In many patients, this does not result in a recognizable abnormality on radiographs or computed tomography (CT).

If an abnormality is visible on CT, the most common abnormality is a solitary nodule, representing a granulomatous reaction to the initial focus of infection (Fig. 14.11A, B). Draining lymph node enlargement may or may not be present; enlarged lymph nodes are commonly low in attenuation. Both the nodule and the abnormal lymph nodes may eventually calcify.

Primary TB may also have a more aggressive course, progressing to a symptomatic infection; this is most typical in children and immunocompromised patients. This tends to appear on CT as a nonspecific lung consolidation, which may be lobar or patchy, a pulmonary nodule, and/or lymphadenopathy. The combination of

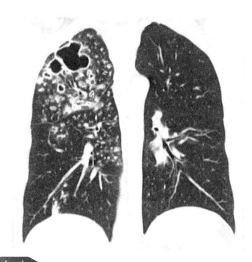

`classic`

FIGURE 14.12 · Reactivation tuberculosis: Classic appearance. Coronal reformatted image shows right-sided upper lobe cavities in association with clustered soft tissue attenuation centrilobular nodules and tree-in-bud opacities.

lung consolidation and lymphadenopathy is most suggestive, as significant lymphadenopathy is unusual with community-acquired bacterial infection.

Postprimary (Reactivation or Secondary) TB

At some point after the initial infection, TB may reactivate, resulting in progressive local disease or dissemination. When this occurs, the infection predominates in regions of the body with a high oxygen tension. The highest oxygen tension within the lungs is in the upper lobes because of a relatively high ventilation to perfusion ratio. As TB thrives in a high oxygen environment, the infection is more likely to recur in this region. If it does, it induces a very pronounced inflammatory reaction characterized by necrosis, scarring, and pleural reaction. The typical HRCT findings of reactivation TB include the following:

1. Consolidation in typical locations (apical and posterior upper lobes and superior segments of lower lobes) (Fig. 14.12)
2. Cavities
3. Endobronchial spread (centrilobular nodules of soft tissue attenuation and TIB)

4. Lung scarring (even relatively early in the course of infection)
5. Pleural effusions and/or thickening

Reactivation TB often results in significant apical fibrosis as a sequela of the active infection. This fibrosis is typically bilateral but asymmetric. The degree of fibrosis caused by TB is usually more severe than that of a bacterial infection.

Other causes of upper lobe cavitary consolidation include fungal infections (particularly coccidioidomycosis and histoplasmosis) and bacterial infections.

Miliary TB

When hematogenous spread of TB is not limited by an immune response, extensive dissemination of organisms may occur, with diffuse lung involvement. This may occur with primary or secondary infection.

On HRCT, miliary TB results in multiple small nodules having a random distribution (Fig. 14.13). Nodules are diffuse and have a uniform distribution in the axial plane. Subpleural nodules are present. The nodules tend to be 1 to 2 mm in size, but without treatment they may grow larger. In some patients, an apical or basal predominance may be seen. The differential of miliary TB includes hematogenous spread of fungal disease (coccidioidomycosis, histoplasmosis, and blastomycosis) or metastatic disease.

Nontuberculous (Atypical) Mycobacteria

The various organisms included in the category of NTMB produce similar abnormalities on HRCT. Of these, MAI, also known as *Mycobacterium avium-intracellulare* complex (MAC), is the most common. MAC infection often presents with chronic symptoms, and its severity may wax and wane over time, as opposed to other infections that are usually acute in presentation and resolve once treated. There are several patterns of disease that may affect either immunocompetent or immunocompromised individuals.

The most common HRCT pattern seen with NTMB (Fig. 14.14) occurs in patients with normal immune status, most frequently elderly women (older than 60 years). The predominant feature is airways disease that predominates in the middle lobe and lingula. Bronchiectasis, airway wall thickening, and mucous impaction

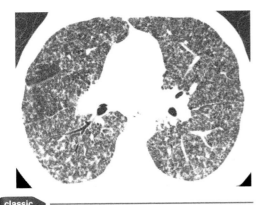

FIGURE 14.13 · **Miliary tuberculosis: Classic appearance.** Diffuse very small discrete nodules are present. They appear evenly distributed. Pleural surfaces, including the fissures, are involved. This indicates a random distribution. The differential diagnosis includes miliary tuberculosis, miliary fungal infection, and hematogenous spread of malignancy.

are typically present. Centrilobular nodules and TIB opacities are also frequently seen. There may be partial or complete collapse of the middle lobe and lingula in severe cases. In most cases, there is a relative paucity of consolidation present. This combination of HRCT abnormalities in an older woman is highly predictive of MAI (MAC) infection. The differential diagnosis includes recurrent bacterial infections or aspiration.

A second manifestation of NTMB occurs in immunocompromised patients, often elderly men. This tends to resemble TB with upper lung consolidation, cavitation, and endobronchial spread of infection.

Uncommon manifestations of NTMB include nonspecific lung consolidation resembling bacterial infection and nodules or masses (Fig. 14.15) resembling fungal infection. These nodules or masses are not infrequently detected as an incidental radiologic abnormality in asymptomatic patients. Extrapulmonary NTMB is most frequently seen in immunocompromised patients, particularly those with AIDS. Enhancing, necrotic lymphadenopathy is typical of extrapulmonary NTMB (Fig. 14.16).

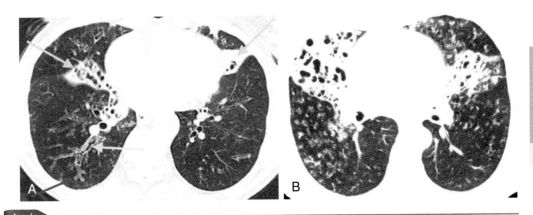

FIGURE 14.14 · **Nontuberculous mycobacterial (*Mycobacterium avium-intracellulare* complex, MAC) infection in two patients: Classic appearance. A.** Extensive airways inflammation with wall thickening is present in this patient with Mycobacterium avium-intracellulare infection. Varicose bronchiectasis (*yellow arrow*), bronchiolar wall thickening (*red arrow*), and near-complete collapse of the middle lobe and lingula (*blue arrows*) are strongly suggestive of an atypical mycobacterial infection. **B.** In a 67-year-old woman with cough, there is severe bronchiectasis involving the middle lobe and lingual, and numerous centrilobular nodules and examples of tree-in-bud are visible. In a woman of this age, this appearance is a strong evidence that MAC infection is present.

FUNGAL INFECTION

Fungal infection has a wide variety of different manifestations, and findings show a significant overlap with those associated with bacterial and mycobacterial infections. Different fungal organisms tend to affect immunocompetent versus immunocompromised patients.

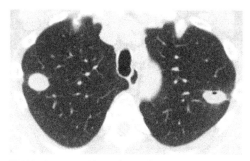

FIGURE 14.15 · **Nontuberculous mycobacterial infection.** Discrete, isolated nodules are present bilaterally. A small area of cavitation is seen in the left-sided nodule. This pattern is most commonly seen with fungal infection or septic emboli; however, atypical mycobacterial infection can occasionally have this appearance.

HRCT Findings

Several patterns may be present with fungal infection (Table 14.4).

Upper Lobe Cavitary Consolidation

Cavitary upper lobe consolidation may resemble reactivation TB (Fig. 14.17). It is most typical of coccidioidomycosis, histoplasmosis, blastomycosis, and chronic aspergillosis. The mechanism of spread to the upper lungs is very similar to TB. Typical findings include consolidation affecting the upper lobes or superior segments of the lower lobes with cavitation and sometimes endobronchial spread. Pleural effusion and/or pleural thickening may also be present. These abnormalities may eventually lead to significant upper lung fibrosis and volume loss.

Solitary Pulmonary Nodule and/or Lymphadenopathy

This manifestation of fungal infection resembles primary TB but is significantly more common with fungal disease. The most common fungi to produce this pattern include coccidioidomycosis, histoplasmosis,

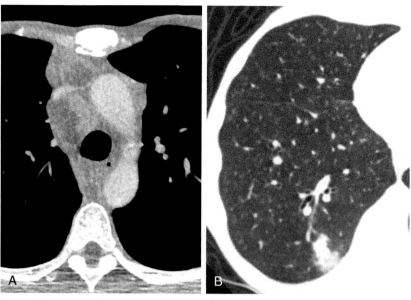

FIGURE 14.16 · **Nontuberculous mycobacterial infection.** Necrotic mediastinal lymphadenopathy **(A)** is seen as the primary manifestation of extrapulmonary nontuberculous mycobacterial infection in a patient with acquired immunodeficiency syndrome. The lungs were clear except for a small region of consolidation **(B)**.

blastomycosis, and cryptococcosis. An isolated pulmonary nodule (Fig. 14.18A–C) is the most common manifestation. Hilar and mediastinal lymphadenopathy may be seen in association with the nodule or as an isolated abnormality. The nodule typically cavitates and often develops a thin wall over time. These patients are often asymptomatic, so the primary differential diagnosis in these cases is malignancy.

Bronchopneumonia or Lobar Pneumonia

Bronchopneumonia associated with fungal disease may be indistinguishable from a typical bacterial infection (Fig. 14.19A,

B). Patchy unilateral or bilateral, asymmetric segmental consolidation with centrilobular nodules and airway inflammation may resemble bacterial bronchopneumonia. A nonsegmental region of consolidation involving a single lobe may resemble a bacterial lobar pneumonia. This is not a common manifestation of fungal infection and is usually seen with primary infections.

TABLE 14.4	HRCT manifestations of fungal infection

Upper lobe cavitary consolidation
Solitary pulmonary nodule
Lymphadenopathy
Bronchopneumonia or lobar pneumonia
Nodular or mass-like consolidation
Random distribution of small nodules

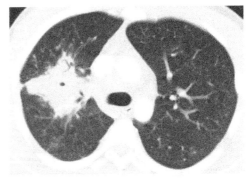

FIGURE 14.17 · **Coccidioidomycosis.** Right upper lobe cavitary consolidation is present with scattered nodules at the periphery of the large mass. Fungal and mycobacterial infections may show significant overlap in the HRCT findings.

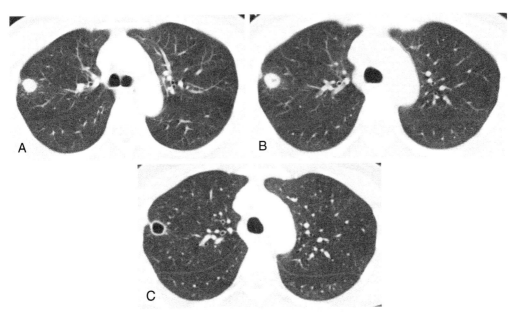

FIGURE 14.18 · **Coccidioidomycosis. A.** An isolated, soft tissue attenuation pulmonary nodule is seen in the right upper lobe in an asymptomatic patient. This finding is nonspecific, but when it represents infection, either fungal or mycobacterial infections are most likely. **B** and **C.** Over time, this nodule cavitates **(B)** and eventually develops a thin wall **(C)**.

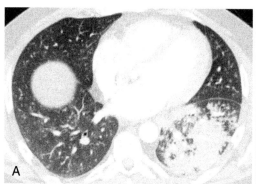
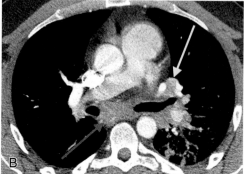

FIGURE 14.19 · **Coccidioidomycosis. A** and **B.** Focal consolidation is seen in the left lower lobe (**A**). While this finding is nonspecific with regard to the type of infection, there is extensive associated lymphadenopathy (**B**) in the left hilum (*yellow arrow*, **B**) and mediastinum (*red arrow*, **B**). Lymphadenopathy is unusual in uncomplicated bacterial infection and suggests fungal or mycobacterial organisms as an etiology.

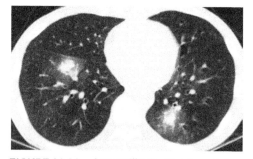

FIGURE 14.20 · **Aspergillosis.** Focal, nodular areas of consolidation are seen with adjacent ground glass opacity (i.e., the halo sign is present) in a neutropenic patient. In this clinical setting, fungal infection such as angioinvasive aspergillosis is the most likely etiology.

As with bacterial infections, an overlap of bronchopneumonia and lobar pneumonia may be present.

Nodular or Mass-Like Areas of Consolidation

Multiple, bilateral, nodular or mass-like regions of consolidation (Fig. 14.20) are a common manifestation of fungal infection in immunocompromised patients. This pattern is characteristic of aspergillus, mucormycosis, *Candida*, and *Cryptococcus* infections. The abnormalities tend to be scattered bilaterally with large (>1 cm) focal regions of rounded consolidation with ill-defined margins. The lung in between the nodules is relatively

unaffected, and endobronchial spread is not a typical manifestation of disease. A halo of ground glass opacity may be seen surrounding nodules, the so-called *halo sign*. In an immunosuppressed patient with neutropenia, the halo sign suggests angioinvasive aspergillosis infection, but otherwise the halo sign is not specific for any one organism. The atoll sign, or reversed halo sign, may also be seen. In the setting of neutropenia this finding is highly suggestive of an angioinvasive fungal infection, particularly mucormycosis (Fig. 14.21).

In immunocompromised patients, the differential diagnosis includes organizing pneumonia (e.g., from drug reaction or graft vs. host disease), lymphoproliferative disease, and infarcts from pulmonary emboli. Other etiologies that may resemble this pattern include invasive mucinous adenocarcinoma, eosinophilic pneumonia, and sarcoidosis; however, the clinical presentation of these diseases is quite different.

Random Distribution of Small Pulmonary Nodules

A pattern of small nodules with a random distribution may be present with fungal infection. This closely resembles miliary TB. Random nodules may be seen in association with the other patterns described above and represents diffuse hematogenous spread of infection to the lungs. This pattern is not only

14

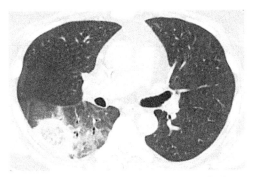

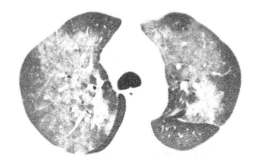

FIGURE 14.21 · **Mucormycosis.** A rounded area of consolidation with central ground glass opacity is seen in the right lower lobe in a neutropenic patient. The atoll or reversed halo sign in this clinical setting is most suggestive of angioinvasive fungal infection, specifically mucormycosis.

FIGURE 14.22 · **Atypical pneumonia.** Extensive bilateral ground glass opacity and consolidation are present. The bilateral distribution and presence of ground glass favor atypical pneumonias such as viral, atypical bacterial, and *Pneumocystis jiroveci*. This patient was diagnosed with adenovirus infection.

TABLE 14.5	Features of atypical infections
Organisms	Viral infections
	Atypical bacterial organisms
	(*Mycoplasma pneumoniae,*
	Chlamydia pneumoniae,
	Legionella pneumophila)
	Pneumocystis jiroveci
HRCT findings	Airway wall thickening
	Mild bronchial dilatation
	Centrilobular nodules
	Mosaic/perfusion air trapping
	Symmetric or diffuse ground
	glass opacity and consolidation

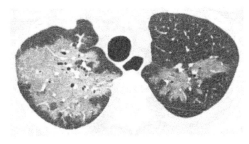

`classic`

FIGURE 14.23 · **Atypical pneumonia: Classic appearance.** Extensive bilateral ground glass opacity is present in a patient with cytomegalovirus pneumonia. The bilateral distribution and presence of ground glass as a significant abnormality makes atypical infections the most likely infectious etiology.

most typical of coccidioidomycosis, histoplasmosis, and blastomycosis but can also be seen with candidiasis.

ATYPICAL INFECTIONS

Included in this category are atypical bacterial infections, viral infections, and infection with *P. jiroveci* (Table 14.5). The most common atypical bacterial organisms within this category include *M. pneumoniae, Chlamydia pneumoniae*, and *Legionella pneumophila*.

Atypical infections share clinical and radiographic features that distinguish them from typical bacterial infections such as *Streptococcus*, TB, and fungal infections. Symptoms attributable to the respiratory system tend to be milder than those in patients

with other infections. Extrapulmonary symptoms are more frequent and severe, and leukocytosis is often absent. Moreover, these organisms are often not responsive to antibiotics given to treat typical bacterial organisms.

Atypical infections may be associated with patchy, diffuse, or centrilobular ground glass opacity (Figs. 14.22 and 14.23). This appearance is most typical of viral infections and *Pneumocystis*. The presence of ground glass opacity and air-filled cysts (pneumatoceles) in an immunosuppressed patient suggests *Pneumocystis*.

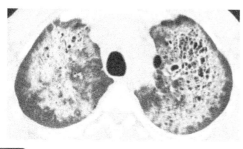

**FIGURE 14.24 · *Pneumocystis jiroveci*
pneumonia in a patient with HIV: Classic
appearance.** Symmetric ground glass opacity
and consolidation are seen in association with
cysts (i.e., pneumatoceles). Pneumatoceles
are most commonly seen with *Pneumocystis
jiroveci*, viral, and bacterial infections.
The distribution and history of human
immunodeficiency virus infection favor
Pneumocystis jiroveci infection.

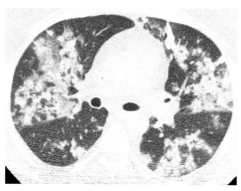

FIGURE 14.25 · Varicella pneumonia.
Extensive bilateral soft tissue attenuation
nodules and consolidation are present. The
nodules have a centrilobular distribution.
Soft tissue attenuation nodules may be seen
with any type of infection, but the bilateral
distribution in this case favors an atypical
infection.

Cysts are more likely of *P. jiroveci* infection
than other atypical infections (Fig. 14.24).

Atypical infections also may have findings similar to bronchopneumonia (Fig.
14.25). Initially, these produce inflammation of airway walls and the peribronchiolar
interstitium with limited airway impaction.
As the infection progresses, areas of bronchiolar impaction, centrilobular nodules, and
peribronchiolar consolidation may develop.

Early, the centrilobular nodules are often of
ground glass opacity, but they may evolve
and be of soft tissue attenuation. More extensive areas of ground glass opacity and consolidation may appear. Pathologically, these
represent areas of diffuse alveolar damage.
Associated mosaic perfusion and/or air trapping reflects narrowing of small airways by
inflammation. Typical HRCT findings in
patients with this pattern of infection include
the following:

1. Airway wall thickening with or without
   dilatation
2. Centrilobular nodules (ground glass opacity, early; soft tissue attenuation, late)
3. Mosaic perfusion and/or air trapping
4. Symmetric or diffuse ground glass opacity
   and consolidation

In patients with an infection, HRCT
is most accurate in distinguishing atypical
infections from other types. Atypical infections often present with abnormalities that
are bilateral and extensive in distribution.
Ground glass opacity is more commonly
seen with atypical infections as compared
with bacterial, mycobacterial, and fungal
infections.

Viral and atypical bacterial infections
also may be associated with airway thickening, impaction, centrilobular nodules (Fig.
14.25), and TIB opacities. These abnormalities also tend to be symmetric in distribution.
Mosaic perfusion and/or air trapping may
also be present, underlying the airway-centric
nature of this process. Airways inflammation
is not typical of *P. jiroveci* infection.

FURTHER READING

Brecher CW, Aviram G, Boiselle PM. CT and radiography
of bacterial respiratory infections in AIDS patients.
AJR Am J Roentgenol. 2003;180:1203-1209.
Cattamanchi A, Nahid P, Marras TK, et al. Detailed analysis of the radiographic presentation of *Mycobacterium
kansasii* lung disease in patients with HIV infection.
Chest. 2008;133:875-880.
Elicker BM, Schwartz BS, Liu C, et al. Thoracic CT
findings of novel influenza A (H1N1) infection
in immunocompromised patients. *Emerg Radiol.*
2010;17:299-307.

14

Erasmus JJ, McAdams HP, Farrell MA, Patz EF Jr. Pulmonary nontuberculous mycobacterial infection: radiologic manifestations. *Radiographics*. 1999;19:1487-1505.

Franquet T, Müller NL, Gimenez A, et al. Spectrum of pulmonary aspergillosis: histologic, clinical, and radiologic findings. *Radiographics*. 2001;21:825-837.

Gotway MB, Dawn SK, Caoili EM, et al. The radiologic spectrum of pulmonary *Aspergillus* infections. *J Comput Assist Tomogr*. 2002;26:159-173.

Gruden JF, Huang L, Turner J, et al. High-resolution CT in the evaluation of clinically suspected *Pneumocystis carinii* pneumonia in AIDS patients with normal, equivocal, or nonspecific radiographic findings. *AJR Am J Roentgenol*. 1997;169:967-975.

Im JG, Itoh H, Shim YS, et al. Pulmonary tuberculosis: CT findings—early active disease and sequential change with antituberculous therapy. *Radiology*. 1993;186:653-660.

Kim EA, Lee KS, Primack SL, et al. Viral pneumonias in adults: radiologic and pathologic findings. *Radiographics*. 2002;22:S137-S149.

Lee KS, Song KS, Lim TH, Kim PN, Kim IY, Lee BH. Adult-onset pulmonary tuberculosis: findings on chest radiographs and CT scans. *AJR Am J Roentgenol*. 1993;160:753-758.

Leung AN. Pulmonary tuberculosis: the essentials. *Radiology*. 1999;210:307-322.

Leung AN, Brauner MW, Gamsu G, et al. Pulmonary tuberculosis: comparison of CT findings in HIV seropositive and HIV seronegative patients. *Radiology*. 1996;198:687-691.

Lieberman D, Porath A, Schlaeffer F, Boldur I. *Legionella* species community-acquired pneumonia. A review of 56 hospitalized adult patients. *Chest*. 1996;109:1243-1249.

Lynch DA, Simone PM, Fox MA, Bucher BL, Heinig MJ. CT features of pulmonary Mycobacterium avium complex infection. *J Comput Assist Tomogr*. 1995;19:353-360.

McAdams HP, Rosado de Christenson ML, Lesar M, Templeton PA, Moran CA. Thoracic mycoses from endemic fungi: radiologic-pathologic correlation. *Radiographics*. 1995;15:255-270.

McAdams HP, Rosado de Christenson ML, Templeton PA, et al. Thoracic mycoses from opportunistic fungi: radiologic-pathologic correlation. *Radiographics*. 1995;15:271-286.

Primack SL, Logan PM, Hartman TE, Lee KS, Müller NL. Pulmonary tuberculosis and Mycobacterium avium-intracellulare: a comparison of CT findings. *Radiology*. 1995;194:413-417.

Reittner P, Muller NL, Heyneman L, et al. Mycoplasma pneumoniae pneumonia: radiographic and high-resolution CT features in 28 patients. *AJR Am J Roentgenol*. 2000;174:37-41.

Saurborn DP, Fishman JE, Boiselle PM. The imaging spectrum of pulmonary tuberculosis in AIDS. *J Thorac Imaging*. 2002;17:28-33.

14

15

Complications of Medical Treatment: Drug-Induced Lung Disease and Radiation

DRUG-INDUCED LUNG DISEASE

Drug-induced lung disease is often overlooked or misdiagnosed. The most common categories of drugs that result in lung disease include chemotherapeutic agents, cardiac medications, and antibiotics.

Drug-induced diffuse lung disease may be associated with a number of possible appearances on high-resolution computed tomography (HRCT) (Table 15.1). These appearances reflect the typical manifestations of different patterns of lung injury reviewed in other parts of this book and include many of the interstitial pneumonias reviewed in Chapter 9.

The most common patterns of lung injury associated with drug toxicity include pulmonary edema and pulmonary hemorrhage, diffuse alveolar damage (DAD), organizing pneumonia (OP), nonspecific interstitial pneumonia (NSIP), usual interstitial pneumonia (UIP), and eosinophilic pneumonia. Less common patterns of drug toxicity include hypersensitivity pneumonitis (HP), a sarcoid-like reaction, constrictive bronchiolitis, pulmonary vasculitis and pulmonary hypertension, desquamative interstitial pneumonia, and lymphoid interstitial pneumonia.

There are no HRCT findings that specifically suggest drug toxicity. Drug reactions must be considered in the differential diagnosis of the various patterns described above. A high degree of suspicion and correlation with medication history is necessary to make a confident diagnosis. The patterns of lung disease related to drugs are reviewed below.

The website http://www.pneumotox.com provides a comprehensive database for determining the types of drug reactions associated with a specific drug or the drugs capable of producing a specific toxic reaction. It is highly recommended as a reference if pulmonary drug toxicity is suspected based on computed tomography (CT) findings and/or clinical history. It is important to note that each drug listed is generally associated with a wide variety of different patterns. Some of these associations are well documented in the literature whereas others are based solely on a single case report. The strength of this association needs to be considered when deciding if a drug is the most likely etiology of lung disease. The timing of the exposure in relation to the onset of symptoms and radiographic abnormalities is also an important consideration. The clinical manifestations of drug-induced lung disease most commonly begin within weeks or months after the start of drug treatment; however, the onset of symptoms may range from minutes to years after the initiation of treatment. Preexisting lung disease places patients at higher risk for drug-induced lung disease; thus, the presence of diffuse lung disease (often mild and subclinical) before the start of an offending drug is not uncommon.

Pulmonary Edema

Hydrostatic pulmonary edema may result from drugs that affect the heart or systemic vasculature. An example is cocaine. HRCT findings are typical of any cause of hydrostatic edema (Fig. 15.1). Pleural effusion may be present.

TABLE 15.1	Patterns of drug-induced lung disease and the most common offending agents
Pattern	**Drugs**
Pulmonary edema	Aspirin, nitrofurantoin, heroin, methotrexate, cyclophosphamide, carmustine, interleukin-2
Pulmonary hemorrhage	Anticoagulants, cyclophosphamide, penicillamine
Diffuse alveolar damage	Carmustine, busulfan, cyclophosphamide, bleomycin, amiodarone, methotrexate, aspirin, narcotics, cocaine
Organizing pneumonia	Carmustine, bleomycin, doxorubicin, cyclophosphamide, amiodarone, nitrofurantoin, cephalosporins, tetracycline, amphotericin B, gold salts, phenytoin, sulfasalazine, cocaine
Nonspecific interstitial pneumonia	Bleomycin, busulfan, cyclophosphamide, methotrexate, amiodarone, nitrofurantoin, hydrochlorothiazide, statins, phenytoin, gold
Usual interstitial pneumonia	Cyclophosphamide, chlorambucil, nitrofurantoin, pindolol
Eosinophilic pneumonia	Bleomycin, amiodarone, nitrofurantoin, antidepressants, beta-blockers, hydrochlorothiazide, nonsteroidal anti-inflammatory drugs, phenytoin, sulfasalazine, cocaine
Hypersensitivity pneumonitis	Methotrexate, cyclophosphamide, mesalamine, fluoxetine, amitriptyline, paclitaxel
Sarcoid-like reaction	Interferon
Vasculitis and pulmonary hypertension	Fenfluramine, busulfan, methylphenidate, and methadone
Constrictive bronchiolitis	Penicillamine and sulfasalazine

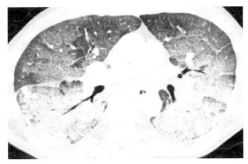

FIGURE 15.1 · Pulmonary edema with cocaine use. Diffuse ground glass opacity and smooth interlobular septal thickening is present, representing the *crazy paving* pattern. This patient had an acute onset of pulmonary edema after the inhalational use of cocaine.

Increased permeability pulmonary edema also may occur with drug treatment. Onset is usually sudden. HRCT findings are typical of pulmonary edema, including interlobular septal thickening, ground glass opacity, and, to a lesser extent, consolidation. This occurrence is typical of interleukin-2, but many other drugs are capable of causing increased permeability pulmonary edema. These include aspirin, nitrofurantoin, heroin, and cytotoxic agents such as methotrexate,

cyclophosphamide, and carmustine. Unlike hydrostatic edema, pleural effusion is typically absent. Prompt resolution may occur with appropriate treatment.

Pulmonary Hemorrhage

Drug-related diffuse pulmonary hemorrhage is uncommon. Typical causes include anticoagulants, cyclophosphamide, and penicillamine. Hemoptysis may or may not be present. HRCT findings are typical of pulmonary hemorrhage with bilateral patchy ground glass opacity or consolidation. Pleural effusion is typically absent.

Diffuse Alveolar Damage

DAD, the histologic pattern associated with acute lung injury (ALI) and, in severe cases, acute respiratory distress syndrome (ARDS), is a common manifestation of drug toxicity. DAD is characterized by edema, intra-alveolar hyaline membranes, and acute interstitial inflammation, eventually followed in some cases by fibroblast proliferation and progressive fibrosis with collagen deposition.

Not all patients with DAD meet the clinical criteria for ARDS (see Chapter 8); this is particularly true in the setting of drug toxicity.

15

The most common drugs associated with this pattern include carmustine, busulfan, cyclophosphamide, bleomycin, amiodarone, methotrexate, aspirin, narcotics, and cocaine.

HRCT findings are identical to those of DAD from other causes. Diffuse ground glass opacity and consolidation are present (Fig. 15.2). Early, this may have a peripheral distribution, but the abnormalities quickly become diffuse. If early treatment is instituted, complete resolution of findings may be seen; otherwise patients may progress to ARDS. Eventually fibrosis may develop, often peripherally, and is anterior in distribution.

Organizing Pneumonia

OP is a common pattern associated with drug toxicity. Conversely, drug toxicity is one of the most common causes of OP. This pattern is most frequently associated with carmustine, bleomycin, doxorubicin, cyclophosphamide, amiodarone, nitrofurantoin, cephalosporins, tetracycline, amphotericin B, gold salts, phenytoin, sulfasalazine, and cocaine.

The predominant HRCT findings are the same as in other causes of OP, including bilateral patchy, nodular, or mass-like areas of peribronchovascular and subpleural consolidation (Fig. 15.3). The *atoll sign or reversed halo sign*, a peripheral rim of consolidation surrounding a central area of ground glass opacity

(Fig. 15.4), is fairly specific for OP. The findings of drug-related OP are indistinguishable from those of cryptogenic (idiopathic) organizing pneumonia or other causes of this pattern.

Nonspecific Interstitial Pneumonia

Drug toxicity is a known cause of nonspecific interstitial pneumonia (NSIP), although connective tissue disease is more commonly responsible. The most common drugs to cause this pattern include bleomycin, busulfan, cyclophosphamide, methotrexate, amiodarone, nitrofurantoin, hydrochlorothiazide, statins, phenytoin, and gold.

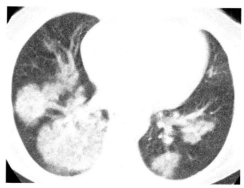

FIGURE 15.3 · **Organizing pneumonia with crack cocaine use.** Patchy, bilateral, mass-like areas of consolidation are seen in a patient presenting with subacute symptoms after the recurrent usage of crack cocaine.

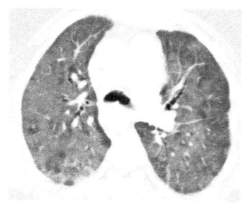

FIGURE 15.2 · **Diffuse alveolar damage due to carmustine treatment.** Diffuse ground glass opacity is present in a patient being treated with carmustine for lymphoma. Pathologically, this corresponded to diffuse alveolar damage. This finding resolved after steroid treatment.

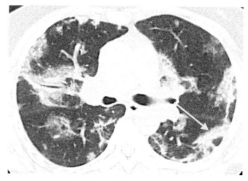

FIGURE 15.4 · **Organizing pneumonia with amiodarone.** Patchy, bilateral, subpleural and peribronchovascular consolidation and ground glass opacity are present without evidence of fibrosis. Note the presence of the *atoll sign* in the left lower lobe (*arrow*). These findings are compatible with organizing pneumonia.

15

NSIP secondary to drugs may be cellular, fibrotic, or a combination of both. HRCT may be helpful in making this distinction; differentiation of cellular and fibrotic NSIP has significant implications for treatment, as cellular NSIP is most likely to respond to treatment and has a better prognosis.

Typical HRCT findings of NSIP include ground glass opacity and/or irregular reticulation with a subpleural and basilar distribution (Fig. 15.5). A peripheral distribution of abnormalities with sparing of the immediate subpleural lung is particularly suggestive of NSIP. The presence of ground glass opacity, with or without reticulation, suggests cellular NSIP. Reticulation associated with traction bronchiectasis suggests the fibrotic subtype of NSIP. Honeycombing is typically absent or minimal in extent but when present indicates fibrotic NSIP.

Usual Interstitial Pneumonia

A UIP pattern may be seen as a manifestation of drug treatment, closely resembling idiopathic pulmonary fibrosis. The most common drugs to present in this manner include cyclophosphamide, chlorambucil, nitrofurantoin, and pindolol. HRCT findings include fibrosis characterized by reticulation, traction bronchiectasis, and honeycombing, with subpleural and basilar predominance (Fig. 15.6).

Eosinophilic Pneumonia

A common cause of eosinophilic lung disease is drug toxicity. Patients with an eosinophilic reaction show a combination of lung abnormalities on HRCT and increased serum or tissue eosinophils. This pattern is most closely associated with bleomycin, amiodarone, nitrofurantoin, antidepressants, beta-blockers, hydrochlorothiazide, nonsteroidal anti-inflammatory drugs, phenytoin, sulfasalazine, and cocaine.

HRCT findings resemble those seen in the idiopathic eosinophilic disorders, particularly chronic eosinophilic pneumonia (see Chapter 13). Peripheral, upper lobe–predominant consolidation is most characteristic, although not commonly seen. Patchy bilateral nodular or mass-like consolidation is a more frequent finding and may closely resemble OP. Eosinophilic pneumonia often shows an upper lobe predominance whereas OP often shows a lower lobe predominance.

Hypersensitivity Pneumonitis

HP is an uncommon pattern associated with drug toxicity but may be seen with methotrexate, cyclophosphamide, mesalamine, fluoxetine, amitriptyline, and paclitaxel.

HRCT findings are similar to those present with inhalational causes of HP, including ground glass opacity, centrilobular nodules, and mosaic perfusion or air trapping (see Chapter 13). If fibrosis is present (Fig. 15.7), it usually presents with irregular reticulation and traction bronchiectasis with a patchy distribution.

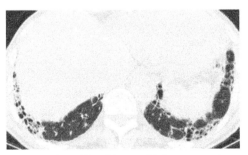

FIGURE 15.6 · **Usual interstitial pneumonia with bleomycin.** Subpleural and basilar fibrosis is present with significant honeycombing. This finding developed during treatment for breast cancer with bleomycin. This appearance is indistinguishable from other causes of usual interstitial pneumonia, such as idiopathic pulmonary fibrosis.

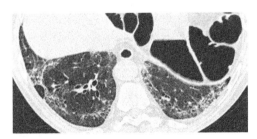

FIGURE 15.5 · **Nonspecific interstitial pneumonia with amiodarone.** Peripheral and basilar irregular reticulation and mild traction bronchiectasis are seen. There is subpleural sparing. After cessation of the drug and treatment with steroids, the majority of these abnormalities resolved.

15

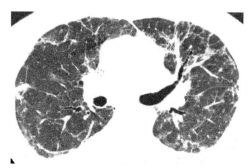

FIGURE 15.7 · Hypersensitivity pneumonitis with infliximab. Patchy, bilateral irregular reticulation is seen in both peripheral and central locations. This finding by itself is nonspecific with regard to pattern but suggests fibrosis. Pathology showed a hypersensitivity reaction.

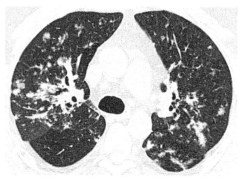

FIGURE 15.8 · Sarcoid-like reaction with interferon. Nodules are noted with a peribronchovascular and subpleural predominance. This perilymphatic distribution is most commonly due to sarcoidosis. These CT abnormalities developed while this patient was on interferon for hepatitis infection.

Sarcoid-Like Reaction

Sarcoidosis is an idiopathic disease, but rarely, a similar reaction may be seen with drug toxicity. This pattern is most commonly associated with interferon treatment. HRCT findings are identical to those typical of sarcoidosis (see Chapter 12), including nodules with a perilymphatic distribution (Fig. 15.8). Fibrosis is not common with drug-induced sarcoidosis.

Pulmonary Vasculitis and Pulmonary Hypertension

The use of various drugs may result in acute or chronic abnormalities of small pulmonary vessels with histologic abnormalities including pulmonary vasculitis, plexogenic arteriopathy (a common histologic finding in pulmonary hypertension), pulmonary capillary hemangiomatosis, and pulmonary veno-occlusive disease. The most common offending medications include fenfluramine, busulfan, methylphenidate, and methadone.

The HRCT appearances of these vary with the specific abnormalities present. Pulmonary vasculitis may result in an appearance similar to that of pulmonary edema or pulmonary hemorrhage with patchy or diffuse consolidation or ground glass opacity. Pulmonary hypertension is associated with enlargement of central pulmonary arteries. Pulmonary veno-occlusive disease and pulmonary capillary hemangiomatosis mimic hydrostatic pulmonary edema but with normal heart size.

Constrictive Bronchiolitis

A rare lung reaction to drugs is constrictive bronchiolitis, a finding primarily described in association with penicillamine therapy for rheumatoid arthritis. However, the role of penicillamine is controversial, as constrictive bronchiolitis can be seen in patients with rheumatoid arthritis who have not been treated with this drug. Constrictive bronchiolitis has also been seen in patients treated with sulfasalazine.

Abnormalities seen on HRCT consist of bronchial wall thickening and a pattern of mosaic perfusion, similar to that seen with other causes of constrictive bronchiolitis (Fig. 15.9); air trapping on expiratory scans is typically present.

RADIATION

Radiation treatment of thoracic malignancies may induce lung inflammation and eventually lead to lung fibrosis. The pattern of radiation-induced lung injury depends primarily on the location (Table 15.2), dose, and type of radiation given. Lung injury due to radiation is most commonly seen with the treatment of breast cancer, lung cancer, lymphoma, esophageal cancer, and neck malignancies.

15

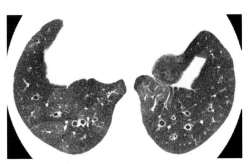

FIGURE 15.9 · **Constrictive bronchiolitis with penicillamine treatment.** Extensive mosaic perfusion is present and associated with bronchiectasis. Pathology confirmed constrictive bronchiolitis. This patient was on penicillamine treatment for rheumatoid arthritis. Both medications and connective tissue disease are causes of this pattern.

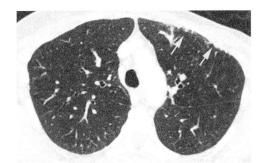

FIGURE 15.10 · **Radiation fibrosis after treatment of breast cancer.** Isolated irregular reticulation is seen in the subpleural region of the left upper lobe (*yellow arrows*). Note volume loss as evidenced by displacement of the major fissure anteriorly (*red arrow*) and superiorly. This is a typical location for fibrosis owing to tangential breast radiation.

TABLE 15.2	Typical locations of radiation-induced lung injury
Location	**Tumor**
Anterior, subpleural lung	Breast cancer, radiation to primary tumor
Unilateral lung apex	Breast cancer, axillary radiation
Bilateral lung apices	Neck malignancy
Paramediastinal	Lymphoma or esophageal cancer

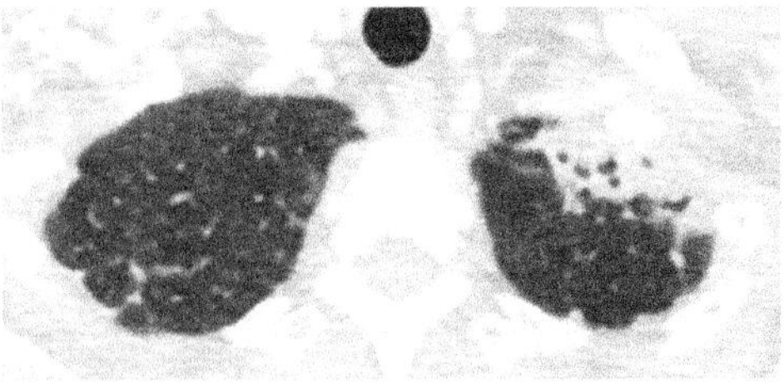

FIGURE 15.11 · **Radiation fibrosis after treatment of breast cancer.** Irregular reticulation and traction bronchiectasis are seen at the left lung apex. When asymmetric, this location is typical of radiation to the axillary or supraclavicular regions.

Radiation injury is divided into two stages: radiation pneumonitis and radiation fibrosis. *Radiation pneumonitis* occurs early, typically less than 6 months after treatment, and is primarily characterized by DAD and OP that is localized to the region of treatment. Over time, *radiation fibrosis* may develop in the same lung regions.

HRCT findings are usually limited to areas of lung that are included in the radiation field. Breast radiation is localized to the anterior subpleural lung just deep to the treated breast (Fig. 15.10). Axillary and supraclavicular radiation manifests with findings in the lung apex on the treated side (Fig. 15.11). Radiation for cancer of the neck shows findings in both lung apices (Fig. 15.12). Mediastinal radiation for lymphoma or esophageal cancer shows abnormalities in the medial lungs, directly adjacent to the mediastinum (Fig. 15.13). Radiation for lung cancer shows abnormalities that surround the radiated tumor (Fig. 15.14). These changes should not be confused with enlargement of the tumor itself.

Newer radiation techniques, such as stereotactic body radiation therapy, limit the effects of radiation on lung uninvolved by tumor. When radiation pneumonitis or fibrosis is seen in this setting, it commonly presents with abnormalities isolated to the regions directly adjacent to the treated tumor.

The HRCT findings present depend on the acuity of radiation-induced lung injury. Radiation pneumonitis presents with ground glass opacity or consolidation in a distribution corresponding to the radiation port. It is usually associated with some volume loss. A combination of ground glass opacity and smooth interlobular septal thickening, the *crazy paving* sign, may be present (Fig. 15.15). In the early

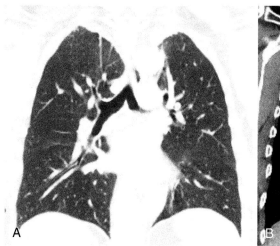

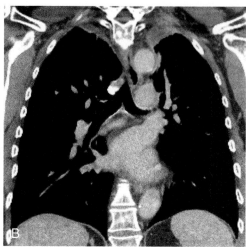

classic

FIGURE 15.12 · **Radiation fibrosis in head and neck cancer. Classic appearance.** Lung **(A)** and mediastinal **(B)** windows from a coronal reformatted CT scan show biapical consolidation, reticulation, and architectural distortion. This is a classic location for fibrosis from radiation treatment of a head and neck malignancy.

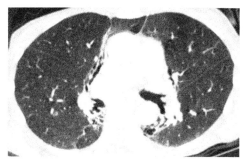

FIGURE 15.13 · **Radiation fibrosis in lymphoma.** Traction bronchiectasis, reticulation, and architectural distortion are seen in a paramediastinal location bilaterally. This patient had a remote history of mediastinal radiation for lymphoma.

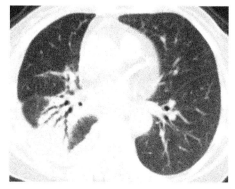

FIGURE 15.14 · **Radiation fibrosis in lung cancer.** This patient with lung cancer was treated with radiation therapy rather than surgery because of his advanced age. After treatment, fibrosis with traction bronchiectasis, consolidation, and architectural distortion are seen predominantly in the right lower lobe, in the region of the tumor.

stages, signs of fibrosis are absent. Over time, radiation pneumonitis may resolve or fibrosis may develop (Fig. 15.16). Regions of radiation fibrosis show a progressive decrease in volume and are associated with architectural distortion, traction bronchiectasis, and irregular reticulation. Regions of fibrosis may show straight edges, reflecting the location of the radiated field. An increase in the severity and extent of these findings may occur for up to 9 to 12 months after the termination of treatment.

In a small percentage of cases, radiation treatment may induce a more generalized lung reaction with abnormalities visible on HRCT outside the area of treatment. Abnormalities usually represent OP or eosinophilic pneumonia. Patchy consolidation is the most common HRCT finding (Fig. 15.17). The consolidation is typically nodular or mass-like and often has a peribronchovascular and subpleural distribution. Clinical history of radiation is important in making the correct diagnosis.

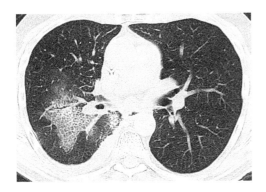

FIGURE 15.15 · **Radiation pneumonitis with crazy paving.** A combination of ground glass opacity and reticulation is noted in the right lower lobe, in the same region as a treated lung cancer. Note the relative lack of architectural distortion or significant signs of fibrosis.

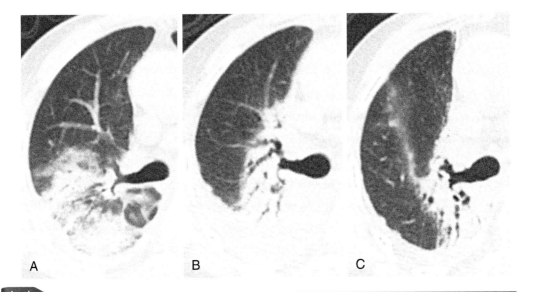

A   B   C

classic

FIGURE 15.16 · **Radiation pneumonitis progressing to fibrosis. Classic appearance. A.** Weeks after radiation treatment for lung cancer, focal ground glass opacity and consolidation are seen in the right upper lobe. **B.** Four months later, traction bronchiectasis, architectural distortion, and volume loss indicate the development of fibrosis. **C.** One year after the baseline CT, there is continued increase in volume loss and architectural distortion.

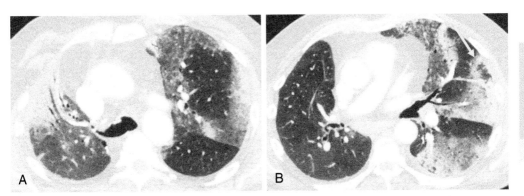

A   B

FIGURE 15.17 · **Images through the upper (A) and mid-lung (B) in a patient who underwent stereotactic body radiation therapy for a right apical lung cancer.** Patchy bilateral ground glass opacity and consolidation is due to diffuse radiation pneumonitis. The reversed halo or atoll sign (*arrow*) is indicative of a component of organizing pneumonia.

15

FURTHER READING

Aquino SL, Webb WR, Golden J. Bronchiolitis obliterans associated with rheumatoid arthritis: findings on HRCT and dynamic expiratory CT. *J Comput Assist Tomogr.* 1994;18:555-558.

Aronchick JM, Gefter WB. Drug-induced pulmonary disorders. *Semin Roentgenol.* 1995;30:18-34.

Bellamy EA, Husband JE, Blaquiere RM, Law MR. Bleomycin-related lung damage: CT evidence. *Radiology.* 1985;156:155-158.

Bush DA, Dunbar RD, Bonnet R, et al. Pulmonary injury from proton and conventional radiotherapy as revealed by CT. *AJR Am J Roentgenol.* 1999;172:735-739.

Cooper JAD, White DA, Matthay RA. Drug induced pulmonary disease, part 1: cytotoxic drugs. *Am Rev Respir Dis.* 1986;133:321-340.

Cooper JAD, White DA, Matthay RA. Drug induced pulmonary disease, part 2: noncytotoxic drugs. *Am Rev Respir Dis.* 1986;133:488-503.

Davis SD, Yankelevitz DF, Henschke CI. Radiation effects on the lung: clinical features, pathology, and imaging findings. *AJR Am J Roentgenol.* 1992;159:1157-1164.

Gotway MB, Marder SR, Hanks DK, et al. Thoracic complications of illicit drug use: an organ system approach. *Radiographics.* 2002;22:119-135.

Huang K, Palma DA. Follow-up of patients after stereotactic radiation for lung cancer: a primer for the non-radiation oncologist. *J Thorac Oncol.* 2015;10:412-419

Huang K, Dahele M, Senan S, et al. Radiographic changes after lung stereotactic ablative radiotherapy (SABR)-can we distinguish recurrence from fibrosis? A systematic review of the literature. *Radiother Oncol.* 2012;102:335-342.

Huang K, Senthi S, Palma DA, et al. High-risk CT features for detection of local recurrence after stereotactic ablative radiotherapy for lung cancer. *Radiother Oncol.* 2013;109:51-57.

Kang KH, Okoye CC, Patel RB, et al. Complications from stereotactic body radiotherapy for lung cancer. *Cancers.* 2015;15:981-1004.

Kuhlman JE. The role of chest computed tomography in the diagnosis of drug-related reactions. *J Thorac Imaging.* 1991;6:52-61.

Kuhlman JE, Teigen C, Ren H, et al. Amiodarone pulmonary toxicity: CT findings in symptomatic patients. *Radiology.* 1990;177:121-125.

Logan PM. Thoracic manifestations of external beam radiotherapy. *AJR Am J Roentgenol.* 1998;171:569-577.

Padley SPG, Adler B, Hansell DM, Müller NL. High-resolution computed tomography of drug-induced lung disease. *Clin Radiol.* 1992;46:232-236.

Pietra GG. Pathologic mechanisms of drug-induced lung disorders. *J Thorac Imaging.* 1991;6:1-7.

Rosenow EC, Myers JL, Swensen SJ, Pisani RJ. Drug-induced pulmonary disease: an update. *Chest.* 1992;102:239-250.

Rossi SE, Erasmus JJ, McAdams HP, et al. Pulmonary drug toxicity: radiologic and pathologic manifestations. *Radiographics.* 2000;20:1245-1259.

15

Pneumocconioses

INTRODUCTION

The incidence of pneumoconioses has decreased in relation to other diffuse lung diseases because of a greater emphasis on prevention in high-risk occupations, although their prevalence is still high in certain high-risk occupations. Because they often have high-resolution computed tomography (HRCT) findings that resemble other diseases, such as sarcoidosis or idiopathic pulmonary fibrosis (IPF), a clinical history of exposure is vital in suggesting the correct diagnosis of pneumoconiosis.

GENERAL APPROACH TO DIAGNOSIS

Pneumoconiosis is defined as a lung disease associated with environmental dust inhalation. Most patients with pneumoconiosis have an identifiable long-term occupational exposure to a known offending agent. However, without knowledge of the exposure history, HRCT findings are commonly mistaken for another disease.

The most common HRCT abnormalities of pneumoconioses include nodules, fibrosis, and lymphadenopathy. Nodules may be perilymphatic or centrilobular in distribution. Fibrosis may appear on HRCT as honeycombing, irregular reticulation, traction bronchiectasis, and consolidation with architectural distortion, so-called progressive massive fibrosis (PMF).

There are several characteristic patterns of pneumoconiosis, each of which may be associated with one or more possible dust exposures. The archetype of each of these patterns is discussed in detail below, with a review of other dust exposures that are associated with a similar appearance.

PNEUMOCONIOSIS PATTERNS ON HRCT

Silicosis and the "Silicosis Pattern"

Silicosis (Table 16.1) is caused by chronic inhalation of silicon dioxide and is associated with professions such as glass manufacturing, sandblasting, mining, stonecutting, and quarrying. Silicosis results from inhalation of dust and subsequent drainage via the lymphatics. It is primarily characterized by nodules, lymphadenopathy, and fibrosis. Silicosis associated with chronic exposure is usually classified as either *simple silicosis* or *complicated silicosis*. A third form of silicosis, *acute silicosis (silicoproteinosis)*, is less frequently seen.

HRCT Findings

Simple silicosis is characterized by scattered nodules (Fig. 16.1). These predominate in the posterior upper lungs and demonstrate a perilymphatic distribution, affecting the centrilobular regions, peribronchovascular interstitium, interlobular septa, and subpleural interstitium (Fig. 16.2). As opposed to other causes of perilymphatic nodules, a predominance of centrilobular nodules (Fig. 16.3) may be present. Lung involvement is usually bilateral and symmetrical. The nodules are usually a few millimeters in diameter, of soft tissue attenuation, well defined, and may calcify.

Hilar and mediastinal lymphadenopathy may also be present (Fig. 16.4). Similar to sarcoidosis, the distribution of adenopathy is usually symmetric. Calcification of nodes may be present and may be diffuse or have a so-called eggshell pattern, involving the periphery of the node.

Some patients with chronic exposure develop progressive fibrosis, termed

TABLE 16.1	Features of silicosis and a "silicosis pattern"
HRCT findings	Perilymphatic nodules, posterior/upper lung distribution, bilateral and symmetrical Fibrosis, upper/central lung distribution Progressive massive fibrosis Lymphadenopathy and/or calcification
Differential diagnosis	Other pneumoconioses: Coal worker's pneumoconiosis Talcosis Berylliosis Other diseases: Sarcoidosis and other causes of perilymphati nodules or upper lobe fibrosis
Complications	Tuberculosis Primary bronchogenic carcinoma

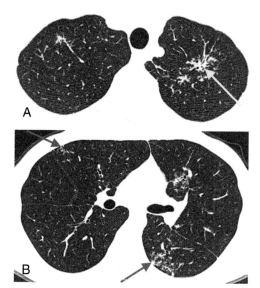

FIGURE 16.2 · **Perilymphatic nodules in silicosis.** HRCT through the lung apices **(A)** and mid-lungs **(B)** shows patchy, clustered nodules. The nodules are predominantly located within the peribronchovascular (*yellow arrow*, **A**) and subpleural interstitium (*red arrows*, **B**).

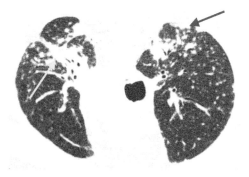

FIGURE 16.1 · **Perilymphatic nodules in silicosis.** Prone HRCT shows nodules clustered in relation to the peribronchovascular (*yellow arrow*) and subpleural interstitium (*red arrow*). This appearance is indistinguishable from sarcoidosis.

complicated silicosis. Fibrosis may be seen in association with perilymphatic nodules (Fig. 16.5) or as an isolated abnormality. Fibrosis is manifested by irregular reticulation and traction bronchiectasis with an upper lobe and peribronchovascular distribution. Confluent areas of fibrosis may produce consolidation with architectural distortion and traction bronchiectasis (Fig. 16.6). This is termed *progressive massive fibrosis* or *PMF*. As PMF develops, the number of small nodules decreases because they are incorporated into the fibrotic mass. Masses of PMF may show calcification.

Silicosis progresses to PMF more frequently than does sarcoidosis.

Acute exposure to large amounts of silica dust can result in a clinical syndrome and HRCT appearance that is markedly different from classic silicosis. In these cases, the exposure results in alveolar filling that closely resembles pulmonary alveolar proteinosis (PAP), both pathologically and on HRCT. This is termed *acute silicosis* or *silicoproteinosis*. The HRCT manifestations include extensive or diffuse bilateral ground glass opacity and consolidation. The combination of ground glass opacity and interlobular septal thickening in the same lung regions (i.e., *crazy paving*) is typical and indistinguishable from other causes of PAP (Fig. 16.7). Centrilobular nodules may also be seen, reflecting the inhaled nature of this disease.

Differential Diagnosis of a Silicosis Pattern

Other pneumoconioses that may show HRCT abnormalities similar to those of silicosis include coal worker's pneumoconiosis (CWP), talcosis, berylliosis (Fig. 16.8), and rare dusts such as cerium. Exposure history

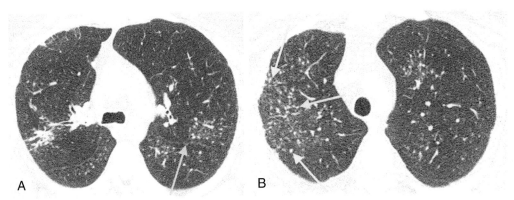

FIGURE 16.3 · **Perilymphatic nodules in silicosis. A.** A perilymphatic distribution of nodules is present, with nodules seen in the peribronchovascular (*red arrow*) and subpleural regions (*blue arrow*). **B.** A number of centrilobular nodules (region delineated by *yellow arrows*) are present, reflecting the inhaled nature of the disease.

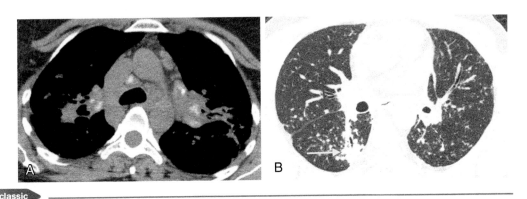

classic

FIGURE 16.4 · **Silicosis with lymphadenopathy: Classic appearance.** Symmetric mediastinal and hilar lymphadenopathy with calcification is present **(A)** indistinguishable from that seen in sarcoidosis. Lung window **(B)** shows peribronchovascular (*yellow arrow*) and subpleural nodules (*red arrow*).

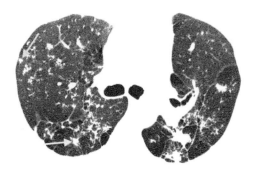

FIGURE 16.5 · **Silicosis with perilymphatic nodules and fibrosis.** HRCT through the upper lobes shows fibrosis with architectural distortion, volume loss, and traction bronchiectasis. Nodules are also present. Note the clustered peribronchovascular (*yellow arrow*), subpleural (*red arrow*), and centrilobular (*blue arrow*) nodules.

is more important than HRCT findings in differentiating these causes of lung abnormalities. Pathology also shows significant overlapping findings. The different pneumoconioses in this category may be difficult to distinguish from one another and from sarcoidosis. Other tests may be required to confirm a specific diagnosis in challenging cases, such as the lymphocyte proliferation test (see below in the section on Berylliosis).

Coal Worker's Pneumoconiosis
CWP exposure occurs in patients with an appropriate coal-mining history. The nodules of CWP are less well defined than those of silicosis, and calcification tends to be less common and central in location. Eggshell

16

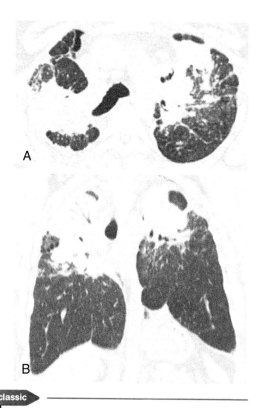

A

B

FIGURE 16.6 **Progressive massive fibrosis in silicosis: Classic appearance.** Axial **(A)** and coronal reformatted **(B)** images demonstrate upper lung, mass-like conglomerates of central fibrosis associated with architectural distortion and bronchiectasis. This appearance is most characteristic of silicosis but can be seen with other pneumoconioses and sarcoidosis.

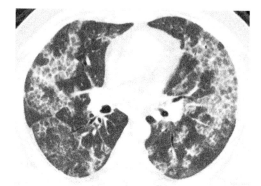

FIGURE 16.7 **Silicoproteinosis.** After an acute exposure to large amounts of silica dust, this patient presented with dyspnea and cough. HRCT showed a combination of ground glass opacity and interlobular septal thickening in the same lung regions. This "crazy paving" pattern is identical to that seen with alveolar proteinosis.

production. Berylliosis is radiographically and pathologically identical to sarcoidosis (Fig. 16.8). The distinction between these two diseases may be made using a lymphocyte proliferation test that examines the sensitivity of plasma lymphocytes for beryllium.

Complications of Silicosis

Patients with silicosis and other pneumoconioses have an increased risk of developing tuberculosis. The diagnosis of tuberculosis may be challenging because both diseases may produce nodules, consolidation, and fibrosis. The presence of cavitation with a mass of PMF should raise the possibility of tuberculosis (Fig. 16.9), although, occasionally, silicosis by itself may result in necrosis of fibrotic masses.

Primary bronchogenic carcinoma has an increased incidence in patients with silicosis. It may be difficult to differentiate areas of PMF from malignancy. Positron emission tomography or magnetic resonance imaging may be helpful in making this distinction.

Asbestosis and the "Asbestosis Pattern"

Asbestos (Table 16.2) exposure occurs in occupations such as mining, shipbuilding, construction, textiles manufacturing, manufacture of brake linings, and exposure to insulation materials containing asbestos. This

calcification is unusual in CWP. Fibrosis is less severe with CWP than with complicated silicosis, but conglomerate masses may be seen.

Talcosis
Talcosis is acquired through high-risk occupations such as the production of textiles, paper, and rubber. Talc is commonly mixed with other dusts such as silica and asbestos; thus, a mix of different patterns may be present. Inhaled talcosis, which resembles silicosis, should be distinguished from the intravenous injection of talc, which has a distinct appearance and is discussed in Chapter 7.

Berylliosis
Berylliosis is acquired in the aerospace and ceramic industries and in nuclear weapons

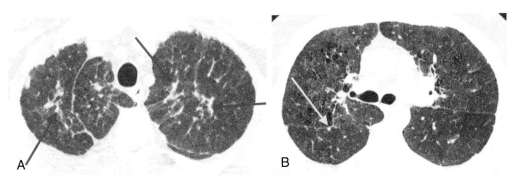

FIGURE 16.8 · **Fibrosis in berylliosis.** Upper lobe–predominant irregular reticulation is present in a central, peribronchovascular distribution (*arrows*, **A**). Minimal nodularity is present, predominantly in the subpleural interstitium (*arrow*, **B**).

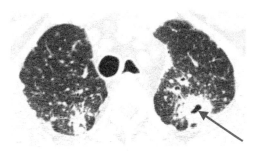

FIGURE 16.9 · **Silicosis with cavitation.** Cavitation (*arrow*) in a patient with a known silicosis should raise the possibility of infection, particularly tuberculosis, to which these patients are predisposed. Rarely cavitation can be seen in uncomplicated pneumoconioses without evidence of infection. Note typical nodules with a perilymphatic distribution.

TABLE 16.2	Features of asbestosis and an "asbestosis pattern"
HRCT findings	Honeycombing with a usual interstitial pneumonia pattern Other signs of fibrosis (irregular reticulation, traction bronchiectasis) Subpleural and basilar distribution 90% associated with typical pleural disease (plaques, calcification)
Differential diagnosis	Other pneumoconioses: Mixed dust pneumoconiosis containing asbestos Other diseases: Lung disease indistinguishable from other causes of usual interstitial pneumonia (idiopathic pulmonary fibrosis, connective tissue disease, drug toxicity)
Complications	Bronchogenic carcinoma Mesothelioma

exposure may result in various abnormalities, including pleural disease, interstitial lung disease, and malignancy.

HRCT Findings

The earliest manifestation of asbestos exposure may be a pleural effusion, unilateral or bilateral. Effusions are commonly exudative, and thus, pleural thickening, enhancement, and loculation may be associated. They may resolve spontaneously or may persist for many years.

Pleural plaques are a characteristic feature of asbestos exposure, occurring after a latent period of many years. Plaques represent focal areas of pleural thickening that are variable in size but often 1 to 2 cm in diameter. The edges of plaques are often elevated, as opposed to the tapered thickening that occurs at the edges

of other benign causes of pleural thickening. Plaques commonly calcify, but even when they are not calcified, they are often high in attenuation because of the mineral they contain. Plaques are typically seen adjacent to ribs, spare the costophrenic angles, and may involve the diaphragmatic pleura. Diffuse pleural thickening is an uncommon finding in patients with asbestos exposure but may be seen.

Asbestosis is the interstitial lung disease associated with asbestos exposure. It is predominantly fibrotic. A peripheral and basilar distribution of fibrosis is typical (Fig. 16.10), while other pneumoconioses are usually upper

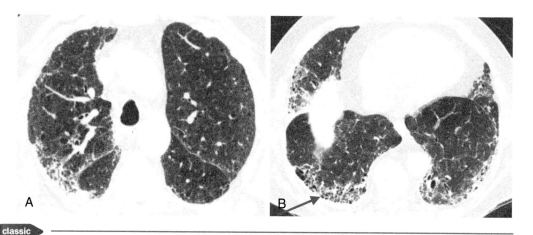

classic

FIGURE 16.10 · **Asbestosis: Classic appearance. A** and **B.** Peripheral and basilar predominant fibrosis is present, with mild honeycombing (**B**, *blue arrow*), irregular reticulation, and traction bronchiectasis (**B**, *red arrow*). This pattern is indistinguishable in most cases from idiopathic pulmonary fibrosis.

lobe predominant. Except for the presence of asbestos fibers (asbestos bodies), biopsy is consistent with usual interstitial pneumonia (UIP).

HRCT abnormalities common in asbestosis result in a UIP pattern (see Chapter 9). These include irregular reticulation, traction bronchiectasis, and honeycombing occurring in the peripheral, posterior, and subpleural lung, typically the lower lobes. The costophrenic angles are usually involved. An absence of ground glass opacity, nodules, and mosaic perfusion/air trapping is characteristic. Rarely, small ill-defined centrilobular nodules are seen in the peripheral lung (Fig. 16.11); these tend to be seen in early disease and reflect the presence of peribronchiolar fibrosis.

Differential Diagnosis of an Asbestosis Pattern

The HRCT pattern of lung disease present with asbestosis is nearly indistinguishable from other causes of UIP. As approximately 90% of patients with asbestosis demonstrate pleural plaques on computed tomography (CT), this may be a helpful distinguishing feature (Fig. 16.12). Otherwise, exposure history is most helpful in making the distinction between asbestosis and the other causes of UIP, such as IPF.

Small centrilobular nodules in the peripheral lung have been described as a differentiating feature of asbestosis, but these are only seen rarely. Longitudinal evaluation of the

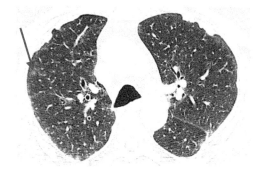

FIGURE 16.11 · **Asbestosis. Peripheral ground glass is seen in a patient with early, biopsy-proven asbestosis.** Note ground glass opacity centrilobular nodules (*arrow*) in the peripheral lung. Centrilobular arteries are seen to be associated with some of these nodules. Pleural plaques are present anteriorly.

progression of lung disease may also be helpful in distinguishing asbestosis from IPF. IPF often shows progression of lung abnormalities over a period of several years, but asbestosis may show long-term stability.

Complimcations

Of the pneumoconioses, asbestosis is associated with the highest risk of malignancy (Fig. 16.13). Because of the lung distortion associated with fibrosis, malignancies often have an atypical appearance; they may be ill-defined or may mimic consolidation. Rounded nodules or masses in the peripheral

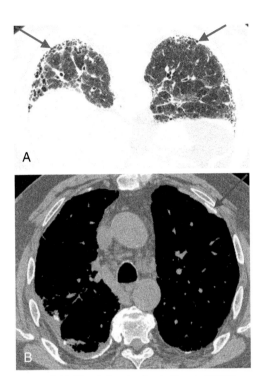

A

B

FIGURE 16.12 · Asbestosis. A. Prone HRCT shows a typical pattern of usual interstitial pneumonia (UIP) with peripheral areas of honeycombing (*arrows*). **B.** The lung fibrosis is associated with pleural plaques, some of which are calcified (*arrow*). This combination indicates asbestosis as the likely cause of the UIP pattern.

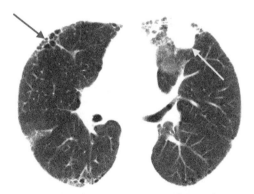

FIGURE 16.13 · Malignancy in asbestosis. eripheral honeycombing (*red arrow*) is present in a patient with asbestosis complicated by a lung cancer (*yellow arrow*).

lung may also be a manifestation of *rounded atelectasis*. Distinguishing rounded atelectasis from malignancy may be challenging. Rounded atelectasis often has typical features of volume loss in association with "swirling" of

TABLE 16.3	Features of siderosis and a "siderosis pattern"
HRCT findings	Centrilobular nodules of ground glass opacity
	Ground glass opacity
	Mild mosaic perfusion/air trapping
	Fibrosis is rare except with a mixed dust exposure
Differential diagnosis	Other pneumoconioses:
	Baritosis
	Stannosis
	Hard metal pneumoconiosis
	Other diseases:
	Hypersensitivity pneumonitis and other causes of centrilobular ground glass nodules
Complications	Rare
	Primary bronchogenic carcinoma (mixed dust exposures)

vessels and bronchi. Positron emission tomography may be required when the distinction between these two entities is challenging.

Asbestos exposure also places a patient at risk for mesothelioma. It may be difficult to distinguish early mesothelioma from benign pleural abnormalities associated with asbestos exposure. Features that suggest malignant mesothelioma include pleural thickening >1 cm, significant mediastinal pleural involvement, concentric pleural thickening, and development of a new pleural effusion.

Siderosis and the "Siderosis Pattern"

Siderosis (Table 16.3) is caused by inhalation of iron oxide, most commonly due to exposure during welding. Iron oxide is a material that, in general, does not elicit a significant granulomatous or inflammatory reaction. When inhaled, the dust is deposited around the small airways, but there is minimal associated reaction. Mixed dusts, particularly a combination of iron oxide and silica, may be inhaled. Mixed dusts may result in a mixed pattern.

HRCT Findings

Typical HRCT findings resemble subacute hypersensitivity pneumonitis and include centrilobular nodules of ground glass opacity (Fig. 16.14) or more generalized patchy ground glass opacity owing to the presence

16

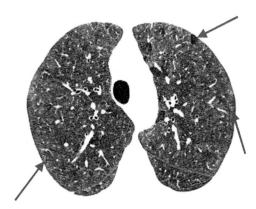

FIGURE 16.14 · **Siderosis.** Centrilobular ground glass nodules (*blue arrows*), ground glass opacity, and minimal mosaic perfusion (*red arrow*) are typical manifestations of siderosis and other pneumoconioses that do not elicit a prominent fibrotic reaction.

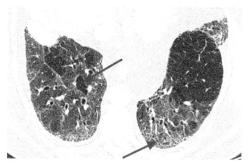

FIGURE 16.15 · **Hard metal pneumoconiosis.** Patchy ground glass opacity is present at the lung bases and associated with patchy mosaic perfusion (*blue arrow*). There is also mild fibrosis in the posterior peripheral lung regions with irregular reticulation and traction bronchiectasis (*red arrow*).

of the dust itself. Associated mosaic and perfusion air trapping may be present, but these tend to be mild in severity.

These abnormalities rarely progress to fibrosis. This primarily occurs in patients with a mixed dust exposure, including silica. In these cases, traction bronchiectasis, irregular reticulation, and PMF may be present. Cases in which fibrosis is present may closely resemble an interstitial pneumonia, particularly nonspecific interstitial pneumonia or UIP.

Differential Diagnosis

Other rare pneumoconioses may closely resemble siderosis. These include *baritosis* (exposure to barium sulfate) and *stannosis* (exposure to tin oxide). These may result in high attenuation opacities, sometimes branching and related to small airways.

Hard metal pneumonconiosis, an alloy of tungsten, cobalt, and various other materials, may also resemble siderosis with centrilobular nodules of ground glass opacity, ground glass opacity, and mosaic perfusion/air trapping (Fig. 16.15). Hard metal pneumoconiosis more commonly progresses to fibrosis in patients with chronic exposure and may show irregular reticulation, traction bronchiectasis, and honeycombing.

The subacute type of hypersensitivity pneumonitis closely resembles siderosis and

its mimics. There are likely no accurate distinguishing HRCT features, and exposure history is paramount in differentiating these two entities. The air trapping in siderosis tends not to be as severe as in certain patients with hypersensitivity pneumonitis. Other causes of chronic centrilobular nodules of ground glass opacity include respiratory bronchiolitis and follicular bronchiolitis.

Complications

Complications from siderosis are rare, unless silica is also present, in which case malignancy can occur. Given its greater association with fibrosis, hard metal pneumoconiosis is more commonly complicated by bronchogenic carcinoma.

FURTHER READING

Aberle DR, Balmes JR. Computed tomography of asbestos-related pulmonary parenchymal and pleural diseases. *Clin Chest Med.* 1991;12:115-131.

Akira M. Uncommon pneumoconioses: CT and pathologic findings. *Radiology.* 1995;197:403-409.

Akira M. High-resolution CT in the evaluation of occupational and environmental disease. *Radiol Clin North Am.* 2002;40:43-59.

Akira M, Kozuka T, Yamamoto S, et al. Inhalational talc pneumoconiosis: radiographic and CT findings in 14 patients. *AJR Am J Roentgenol.* 2007;188:326-333.

Akira M, Yamamoto S, Yokoyama K, et al. Asbestosis: high-resolution CT-pathologic correlation. *Radiology.* 1990;176:389-394.

Akira M, Yokoyama K, Yamamoto S, et al. Early asbestosis: evaluation with high-resolution CT. *Radiology.* 1991;178:409-416.

Alper F, Akgun M, Onbas O, Araz O. CT findings in silicosis due to denim sandblasting. *Eur Radiol.* 2008;18:2739-2744.

Antao VC, Pinheiro GA, Terra-Filho M, et al. High-resolution CT in silicosis: correlation with radiographic findings and functional impairment. *J Comput Assist Tomogr.* 2005;29:350-356.

Chong S, Lee KS, Chung MJ, et al. Pneumoconiosis: comparison of imaging and pathologic findings. *Radiographics.* 2006;26:59-77.

Copley SJ, Wells AU, Sivakumaran P, et al. Asbestosis and idiopathic pulmonary fibrosis: comparison of thin-section CT features. *Radiology.* 2003;229:731-736.

Henry DA. International Labor Office Classification System in the age of imaging: relevant or redundant. *J Thorac Imaging.* 2002;17:179-188.

Kim KI, Kim CW, Lee MK, et al. Imaging of occupational lung disease. *Radiographics.* 2001;21:1371-1391.

Marchiori E, Souza CA, Barbassa TG, et al. Silicoproteinosis: high-resolution CT findings in 13 patients. *AJR Am J Roentgenol.* 2007;189:1402-1406.

Newman LS, Buschman DL, Newell JD, Lynch DL. Beryllium disease: assessment with CT. *Radiology.* 1994;190:835-840.

Remy-Jardin M, Degreef JM, Beuscart R, et al. Coal worker's pneumoconiosis: CT assessment in exposed workers and correlation with radiographic findings. *Radiology.* 1990;177:363-371.

Savranlar A, Altin R, Mahmutyazicioglu K, et al. Comparison of chest radiography and high-resolution computed tomography findings in early and low-grade coal worker's pneumoconiosis. *Eur J Radiol.* 2004;51:175-180.

Sette A, Neder JA, Nery LE, et al. Thin-section CT abnormalities and pulmonary gas exchange impairment in workers exposed to asbestos. *Radiology.* 2004;232:66-74.

Shida H, Chiyotani K, Honma K, et al. Radiologic and pathologic characteristics of mixed dust pneumoconiosis. *Radiographics.* 1996;16:483-498.

Silva CI, Müller NL, Neder JA, et al. Asbestos-related disease: progression of parenchymal abnormalities on high-resolution CT. *J Thorac Imaging.* 2008;23:251-257.

Ward S, Heyneman LE, Reittner P, et al. Talcosis associated with IV abuse of oral medications: CT findings. *AJR Am J Roentgenol.* 2000;174:789-793.

16

Neoplastic and Lymphoproliferative Diseases

INTRODUCTION

Pulmonary neoplasm and lymphoproliferative disorders may present with diffuse lung abnormalities. The goal of this chapter is to discuss the various patterns of diffuse pulmonary neoplasm and lymphoproliferative disease and when these entities should be considered in the differential diagnosis.

PULMONARY MALIGNANCIES: MECHANISM OF SPREAD

Neoplasms may result in diffuse lung abnormalities by several different mechanisms (Table 17.1). These result in different appearances on high-resolution computed tomography (HRCT).

Hematogenous Spread with Random Nodules

The primary HRCT manifestation of diffuse lung involvement by metastatic tumor is that of randomly distributed pulmonary nodules. This results from hematogenous spread of tumor (see Chapter 3; Fig. 17.1).

Nodules involve the entire lung, with a random distribution relative to lung structures, because they are distributed on the basis of blood flow. They tend to have a diffuse and uniform distribution, although they may show a lower lobe predominance because of greater blood flow to this location.

Nodules are usually of soft tissue attenuation and may range in size from a few millimeters in size, when first recognized, to many centimeters. The nodules tend to be similar in size.

The differential diagnosis of this appearance includes other causes of random nodules, including miliary tuberculosis and miliary fungal infection. Clinical history is often helpful in distinguishing infections from neoplasm.

Moreover, the size of nodules may be helpful when the clinical presentation is unclear. Large nodules are more likely to represent metastases. Miliary infections uncommonly produce nodules larger than 5 mm.

Intravascular Metastases

In occasional patients, tumor embolism to small pulmonary arteries results in intravascular metastases and tumor deposits that grow within the lumen of the arteries. These may be seen with various neoplasms but are most common with very vascular primary tumors (e.g., sarcomas) and tumors that result in invasion of large veins (e.g., hepatoma and renal cell carcinoma).

Intravascular metastases result in focally dilated, nodular, beaded, or lobulated small pulmonary artery branches (Fig. 17.2). Intravascular filling defects may be visible if contrast agent is injected. This appearance may mimic pulmonary embolism, but smooth luminal filling defects, resembling thrombotic pulmonary emboli, are rare as an isolated finding.

Lymphangitic Spread

Pulmonary lymphatics predominate in the parahilar peribronchovascular interstitium, centrilobular regions, interlobular septa, and subpleural interstitium. Tumors that spread via the lymphatics, or involve the lymphatics secondary to hematogenous metastasis, may demonstrate abnormalities associated with these structures, particularly the interlobular septa and peribronchovascular interstitium (Fig. 17.3). Thickening of these structures may be smooth or nodular in the presence of metastasis.

The most common tumors to produce this pattern include lymphoma and cancers of the lung, breast, thyroid gland, stomach, pancreas, prostate, and head and neck. In many cases, lymphangitic spread occurs as a result

of hematogenous dissemination to small vessels, with tumor invasion of the interstitium. Thus, an overlap between the appearance of hematogenous spread and lymphangitic spread may be seen in some patients.

TABLE 17.1	Mechanisms of spread of pulmonary malignancies
Type of spread	**HRCT finding(s)**
Hematogenous spread	Random distribution of nodules
Intravascular metastases	Dilated, nodular, unopacified pulmonary arterial branches
Lymphangitic spread	Smooth or nodular thickening of the interlobular septa or peribronchovascular interstitium
Endobronchial spread	Centrilobular nodules

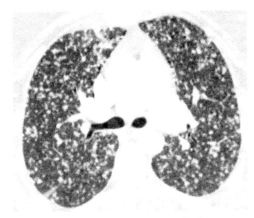

FIGURE 17.1 · Hematogenous metastases. HRCT in a patient with metastatic medullary thyroid carcinoma shows diffuse nodules, less than 1 cm in diameter, with a random distribution. The random distribution reflects hematogenous spread of tumor to the lungs.

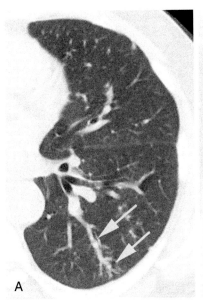

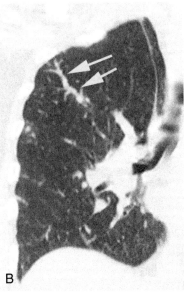

A   **B**

classic

FIGURE 17.2 · Intravascular metastases. Classic appearance. A. A dilated, nodular, branching, lower lobe pulmonary artery (*arrows*) reflects intravascular metastases in a patient with transitional cell carcinoma. Several nodular metastases are also visible. **B.** Coronal reformatted image shows a dilated and nodular upper lobe artery (*arrows*).

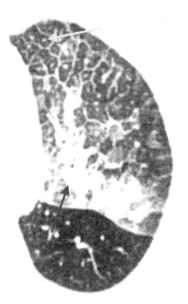

FIGURE 17.3 · Lymphangitic metastases. Focal smooth interlobular septal thickening is noted in the left upper lobe in a patient with lung cancer. Note the polygonal lobules outlined by the thickened septa. Centrilobular arteries are visible in their centers (*yellow arrow*). Central peribronchovascular interstitial thickening is also present (*red arrow*).

Interlobular septal thickening is the result of direct invasion of the pulmonary lymphatics and interstitium by a lung metastasis or primary tumor. Peribronchovascular interstitial thickening is most commonly seen in patients with mediastinal metastases that spread peripherally via lymphatics.

The differential diagnosis of nodular interlobular septal and peribronchovascular interstitial thickening includes other causes of perilymphatic disease including sarcoidosis, pneumoconioses, amyloidosis, and lymphoid interstitial pneumonia (LIP). When smooth thickening of these structures is present, the primary differential consideration is pulmonary edema.

Endobronchial Spread of Tumor

Endobronchial spread of tumor is rare with extrathoracic malignancies. It is more commonly seen with primary lung carcinomas, particularly invasive mucinous adenocarcinoma or squamous cell carcinoma.

Endobronchial spread of tumor may be associated with multiple lung nodules or

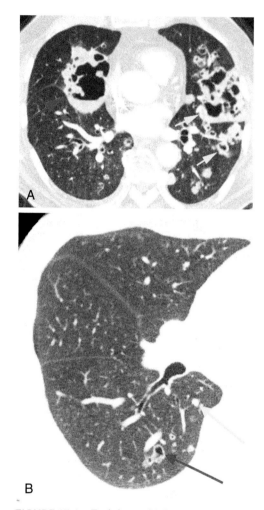

B

FIGURE 17.4 · Endobronchial spread of tumor in two patients. A. In a patient with a cavitary squamous cell carcinoma, HRCT shows nodular thickening of bronchial walls (yellow arrows) and thick-walled cavities (red arrow). Extensive endobronchial tumor was visible at bronchoscopy. **B.** In a patient with tracheobronchial papillomatosis, HRCT shows nodules (*yellow arrow*) and a thick-walled cavitary nodule or cyst (*red arrow*).

bronchial wall thickening, endobronchial nodules, and/or bronchial obstruction (Fig. 17.4A, B) or may closely resemble bronchopneumonia with airway impaction and centrilobular nodules. Consolidation or ground glass opacity may be due to atelectasis or postobstructive pneumonia.

The most common extrathoracic primaries to show endobronchial spread include melanoma, breast, renal, pancreatic, and colon cancers. Tracheobronchial papillomatosis is associated with infection by the human papilloma virus. Papillomas involving the larynx may spread via the airways to involve the trachea, bronchi, and lung parenchyma. Squamous cell carcinoma may result. HRCT may show cysts, nodules, cavitary nodules, and endobronchial lesions (Fig. 17.4B). Papillomas may be seen within cysts.

INVASIVE MUCINOUS ADENOCARCINOMA

Invasive mucinous adenocarcinoma (IMA; formerly termed diffuse bronchioloalveolar carcinoma or BAC) is a subtype of pulmonary adenocarcinoma, characterized by endobronchial spread and diffuse or multifocal lung involvement. The nonmucinous subtype of adenocarcinoma is much less likely to result in this type of dissemination; it more frequently appears as a solitary nodule, often of ground glass opacity.

The HRCT findings of IMA often resemble lobar pneumonia or patchy bronchopneumonia. Consolidation and ground glass are the most frequent abnormalities; these abnormalities often result from filling of alveoli by mucin or fluid secreted by the tumor. The tumor itself is characterized by *lepidic growth* or growth along alveolar walls, without filling or replacement of the alveolar spaces by tumor.

Abnormalities may be unilateral, bilateral, asymmetric, or symmetric and may be focal, patchy, or diffuse (Fig. 17.5). When intravenous contrast is administered, the vessels within areas of consolidation may appear dense compared with the low-density consolidation. This is called the *computed tomography (CT) angiogram sign* and is common with invasive mucinous adenocarcinomas.

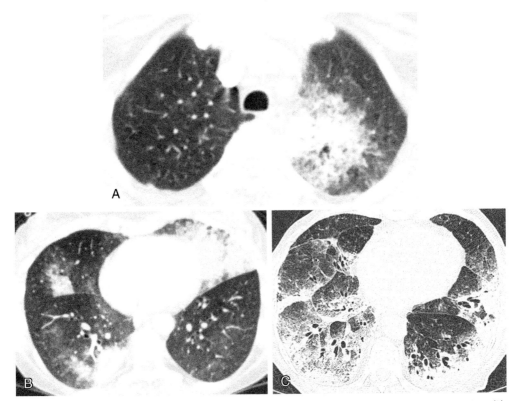

FIGURE 17.5 · **Invasive mucinous adenocarcinoma (IMA) in two patients.** IMA may present with consolidation or ground glass opacity (GGO) that is focal **(A)**, patchy, or bilateral **(B)**. In another patient **(C)**, IMA appears extensive and diffuse. These appearances may resemble a variety of other diseases, and IMA should always be considered in the setting of chronic consolidation and GGO.

However, this sign is nonspecific and may be seen in many causes of consolidation.

Centrilobular nodules may also be present, reflecting endobronchial spread of tumor (Fig. 17.6). Similar to bronchopneumonia, the nodules are often heterogeneous in size, with variable spread into the alveoli surrounding the centrilobular bronchiole. Nodules are most commonly of soft tissue attenuation, but ground glass opacity nodules may also be seen.

Interlobular septal thickening may be present and is typically seen in areas of ground glass opacity. This combination is termed *crazy paving*, and although classically associated with pulmonary alveolar proteinosis, it may be seen with a variety of other acute and chronic lung diseases.

The differential diagnosis of IMA includes infection with endobronchial spread. However, the clinical presentations of these two entities are quite different; pneumonia presents with acute symptoms and mucinous adenocarcinoma presents with chronic progressive symptoms, usually of greater than 3 months' duration. IMA may be associated with *bronchorrhea*, the production of liters of watery sputum each day.

In patients presenting with chronic symptoms, the differential diagnosis of invasive mucinous adenocarcinoma includes other causes of chronic consolidation and ground glass opacity, such as organizing pneumonia, chronic eosinophilic pneumonia, sarcoidosis, lymphoma, lipoid pneumonia, and alveolar proteinosis. Centrilobular nodules are rare with these diseases and relatively common with invasive mucinous adenocarcinoma, although organizing pneumonia and sarcoidosis may rarely have associated centrilobular nodules as a prominent finding. When centrilobular nodules are absent, the various causes of chronic consolidation may be difficult to distinguish from one another.

KAPOSI SARCOMA

Kaposi sarcoma (KS) is a malignancy originally described in elderly men of Mediterranean descent but is most frequently seen in patients with human immunodeficiency virus (HIV) infection. Pulmonary involvement has been seen in up to 50% of HIV patients with KS, but its incidence has significantly declined since the development of highly active antiretroviral therapy. KS is associated with infection by the Kaposi sarcoma–associated herpes virus (KSHV), also known as human herpes virus 8 (HHV-8).

The earliest HRCT manifestation of KS is thickening of the peribronchovascular interstitium (Fig. 17.7), which is visible as

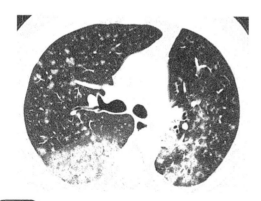

classic

FIGURE 17.6 · **Invasive mucinous adenocarcinoma with centrilobular nodules. Classic appearance.** Patchy, bilateral centrilobular nodules are present, most of which are of soft tissue attenuation. This reflects endobronchial spread of tumor. A more confluent region of lobular consolidation is seen in the right lower lobe reflecting extensive tumor spread.

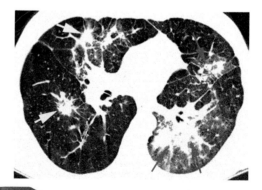

classic

FIGURE 17.7 · **Kaposi sarcoma. Classic appearance.** Peribronchovascular interstitial infiltration, appearaing as bronchial wall thickening or perihilar masses, is noted in the left lung (*red arrows*). Irregular ("flame-shaped") peribronchovascular nodules are visible, along with interlobular septal thickening (*yellow arrows*) in the right lung.

bronchial wall thickening. A later and more suggestive feature of KS is large (more than 1 cm), irregular, or "flame-shaped" nodules (Fig. 17.7). These typically have a peribronchovascular distribution. Other findings include interlobular septal thickening, pleural effusions, and mediastinal lymphadenopathy.

PULMONARY LYMPHOMA

Pulmonary lymphoma may be *primary* (originating in the lung) or *secondary* to extensive, disseminated, or extrathoracic lymphoma.

Lymphatic neoplasms and lymphoid diseases are described using the World Health Organization (WHO) classification (2008), with modifications related to the 2015 WHO classification of primary pulmonary lymphoma.

Non-Hodgkin's lymphoma (NHL) accounts for 75% of thoracic lymphoma, and 25% represent Hodgkin's lymphoma (HL). Most cases are manifested by lymph node enlargement. Primary pulmonary lymphoma almost always represents NHL.

Primary Pulmonary Lymphoma

Pulmonary NHL is considered to be primary to the lung if it shows no evidence of extrathoracic dissemination for at least 3 months after the initial diagnosis. Less than 1% of pulmonary lymphomas are primary.

Primary pulmonary lymphoma arises in pulmonary lymphoid tissue. Many are related to malignant proliferation of submucosal lymphoid follicles distributed along distal bronchi and bronchioles, termed mucosa-associated lymphoid tissue (MALT) or bronchus-associated lymphoid tissue (BALT).

Primary pulmonary lymphoma usually represents (1) extranodal marginal zone B-cell lymphoma arising from MALT (BALT) and termed MALToma or (2) diffuse large B-cell lymphoma (DLBCL). Both are rare.

Solitary or multiple nodules are most common. These may be peribronchial and air bronchograms may be visible within them (Fig. 17.8) Lymph node enlargement may or may not be present. Other manifestations include bilateral consolidation, ground glass opacity, or a diffuse reticulonodular pattern (Fig. 17.9).

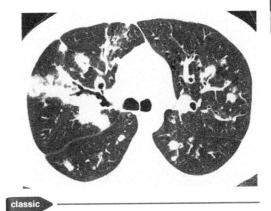

classic

FIGURE 17.8 • **Primary pulmonary lymphoma. Classic appearance.** Peribronchovascular nodules and masses (*arrows*) are visible in relation to or surrounding airways. Air bronchograms are visible within some masses.

MALToma

MALToma accounts for 70 to 90% of primary pulmonary lymphomas but less than 0.5% of all primary lung tumors. These are derived from MALT, hence the term *MALToma* or *MALT lymphoma*. These tumors are indolent, and patients with primary pulmonary B-cell MALT lymphoma have a good prognosis. These tumors are thought to arise because of chronic antigenic stimulation associated with smoking, autoimmune disease (particularly Sjögren's syndrome), or infection. They respond to surgery, if localized, chemotherapy, and radiation, with a 5-year survival of 85 to 95% and a 10-year survival of about 70%.

The most common radiologic manifestation of primary B-cell lymphoma of MALT is a solitary nodule or a focal area of consolidation, ranging in size from a few centimeters to an entire lobe. Multiple nodules or multifocal areas of consolidation may also be present. Air bronchograms are visible in 50% of cases. The parenchymal abnormalities typically show an indolent course with slow growth over months or years. The single or multiple masses or areas of consolidation may appear primarily peribronchial in location. Lymphadenopathy is evident radiographically in 5 to 30% of cases at presentation.

Diffuse Large B-cell Lymphoma

DLBCL account for 5 to 20% of primary pulmonary lymphomas. It is not a single entity but may be associated with various morphologies

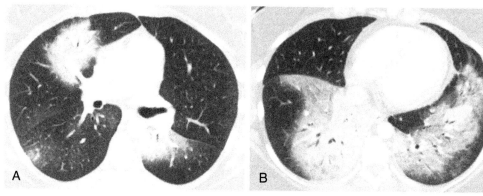

FIGURE 17.9 · **Primary pulmonary lymphoma. A** and **B.** Patchy bilateral consolidation and ground glass opacity, stable for nearly 2 years, are present. Biopsy showed low-grade B-cell lymphoma. Chronic consolidation as a manifestation of lymphoma is most commonly seen with recurrent disease but may occasionally be the presenting abnormality.

and causes. Some tumors occur in patients who have collagen vascular disease, acquired immunodeficiency syndrome (AIDS), organ transplants (posttransplantation lymphoproliferative disorder [PTLD]), Epstein–Barr virus (EBV) infection, or associated with other causes of immunosuppression.

Secondary Pulmonary Lymphoma

Most cases of lymphoma with lung involvement are secondary to a diffuse lymphoma or lymphoma with predominantly extrathoracic disease. Secondary lung involvement may be seen with HL or NHL.

Only 10% of patients with HL have lung involvement at initial presentation, and all show lymph node enlargement in association. Lung involvement is more typical with recurrence.

Lung abnormalities are similar in HL and NHL, consisting of nodules or masses, areas of consolidation or ground glass opacity, or interstitial thickening. Nodules are most common; they are often larger than 1 cm in size (Fig. 17.10) and typically ill-defined (Fig. 17.11). Nodules less than 1 cm may also be seen, but a pattern resembling miliary spread of disease is rare.

Consolidation is also a relatively common pattern (Fig. 17.11). The consolidation may or may not have a mass-like appearance. Air bronchograms may be present within nodules or masses.

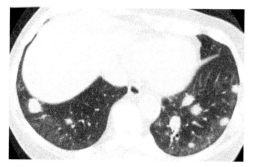

FIGURE 17.10 · **Lymphoma with nodules.** Scattered, bilateral mass-like regions of nodular consolidation are present in a patient with recurrent lymphoma after treatment. This is a typical appearance of lymphoma involving the lungs.

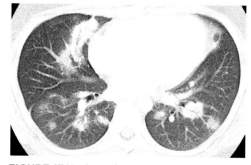

FIGURE 17.11 · **Lymphoma with ill-defined nodules and consolidation.** Ill-defined nodules and patchy mass-like consolidations with air bronchograms are present in a patient with previously treated lymphoma. This appearance is most typical of recurrent secondary lymphoma.

In the setting of known lymphoma, the primary differential diagnosis of consolidation includes infections (particularly fungal infection) and drug reaction presenting with an organizing pneumonia pattern.

LYMPHOPROLIFERATIVE DISEASE

The term *lymphoproliferative disease* is used to describe a spectrum of lymphoid diseases, ranging from lymphoma to benign lymphoid proliferations. It may have a variety of causes or associations and may be described by its clinical associations.

Focal (Nodular) Lymphoid Hyperplasia

Also known as pseudolymphoma, focal lymphoid hyperplasia represents a localized collection of nonneoplastic lymphocytes and other immune cells. This rare disorder usually presents with a solitary nodule or focal area of consolidation. Occasionally, multiple nodules or areas of consolidation may be seen (Fig. 17.12). There is no associated lymphadenopathy. It may occur in association with Sjögren's syndrome.

When presenting as a solitary nodule, focal lymphoid hyperplasia is indistinguishable from primary bronchogenic carcinoma,

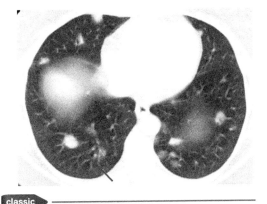

classic

FIGURE 17.12 · **Focal lymphoid hyperplasia. Classic appearance.** Multiple nodules are seen bilaterally, some of which are solid and some of which are of ground glass opacity. Note an air bronchogram in one of the right lower lobe nodules (*arrow*). Lymphoid hyperplasia was confirmed on surgical pathology.

metastasis, granulomas, hamartomas, or other causes of solitary nodules. When presenting as a focal area of consolidation, the differential often includes adenocarcinoma and other causes of chronic consolidation.

Lymphoid Interstitial Pneumonia (LIP) and Follicular Bronchiolitis (FB)

LIP and follicular bronchiolitis (FB) are benign lymphoproliferative disorders characterized pathologically by polyclonal lymphocyte proliferation, predominantly within the interstitium in LIP or in relation to small airways in FB. These two entities show significant clinical, pathologic, and radiographic similarities.

LIP and FB are frequently associated with either immunocompromised states or connective tissue disease. The most common diseases to lead to these patterns include HIV infection, common variable immunodeficiency, and Sjögren's syndrome. A history of an associated disease is vital in making this diagnosis, as LIP and FB are rare and show features that overlap with other, more common, disorders.

FB is also known as hyperplasia of BALT or MALT. FB results from antigenic stimulation of BALT and polyclonal lymphoid hyperplasia. Histologically, FB is characterized by abundant peribronchiolar lymphoid follicles with the lymphoid infiltrate extending into adjacent alveolar interstitium. Although FB lacks the extensive alveolar infiltration of LIP, a distinction between them is somewhat arbitrary.

The most typical HRCT abnormality in FB is centrilobular nodules of ground glass opacity (Fig. 17.13). These nodules are indistinguishable from the nodules seen in hypersensitivity pneumonitis, respiratory bronchiolitis, and atypical infections. Rarely, FB presents with tree-in-bud opacities resembling infection. Mild mosaic perfusion and/or air trapping may be present (Fig. 17.14), but this is rarely as severe as that seen in hypersensitivity pneumonitis.

LIP is characterized histologically by a diffuse interstitial infiltrate of mononuclear cells consisting predominantly of lymphocytes and plasma cells. The findings of LIP are more variable. Ground glass opacity and/or consolidation may be present and is often bilateral and patchy in nature (Fig. 17.15). Both are nonspecific findings. Pulmonary nodules may also be seen. In distinction to FB, these are usually well-defined and have a perilymphatic distribution (Fig. 17.16) resembling sarcoidosis, lymphangitic

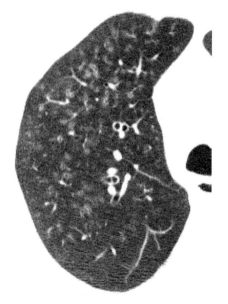

FIGURE 17.13 · **Follicular bronchiolitis.** Centrilobular nodules of ground glass opacity are seen in this patient with follicular bronchiolitis. The centrilobular distribution of nodules reflects the pathologic correlate of lymphoid follicles around the small airways.

spread of malignancy, silicosis, or amyloidosis. Cysts may be seen in association with any of these abnormalities (Fig. 17.17) or may be an isolated finding. Sjögren's syndrome and collagen vascular disease, in particular, may present with cysts as the only abnormality (Fig. 17.18).

The manifestations of LIP and FB (Table 17.2) reflect a spectrum of abnormalities in this disease; an overlap of findings may be present (Fig. 17.19). For instance, there may be centrilobular nodules with more diffuse patchy ground glass opacity. Regardless, this diagnosis is not usually considered unless there is an appropriate clinical history.

IgG4-Related Lung Disease

IgG4-related disease is a systemic disorder in which lymphoplasmocytic infiltrates are present in one or more organs. This disease was originally described in the pancreas as lymphoplasmocytic sclerosing pancreatitis; however, it is now recognized as a multisystem disorder. The most commonly affected organs include the pancreas, liver, lung, and mediastinum. The infiltrates of IgG4-related disease are not neoplastic; however, there may be an association in some patients with lymphoma or other malignancies.

There are several different patterns of lung disease that may be seen on HRCT (Fig. 17.20). One or more nodules or masses may be present. Solitary nodules/masses are typically >1 cm in diameter and may be

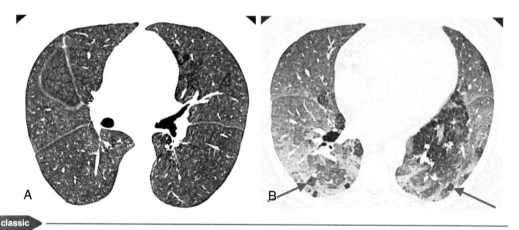

classic

FIGURE 17.14 · **Follicular bronchiolitis. Classic appearance.** A combination of centrilobular nodules of ground glass opacity **(A)** and air trapping (*red arrows* in **B**) is present in a patient with connective tissue disease. Note the sparing of the subpleural lung by the nodules in **A**.

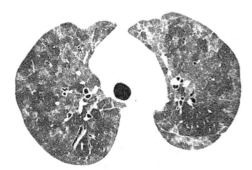

FIGURE 17.15 · **Lymphoid interstitial pneumonia (LIP).** Nonspecific patchy bilateral ground glass opacity is present in a patient with connective tissue disease (CTD). In the presence of chronic symptoms, the differential diagnosis of this pattern in a patient with CTD is limited and includes LIP and an atypical distribution of nonspecific interstitial pneumonia. This represented LIP.

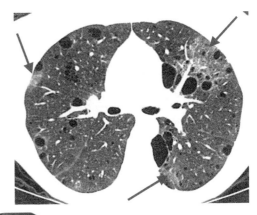

classic

FIGURE 17.17 · **Lymphoid interstitial pneumonia (LIP). Classic appearance.** A combination of cysts and patchy ground glass opacity (*arrows*) is present in a patient with Sjögren's syndrome. While the ground glass opacity is nonspecific, its association with cysts in a patient with connective tissue disease is strongly suggestive of LIP.

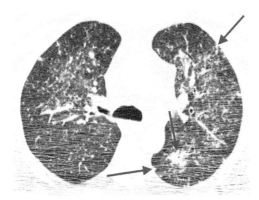

FIGURE 17.16 · **Lymphoid interstitial pneumonia.** Tiny nodules are present in a patient with human immunodeficiency virus infection and chronic, progressive symptoms. The perilymphatic distribution of these nodules is evidenced by their patchy nature and the presence of subpleural (*blue arrows*) and peribronchovascular (*red arrow*) nodules.

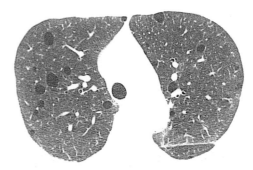

FIGURE 17.18 · **Lymphoid interstitial pneumonia.** Cysts are usually seen as an isolated finding. This is a common manifestation of lymphoid interstitial pneumonia in the setting of Sjögren's syndrome.

as large as 6 cm or more. The differential diagnosis in these cases is primarily malignancy. When multiple nodules are present, they are often ground glass in attenuation, resembling multifocal areas of primary lung adenocarcinoma or adenocarcinoma in situ, although multiple solid nodules are also possible. A lymphatic pattern of peribronchovascular interstitial thickening and/or interlobular septal thickening is another

TABLE 17.2	HRCT findings of lymphoid interstitial pneumonia and follicular bronchiolitis
Follicular bronchiolitis	Centrilobular nodules of ground glass opacity
	Mild mosaic perfusion and air trapping
Lymphoid interstitial pneumonia	Patchy bilateral ground glass opacity and consolidation
	Perilymphatic nodules
	Cysts

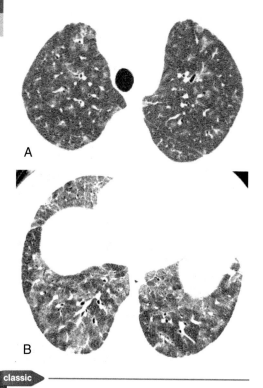

A

B

classic

FIGURE 17.19 · **Follicular bronchiolitis/ lymphoid interstitial pneumonia. Classic appearance.** As these two entities are considered a spectrum of the same disease, an overlap of HRCT findings may be present. This patient with common variable immunodeficiency shows a combination of centrilobular nodules of ground glass attenuation in the upper lobes **(A)** and more generalized ground glass opacity in the lower lobes **(B)**.

common manifestation. The differential diagnosis in these cases includes other lymphatic diseases such as malignancy or sarcoidosis. Last, IgG4-related sclerosing disease may have HRCT findings that overlap with interstitial pneumonias and other causes of interstitial lung disease including ground glass opacity and honeycombing. Hilar and mediastinal lymphadenopathy are the most common nonlung findings in the chest.

Lymphomatoid Granulomatosis

Lymphomatoid granulomatosis (LG) is a rare disease, characterized by an angiocentric, angiodestructive polymorphous lymphoid infiltrate with neoplastic EBV-positive B cells, varying in atypical features, and a large number of reactive T cells. LG is considered to be an EBV-associated B-cell lymphoproliferative disease. It occurs most commonly in immunodeficient patients, and it may be a manifestation of PTLD.

Three grades are thought to exist based on the degree of cytologic atypia, the proportion of EBV-positive cells, presence of necrosis, and their response to treatment. In advanced grades, LG resembles DLBCL, and its prognosis is similar. The lung is the primary site of disease, although other organs, including the skin, brain, kidneys, and heart, may be involved; patients with involvement of other organs have a poorer prognosis.

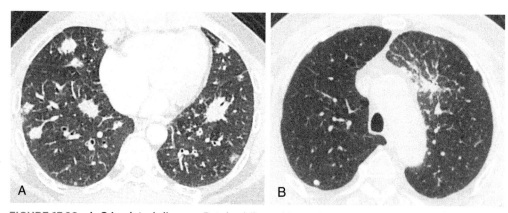

A

B

FIGURE 17.20 · **IgG4-related disease.** Patchy, bilateral irregular nodules are seen, predominantly in a peribronchovascular distribution **(A)**. In another patient **(B)**, left upper lobe peribronchovascular consolidation and interlobular septal thickening suggest a lymphatic distribution of abnormalities.

HRCT findings consist primarily of bilateral, poorly defined nodular lesions, ranging from 0.5 to 8 cm in diameter, with a basal predominance (Fig. 17.21). Lesions may progress rapidly and cavitate, mimicking granulomatosis with polyangitis (Wegener's granulomatosis).

Posttransplant Lymphoproliferative Disorders

PTLD may occur with solid organ or bone marrow transplantation. PTLD represents a spectrum of disease from benign proliferation of nonneoplastic lymphocytes to malignant lymphoma, either HL or NHL. Development

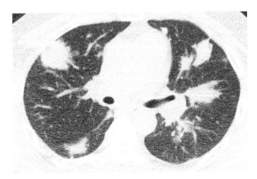

FIGURE 17.21 · **Lymphomatoid granulomatosis.** Large, irregular nodules are seen bilaterally in a patient with lymphomatoid granulomatosis. This is a typical manifestation of this rare disease, but there are many other more common causes in the setting of chronic symptoms, including tumor, organizing pneumonia, eosinophilic pneumonia, and sarcoidosis.

of PTLD is closely correlated with EBV infection. In general, the likelihood of developing PTLD is associated with the severity of immunosuppression, but this may be affected by chronic antiviral therapy. Presentation within 1 year of transplantation is most typical.

The HRCT findings of PTLD resemble primary or secondary pulmonary lymphoma. Single or multiple pulmonary nodules, masses, or areas of consolidation may be present. These are often associated with mediastinal and/or hilar lymphadenopathy (Fig. 17.22). In transplant patients, the differential diagnosis predominantly includes infections, particularly fungal infection. Organizing pneumonia from drugs or graft-versus-host disease may also closely resemble PTLD.

LEUKEMIA

Lung abnormalities in patients with leukemia are not uncommon, but many are due to non-neoplastic diseases such as pneumonia, drug reaction, edema, or hemorrhage. Leukemic infiltration occurs in approximately 15% of patients with significant HRCT abnormalities.

On HRCT, leukemic lung infiltration often shows lymphatic dissemination. Thus, thickening of the interlobular septa and peribronchovascular interstitium are common. Small nodules may also be present and are typically perilymphatic or random in distribution. The presence of centrilobular nodules favors a nonneoplastic cause, such as pneumonia. Ground glass opacity and

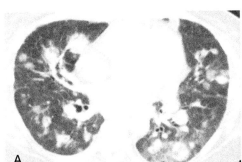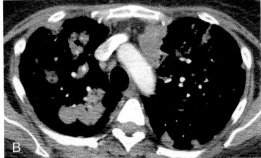

FIGURE 17.22 · **Posttransplant lymphoproliferative disorder.** Multiple nodules and masses are seen bilaterally **(A)** in this patient with a history of renal transplantation. **B.** These findings are associated with mediastinal lymphadenopathy.

consolidation are uncommon findings of leukemic infiltration and more likely represent pneumonia, diffuse alveolar damage, edema, or hemorrhage.

FURTHER READING

Akira M, Atagi S, Kawahara M, Iuchi K, Johkoh T. High-resolution CT findings of diffuse bronchioloalveolar carcinoma in 38 patients. *AJR Am J Roentgenol.* 1999;173:1623-1629.

Aquino S. Imaging of metastatic disease to the thorax. *Radiol Clin North Am.* 2005;43:481-495.

Bae YA, Lee KS. Cross-sectional evaluation of thoracic lymphoma. *Radiol Clin North Am.* 2008;46:253-264.

Borhani AA, Hosseinzadeh K, Almusa O, Furlan A, Nalesnik M. Imaging of posttransplantation lymphoproliferative disorder after solid organ transplantation. *Radiographics.* 2009;29:981-1000.

Bragg DG, Chor PJ, Murray KA, Kjeldsberg CR. Lymphoproliferative disorders of the lung: histopathology, clinical manifestations, and imaging features. *AJR Am J Roentgenol.* 1994;163:273-281.

Camacho JC, Moreno CC, Harri PA, Aguirre DA, Torres WE, Mittal PK. Posttransplantation lymphoproliferative disease: proposed imaging classification. *Radiographics.* 2014;34:2025-2038.

Campo E, Swerdlow SH, Harris NL, Pileri S, Stein H, Jaffe ES. The 2008 WHO classification of lymphoid neoplasms and beyond: evolving concepts and practical applications. *Blood.* 2011;117:5019-5032.

Carignan S, Staples CA, Müller NL. Intrathoracic lymphoproliferative disorders in the immunocompromised patient: CT findings. *Radiology.* 1995;197:53-58.

Chou SHS, Prabhu SJ, Crothers K, et al. Thoracic diseases associated with HIV infection in the era of antiretroviral therapy: clinical and imaging findings. *Radiographics.* 2014;34:895-911.

Collins J, Müller NL, Leung AN, et al. EpsteinBarr virus–associated lymphoproliferative disease of the lung: CT and histologic findings. *Radiology.* 1998;208:749-759.

Do KH, Lee JS, Seo JB, et al. Pulmonary parenchymal involvement of low-grade lymphoproliferative disorders. *J Comput Assist Tomogr.* 2005;29:825-830.

Dodd G, Ledesma-Medina J, Baron RL, Fuhrman CR. Posttransplant lymphoproliferative disorder: intrathoracic manifestations. *Radiology.* 1992;184:65-69.

Eisner MD, Kaplan LD, Herndier B, Stulbarg MS. The pulmonary manifestations of AIDS related non Hodgkin's lymphoma. *Chest.* 1996;110:729-736.

Gibson M, Hansell DM. Lymphocytic disorders of the chest: pathology and imaging. *Clin Radiol.* 1998;53:469-480.

Gruden JF, Huang L, Webb WR, et al. AIDS-related Kaposi sarcoma of the lung: radiographic findings and staging system with bronchoscopic correlation. *Radiology.* 1995;195:545-552.

Hartman TE, Primack SL, Müller NL, Staples CA. Diagnosis of thoracic complications in AIDS: accuracy of CT. *AJR Am J Roentgenol.* 1994;162:547-553.

Heyneman LE, Johkoh T, Ward S, et al. Pulmonary leukemic infiltrates: high resolution CT findings in 10 patients. *AJR Am J Roentgenol.* 2000;174:517-521.

Howling SJ, Hansell DM, Wells AU, et al. Follicular bronchiolitis: thin-section CT and histologic findings. *Radiology.* 1999;212:637-642.

Johkoh T, Ikezoe J, Tomiyama N, et al. CT findings in lymphangitic carcinomatosis of the lung: correlation with histologic findings and pulmonary function tests. *AJR Am J Roentgenol.* 1992;158:1217-1222.

Johkoh T, Müller NL, Pickford HA, et al. Lymphocytic interstitial pneumonia: thin section CT findings in 22 patients. *Radiology.* 1999;212:567-572.

Knisely BL, Mastey LA, Mergo PJ, et al. Pulmonary mucosa-associated lymphoid tissue lymphoma: CT and pathologic findings. *AJR Am J Roentgenol.* 1999;172:1321-1326.

Lee DK, Im JG, Lee KS, et al. Bcell lymphoma of bronchus-associated lymphoid tissue (BALT): CT features in 10 patients. *J Comput Assist Tomogr.* 2000;24:30-34.

Lee KS, Kim Y, Primack SL. Imaging of pulmonary lymphomas. *AJR Am J Roentgenol.* 1997;168:339-345.

Lee WK, Duddalwar VA, Rouse HC, Lau EW, Bekhit E, Hennessy OF. Extranodal lymphoma in the thorax: cross-sectional imaging findings. *Clin Radiol.* 2009;64:542-549.

Lynch DA, Travis WD, Muller NL, et al. Idiopathic interstitial pneumonias: CT features. *Radiology.* 2005;236:10-21.

Munk PL, Müller NL, Miller RR, Ostrow DN. Pulmonary lymphangitic carcinomatosis: CT and pathologic findings. *Radiology.* 1988;166:705-709.

Naidich DP, Tarras M, Garay SM, et al. Kaposi sarcoma: CT radiographic correlation. *Chest.* 1989;96:723-728.

Okada F, Ando Y, Kondo Y, Matsumoto S, Maeda T, Mori H. Thoracic CT findings of adult T-cell leukemia or lymphoma. *AJR Am J Roentgenol.* 2004;182:761-767.

Rappaport DC, Chamberlain DW, Shepherd FA, Hutcheon MA. Lymphoproliferative disorders after lung transplantation: imaging features. *Radiology.* 1998;206:519-524.

Silva CI, Flint JD, Levy RD, Müller NL. Diffuse lung cysts in lymphoid interstitial pneumonia: high-resolution CT and pathologic findings. *J Thorac Imaging.* 2006;21:241-244.

Stein MG, Mayo J, Müller N, et al. Pulmonary lymphangitic spread of carcinoma: appearance on CT scans. *Radiology.* 1987;162:371-375.

Travis WD, Brambilla E, Noguchi M, et al. International Association for the Study of Lung Cancer/American Thoracic Society/European Respiratory Society International Multidisciplinary Classification of Lung Adenocarcinoma. *J Thorac Oncol.* 2011;6:244-285.

Travis WD, Garg K, Franklin WA, et al. Evolving concepts in the pathology and computed tomography imaging of lung adenocarcinoma and bronchioloalveolar carcinoma. *J Clin Oncol.* 2005;23:3279-3287.

Travis WD, Galvin JR. Non-neoplastic pulmonary lymphoid lesions. *Thorax.* 2001; 56:964-971.

Travis WD, Brambilla E, Burke AP, Marx A, Nicholson AG, eds. *WHO Classification of Tumours of the Lung, Pleura, Thymus and Heart.* Geneva: WHO Press; 2015.

CHAPTER 18

Rare Diseases

PULMONARY ALVEOLAR PROTEINOSIS

Pulmonary alveolar proteinosis (PAP) is a rare disorder characterized pathologically by the accumulation of lipoprotein within alveoli. There are three different forms of the disease. *Congenital PAP* results from mutations in genes encoding surfactant B or C or granulocyte–macrophage colony-stimulating factor (GM-CSF). *Secondary PAP* occurs in association with a wide variety of disorders, including acute silicosis (silicoproteinosis), infections, and hematologic and lymphatic malignancy. *Idiopathic PAP* accounts for nearly 90% of cases. It is an autoimmune disease in which antibodies to GM-CSF interfere with the degradation or clearance of surfactant.

Men with PAP outnumber women. Patients range in age from a few months to more than 70 years, with two-thirds of patients being between 30 and 50 years old. Symptoms are usually mild and of insidious onset. They include cough, fever, and mild dyspnea. About 30% of patients are asymptomatic.

HRCT abnormalities are typically diffuse, bilateral, and often symmetric (Table 18.1). The characteristic HRCT abnormality consists of geographic regions of ground glass opacity and smooth interlobular septal thickening in the same lung regions. This is termed the *crazy paving* pattern (Figs. 18.1 and 18.2). Consolidation or ill-defined nodules may also be present but are not particularly common. The differential diagnosis of the *crazy paving* pattern in patients with chronic symptoms is long and includes interstitial pneumonias, organizing pneumonia, eosinophilic pneumonia, hypersensitivity pneumonitis, lipoid pneumonia, and invasive mucinous adenocarcinoma.

HRCT may be used to monitor treatment (Fig. 18.2). Large volume bronchoalveolar lavage is used for treatment in an attempt to clear the proteinaceous material from the alveolar spaces. HRCT can help target appropriate regions of the lung for bronchoalveolar lavage and to confirm successful treatment. With lavage, ground glass opacities improve or resolve. Septal thickening may sometimes persist (Fig. 18.2B).

LIPOID PNEUMONIA

Lipoid pneumonia reflects the accumulation of fats within the lung parenchyma. It may be endogenous or exogenous. Endogenous lipoid pneumonia is characterized by lipid-laden macrophages within consolidated lung distal to an obstructed airway. HRCT findings are those of a postobstructive pneumonia.

Exogenous lipoid pneumonia is caused by the aspiration of fatty materials such as mineral oil. As a large amount of lipid needs to be aspirated over a long period, patients usually present with chronic symptoms. Also, CT abnormalities may be incidentally discovered in asymptomatic patients.

The HRCT findings of exogenous lipoid pneumonia include ground glass opacity or consolidation that is patchy, focal, or mass-like (Table 18.2). A combination of ground glass opacity and interlobular septal thickening, the *crazy paving* pattern, is not uncommon. Soft tissue windows may show low-attenuation regions within areas of consolidation, with

Hounsfield unit measurements consistent with fat (Fig. 18.3). Masses or regions of consolidation may be round or irregular in shape.

Findings are often most severe in the dependent lung regions, reflecting the typical distribution of aspiration. Associated fibrosis may be present, although this is usually not a significant component of disease.

AMYLOIDOSIS

Amyloidosis reflects the accumulation of an extracellular protein in multiple organs. The most commonly involved organs include the kidneys, heart, nervous system, and liver.

There are two types of amyloid that may be deposited in the lungs, amyloid L (light chain) and amyloid A. The former is responsible for the large majority of patients with symptomatic lung involvement; it may be idiopathic or associated with myeloma or lymphoma. *Amyloidosis A* is associated with rheumatoid arthritis, inflammatory bowel disease, chronic inflammatory disorders (e.g., osteomyelitis), and chronic pulmonary infections (e.g., tuberculosis) and rarely leads to symptoms.

Amyloidosis may involve the lung parenchyma or airways (Table 18.3). Lung parenchymal involvement may be focal or diffuse. Lymphadenopathy may be associated with any of the above patterns of amyloid or as an isolated abnormality. Calcification is often present in mediastinal or hilar lymph nodes.

TABLE 18.1	HRCT findings of pulmonary alveolar proteinosis

Three forms: congenital, secondary, idiopathic (90% of cases)
Diffuse and bilateral
Patchy and geographic regions of GGO and crazy paving
Consolidation less common
GGO decreases with bronchoalveolar lavage

GGO, ground glass opacity.

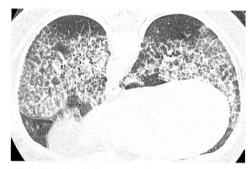

FIGURE 18.1 · **Pulmonary alveolar proteinosis.** Prone HRCT shows a combination of ground glass opacity and interlobular septal thickening in the same lung regions, the *crazy paving* sign. In a patient with chronic symptoms, alveolar proteinosis is one of several diagnoses that can produce this pattern.

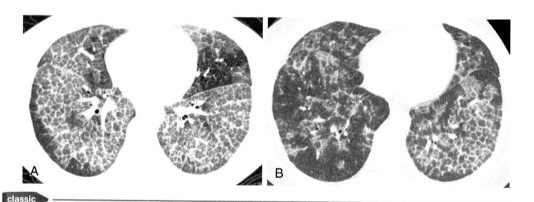

classic

FIGURE 18.2 · **Pulmonary alveolar proteinosis, before and after treatment: Classic appearances.**
A. Typical findings of alveolar proteinosis with crazy paving are present on pretreatment HRCT.
B. After several treatments with large volume bronchoalveolar lavage, there has been significant improvement in the ground glass opacity and septal thickening.

Focal Parenchymal Amyloidosis

Focal parenchymal amyloidosis presents with a single or multiple discrete lung nodules or masses (Fig. 18.4). These may be calcified. They are difficult to differentiate from other causes of nodules such as primary bronchogenic carcinoma, metastases, granulomatous disease, or hamartoma. Associated airway wall thickening may be present in patients with focal parenchymal amyloid.

Diffuse Parenchymal Amyloidosis

Diffuse parenchymal amyloidosis typically presents with diffuse small (<1.5 cm) nodules. These are often calcified and may have a perilymphatic distribution (Fig. 18.5). Other causes of diffuse, small, calcified lung nodules include sarcoidosis, pneumoconioses such as silicosis, granulomatous infections such as tuberculosis, metastatic calcification, and alveolar microlithiasis. Less characteristic findings include diffuse

lung infiltration with consolidation (Fig. 18.6), ground glass opacity, interlobular septal thickening or intralobular interstitial thickening, extensive lung calcification, and fibrosis.

Tracheobronchial Amyloidosis

Involvement of the airways is characterized by diffuse or nodular thickening of the walls of the trachea and/or central bronchi (Fig. 18.7). Calcification may be present. The differential diagnosis of extensive tracheal or central bronchial wall thickening includes relapsing polychondritis, sarcoidosis, Wegener's granulomatosis, inflammatory bowel disease, and infections such as aspergillosis. Tracheobronchopathia osteochondroplastica may result in nodular tracheal and bronchial wall thickening with calcification.

LIGHT CHAIN DEPOSITION DISEASE

Light chain deposition disease (LCDD) is characterized by the deposition of nonamyloid light chains in various tissues and organs. Although the protein deposits are similar to those seen in amyloidosis, they do not bind Congo red as in amyloidosis. About 75% of

TABLE 18.2	HRCT findings of lipoid pneumonia

Aspiration of fatty materials (exogenous lipoid pneumonia)
Patchy and dependent
Ground glass opacity or consolidation
Low-attenuation consolidation

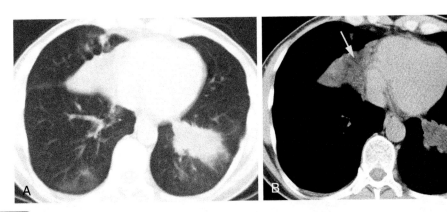

classic

FIGURE 18.3 · Lipoid pneumonia: Classic appearance. A. Lung windows show focal regions of consolidation at both lung bases in a patient with chronic symptoms. This finding is nonspecific. **B.** The presence of low-attenuation fat (*arrows*) within regions of consolidation on the mediastinal windows strongly suggests the diagnosis of lipoid pneumonia.

18

LCDD occur in association with multiple myeloma or a lymphoproliferative disease, especially Waldenström's macroglobulinemia. Renal involvement is a constant feature of LCDD. In addition, the kidneys, the liver, and heart are commonly affected, although lung involvement is very uncommon. HRCT findings include single or multiple nodular lesions of various sizes.

LCDD, almost entirely limited to the lung and not associated with myeloma, is sometimes seen in association with Sjögren's syndrome. Radiographs and CT show nodules and/or scattered cysts, usually up to 2 cm or larger in diameter (Fig. 18.8), closely resembling the apperance of cystic lymphoid interstitial pneumonia (LIP), although deposits of light chains can result in nodular thickening of cyst walls.

TABLE 18.3	HRCT findings of amyloidosis

Focal parenchymal amyloidosis
Single or multiple lung nodules, sometimes calcified
Diffuse parenchymal amyloidosis
Small nodules with a perilymphatic distribution, septal thickening
Consolidation, ground glass opacity, calcification, fibrosis
Tracheobronchial amyloidosis
Diffuse or focal thickening of tracheal and bronchial walls
Calcification common

PULMONARY ALVEOLAR MICROLITHIASIS

Pulmonary alveolar microlithiasis (PAM) is a rare disorder characterized by the accumulation of small calcified *microliths* within the alveolar spaces. It may be sporadic or familial, predominantly affecting siblings. PAM occurs because of a gene mutation, resulting in an abnormal protein, which is normally responsible for sodium-dependent phosphate transport in the lungs. Patients typically have no or mild symptoms in the setting of significant lung abnormalities.

The characteristic HRCT finding is that of very small, pinhead-sized, discrete, calcified nodules. These nodules may be perilymphatic or centrilobular in distribution and are most severe in the posterior and inferior lungs. Ground glass opacity and reticulation may be seen but are not specifically suggestive of PAM. The differential diagnosis includes diffuse parenchymal amyloidosis and metastatic calcification. Granulomatous diseases and pneumoconioses associated with calcification produce nodules larger than those seen in PAM.

ERDHEIM-CHESTER DISEASE

Erdheim–Chester disease (ECD) is a very rare xanthogranulomatous histiocytosis characterized by organ infiltration by lipid-laden (foamy) histiocytes. Some studies suggest it is

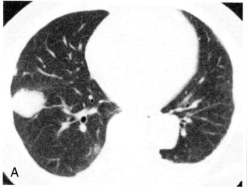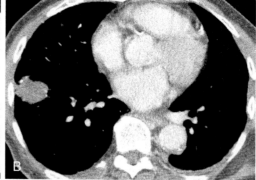

FIGURE 18.4 · Amyloidosis, focal parenchymal. A. A nonspecific nodule is seen in the right lower lobe. **B.** On a soft tissue window, focal areas of calcification are visible within the nodule. Biopsy confirmed amyloidosis in this patient with rheumatoid arthritis.

clonal and associated with specific gene mutations in half of cases. The bones are most commonly affected, but involvement of the central nervous system, heart, kidneys, and lymphatic system may also be present. Pulmonary involvement occurs in 20 to 30% of cases and has a poor prognosis; it consists of interstitial infiltration by histiocytes with resulting fibrosis. ECD classically presents in middle-aged men with chronic dyspnea or cough.

The HRCT findings in ECD have a lymphatic distribution. Smooth interlobular septal and fissural thickening resembling pulmonary edema or lymphangitic carcinomatosis are most characteristic. Small nodules may be present in a centrilobular or perilymphatic distribution (Fig. 18.9). Other lung findings such as ground glass opacity may be present but are not particularly characteristic. Hilar, mediastinal, and axillary lymphadenopathy are commonly present. As ECD is rare, a combination of HRCT findings and other characteristic lesions is most suggestive of the diagnosis. Other characteristic findings include sclerotic bone lesions, diffuse thickening (i.e., "coating) of the aorta and major vessels, and circumferential perinephric soft tissue.

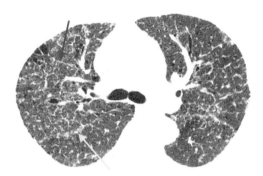

FIGURE 18.5 · Amyloidosis, diffuse parenchymal. HRCT through the upper lobes demonstrates nodules with a perilymphatic distribution. The nodules are clustered along fissures (*yellow arrow*) and in interlobular septa (*red arrow*). Sarcoidosis is the most common cause of this pattern, but this patient was diagnosed with amyloidosis on surgical biopsy.

LYMPHANGIOLEIOMYOMATOSIS

Lymphangioleiomyomatosis (LAM) is a rare disorder characterized by progressive proliferation of perivascular epithelioid cells (PECs) in relation to bronchioles, small pulmonary vessels, and lymphatics in the chest

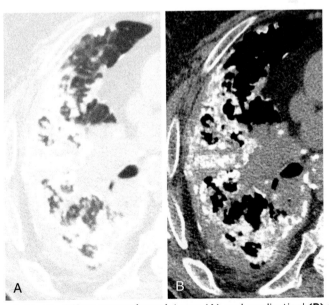

FIGURE 18.6 · Amyloidosis, diffuse parenchymal. Lung **(A)** and mediastinal **(B)** windows demonstrate extensive right lung consolidation with calcification in advanced amyloidosis.

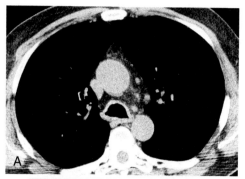

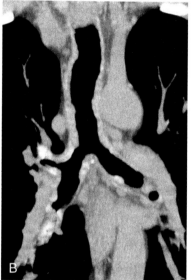

classic

FIGURE 18.7 · Amyloidosis, tracheobronchial: Classic appearance. Axial **(A)** and coronal reformatted **(B)** images are shown in a patient with diffuse tracheal wall thickening and calcification from amyloidosis. There is also involvement of the central bronchi.

and abdomen. It is considered to be a low-grade destructive malignancy. LAM occurs in association with tuberous sclerosis complex (TSC-LAM) or as sporadic LAM (S-LAM). TSC-LAM is linked to mutations in the tuberous sclerosis genes TSC1 and TSC2, while S-LAM is associated with mutations of TSC2. Peribronchiolar PEC infiltration eventually leads to bronchiolar obstruction and destruction of lung parenchyma with formation of isolated lung cysts.

The clinical presentation is quite variable. Patients may present with chronic dyspnea or spontaneous pneumothorax. Occasionally, lung cysts are discovered as an incidental finding. Pulmonary hypertension is not uncommonly associated with LAM but is less common than with pulmonary LCH.

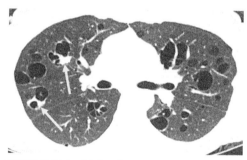

FIGURE 18.8 · Light chain deposition disease. Multiple bilateral cysts are present, some of which show nodular thickening of their walls (*arrows*).

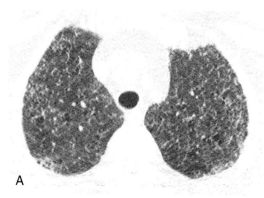

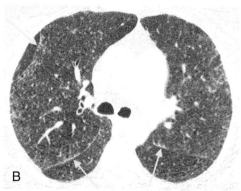

FIGURE 18.9 · Erdheim–Chester disease. A. Tiny nodules are present in a patchy and upper lung distribution. The predominance of subpleural nodules (*arrows*) **(B)** suggests a perilymphatic distribution. This is one possible manifestation of Erdheim–Chester disease.

The principal HRCT finding is the presence of lung cysts (Table 18.4). Cysts tend to be round and thin walled and show uniform involvement of the lung from apex to base. A few scattered cysts may be present (Fig. 18.10) or there may be near-complete replacement of the lung (Fig. 18.11). Associated nodules are rare. Pleural effusions are common and are due to lymphatic obstruction. Patients with tuberous sclerosis and some patients with isolated LAM may show associated abnormalities such as renal angiomyolipomas (Fig. 18.12).

Both LAM and LCH (see Chapter 11) may show extensive cystic lung disease. Demographics are important in distinguishing these diseases, as LAM is seen in females of childbearing age (it is very rare in men), whereas LCH is usually associated with cigarette smoking. Nodules are common with

LCH and rare with LAM. The cysts of LCH tend to be irregular and lobulated in contrast to the round cysts of LAM. Pleural effusions in association with cystic lung disease suggest LAM. Other causes of cystic lung disease, such as LIP, usually show fewer cysts.

BIRT-HOGG-DUBÉ SYNDROME

Birt–Hogg–Dubé syndrome is a rare autosomal-dominant disorder characterized by a combination of (1) fibrofolliculomas distributed over the face, neck, and upper trunk; (2) renal tumors ranging from benign oncocytoma to renal cell carcinoma; and (3) lung cysts. Occasionally, lung cysts are the only manifestation, although the other manifestations may develop later in the course of the disease. It often presents initially with pneumothorax, when a cyst perforates into the pleural space.

The primary HRCT manifestation of Birt–Hogg–Dubé syndrome is lung cysts (Fig. 18.13). These are thin walled and variable in size. The cysts are most numerous in the subpleural and medial lung bases. They are often directly adjacent to the pulmonary veins and arteries. This distribution of cysts may be specifically suggestive of Birt–Hogg–Dubé syndrome, although it is also seen in lymphoid interstitial pneumonia (LIP). The cysts tend

TABLE 18.4	HRCT findings of lymphangioleiomyomatosis

Women of childbearing age, sometimes associated with tuberous sclerosis
Round, thin-walled cysts
Diffuse distribution, lung bases equally involved
Nodules rare
Pleural effusion in some
Associated with renal angiomyolipoma

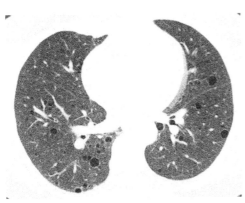

FIGURE 18.10 · **Lymphangioleiomyomatosis (LAM).** A relatively mild case of LAM in a middle-aged woman is depicted, showing scattered round cysts. This was an incidental finding on a CT performed to evaluate possible malignancy.

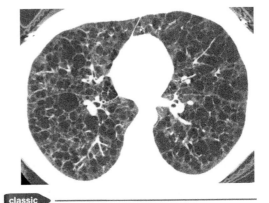

classic

FIGURE 18.11 · **Lymphangioleiomyomatosis (LAM): Classic appearance.** An advanced case of LAM is shown, with extensive replacement of the lung parenchyma by thin-walled cysts. This woman patient presented with dyspnea and pulmonary hypertension.

18

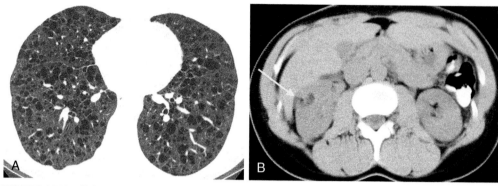

FIGURE 18.12 · **Tuberous sclerosis.** HRCT and pathologic findings of cystic lung disease in tuberous sclerosis are identical to those of isolated lymphangioleiomyomatosis. **A.** HRCT shows a diffuse distribution of thin-walled, round cysts. **B.** CT through the abdomen shows a fat-containing renal mass (*arrow*) compatible with an angiomyolipoma.

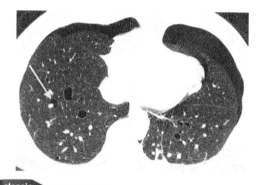

classic

FIGURE 18.13 · **Birt-Hogg-Dubé syndrome: Classic appearance.** Scattered cysts are seen in a patient presenting with bilateral pneumothoraces. Some of the cysts are directly adjacent to pulmonary veins in the lower lobes (*arrow*), a finding that may be suggestive of this syndrome.

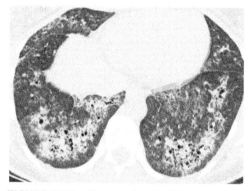

FIGURE 18.14 · **Hermansky–Pudlak syndrome.** HRCT shows peripheral and basilar predominant irregular reticulation, traction bronchiectasis, and consolidation. The presence of subpleural sparing would be suggestive of nonspecific interstitial pneumonia, but the demographics and other associated abnormalities in this patient were compatible with Hermansky–Pudlak syndrome.

to be less numerous than those seen in LAM and LCH. Other causes of lung cysts include LIP, pneumatoceles from prior infection, and neurofibromatosis.

Hermansky–Pudlak Syndrome
Hermansky–Pudlak syndrome is an inherited disorder characterized by albinism, platelet dysfunction, and pulmonary fibrosis. Renal and intestinal abnormalities may also be present, but pulmonary disease is the most common cause of mortality. This disorder is seen with a particularly high prevalence in Puerto Rico.

There are no HRCT findings that specifically suggest Hermansky–Pudlak syndrome;

thus diagnosis is usually made clinically. Fibrosis is the most common finding and manifests as irregular reticulation and traction bronchiectasis (Fig. 18.14). It has a variable distribution but is often peripheral. HRCT performed early in the progression of the disease shows ground glass opacity and mild reticulation.

Minute Pulmonary Meningothelial-like Nodules
Minute pulmonary meningothelial-like nodules are a common incidental finding seen on pathology. They are rarely a cause of clinically

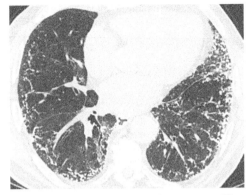

18

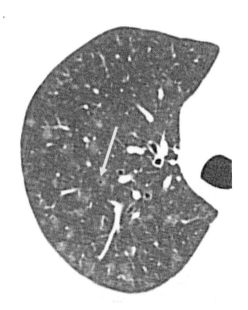

FIGURE 18.15 · **Minute pulmonary meningo-thelial-like nodules.** Multiple discreet ground glass attenuation nodules are seen, at least one of which has a lucency at its center (*arrow*).

FIGURE 18.16 · **Idiopathic pulmonary ossification.** Immunerable calcified nodules with a subpleural predominance are present in the absence of interstitial lung disease.

relevant disease; however, they may be seen in association with thromboembolic disease and smoking-related lung disease. On HRCT bilateral scattered small nodules are seen with well-defined borders. When extensive they demonstrate a random distribution. These nodules are often ground glass in attenuation and some nodules may demonstrate cystic lucencies at their centers (Fig. 18.15).

Pulmonary Ossification

Pulmonary ossification is the presence of mature bone within the pulmonary parenchyma that may be nodular or dendriform in morphology. Ossification is most commonly associated with interstitial lung disease and is often seen in patients with idiopathic pulmonary fibrosis. It is also associated with recurrent/chronic aspiration. Rarely, it is seen as an isolated abnormality. Pulmonary ossification is usually asymptomatic except in extreme cases. Typical HRCT findings include multiple small calcified nodules (Fig. 18.16) seen in association with interstitial lung disease or in isolation. When seen in isolation they often predominate in the subpleural lung.

FURTHER READING

Aberle DR, Hansell DM, Brown K, Tashkin DP. Lymphangiomyomatosis: CT, chest radiographic, and functional correlations. *Radiology.* 1990;176:381-387.

Adriaensen ME, Schaefer-Prokop CM, Duyndam DA, Zonnenberg BA, Prokop M. Radiological evidence of lymphangioleiomyomatosis in female and male patients with tuberous sclerosis complex. *Clin Radiol.* 2011;66:625-628.

Agarwal PP, Gross BH, Holloway BJ, et al. Thoracic CT findings in Birt-Hogg-Dube syndrome. *AJR Am J Roentgenol.* 2011;196:349-352.

Aylwin ACB, Gishen P, Copley SJ. Imaging appearance of thoracic amyloidosis. *J Thorac Imaging.* 2005;20:41-46.

Ayuso MC, Gilabert R, Bombi JA, Salvador A. CT appearance of localized pulmonary amyloidosis. *J Comput Assist Tomogr.* 1987;11:197-199.

Brun AL, Touitou-Gottenberg D, Haroche J, et al. Erdheim-Chester disease: CT findings of thoracic involvement. *Eur Radiol.* 2010;20:2579-2587.

Castellana G, Lamorgese V. Pulmonary alveolar microlithiasis. World cases and review of the literature. *Respiration.* 2003;70:549-555.

Chu SC, Horiba K, Usuki J, et al. Comprehensive evaluation of 35 patients with lymphangioleiomyomatosis. *Chest.* 1999;115:1041-1052.

Cluzel P, Grenier P, Bernadac P, et al. Pulmonary alveolar microlithiasis: CT findings. *J Comput Assist Tomogr.* 1991;15:938-942.

Colombat M, Stern M, Groussard O, et al. Pulmonary cystic disorder related to light chain deposition disease. *Am J Respir Crit Care Med.* 2006;173:777-780.

Czeyda-Pommersheim F, Hwang M, Chen SS, et al. Amyloidosis: modern cross-sectional imaging. *Radiographics.* 2015;35:1381-1392.

Deniz O, Ors F, Tozkoparan E, et al. High resolution computed tomographic features of pulmonary alveolar microlithiasis. *Eur J Radiol.* 2005;55:452-460.

Franquet T, Giménez A, Bordes R, et al. The crazy-paving pattern in exogenous lipoid pneumonia: CT-pathologic correlation. *AJR Am J Roentgenol.* 1998;170:315-317.

18

Furuya M, Nakatani Y. Birt-hogg-dubé syndrome: clinicopathologic features of the lung. *J Clin Pathol.* 2013;66:178-186.

Georgiades CS, Neyman EG, Barish MA, et al. Amyloidosis: review and CT manifestations. *Radiographics.* 2004;24:405-416.

Graham CM, Stern EJ, Finkbeiner WE, Webb WR. High-resolution CT appearance of diffuse alveolar septal amyloidosis. *AJR Am J Roentgenol.* 1992;158:265-267.

Helbich TH, Wojnarovsky C, Wunderbaldinger P, et al. Pulmonary alveolar microlithiasis in children: radiographic and high-resolution CT findings. *AJR Am J Roentgenol.* 1997;168:63-65.

Johkoh T, Itoh H, Müller NL, et al. Crazy-paving appearance at thin-section CT: spectrum of disease and pathologic findings. *Radiology.* 1999;211:155-160.

Johnson SR, Cordier JF, Lazor R, et al. European respiratory society guidelines for the diagnosis and management of lymphangioleiomyomatosis. *Eur Respir J.* 2010;35:14-26.

Kirchner J, Stein A, Viel K, et al. Pulmonary lymphangioleiomyomatosis: high-resolution CT findings. *Eur Radiol.* 1999;9:49-54.

Korn MA, Schurawitzki H, Klepetko W, Burghuber OC. Pulmonary alveolar microlithiasis: findings on high-resolution CT. *AJR Am J Roentgenol.* 1992;158:981-982.

Lee KN, Levin DL, Webb WR, et al. Pulmonary alveolar proteinosis: high-resolution CT, chest radiographic, and functional correlations. *Chest.* 1997;111:989-995.

Lee KS, Müller NL, Hale V, et al. Lipoid pneumonia: CT findings. *J Comput Assist Tomogr.* 1995;19:48-51.

Lenoir S, Grenier P, Brauner MW, et al. Pulmonary lymphangiomyomatosis and tuberous sclerosis: comparison of radiographic and thin-section CT findings. *Radiology.* 1990;175:329-334.

Müller NL, Chiles C, Kullnig P. Pulmonary lymphangiomyomatosis: correlation of CT with radiographic and functional findings. *Radiology.* 1990;175:335-339.

Pickford HA, Swensen SJ, Utz JP. Thoracic cross-sectional imaging of amyloidosis. *AJR Am J Roentgenol.* 1997;168:351-355.

Templeton PA, McLoud TC, Müller NL, et al. Pulmonary lymphangioleiomyomatosis: CT and pathologic findings. *J Comput Assist Tomogr.* 1989;13:54-57.

Tobino K, Hirai T, Johkoh T, et al. Differentiation between Birt Hogg Dube syndrome and lymphangioleiomyomatosis: quantitative analysis of pulmonary cysts on computed tomography of the chest in 66 females. *Eur J Radiol.* 2012;81:1340-1346.

Toro JR, Pautler SE, Stewart L, et al. Lung cysts, spontaneous pneumothorax, and genetic associations in 89 families with Birt-Hogg-Dube syndrome. *Am J Respir Crit Care Med.* 2007;175:1044-1053.

Index

Note: Page numbers followed by "f" indicate figures and "t" indicate tables.